NEUROLOGY BOARD REVIEW

QUESTIONS AND ANSWERS

NEUROLOGY BOARD REVIEW

QUESTIONS AND ANSWERS

BY

Amy McGregor, MD

ASSOCIATE PROFESSOR OF NEUROLOGY AND PEDIATRICS

UNIVERSITY OF TENNESSEE HEALTH SCIENCE CENTER

LE BONHEUR CHILDREN'S HOSPITAL

MEMPHIS, TN

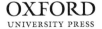
OXFORD
UNIVERSITY PRESS

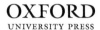

OXFORD
UNIVERSITY PRESS

Oxford University Press is a department of the University of Oxford. It furthers
the University's objective of excellence in research, scholarship, and education
by publishing worldwide. Oxford is a registered trade mark of Oxford University
Press in the UK and certain other countries.

Published in the United States of America by Oxford University Press
198 Madison Avenue, New York, NY 10016, United States of America.

Library of Congress Cataloging-in-Publication Data
Names: McGregor, Amy, author.
Title: Neurology board review : questions and answers / by Amy McGregor.
Description: Oxford; New York: Oxford University Press, [2016] | Includes
bibliographical references and index.
Identifiers: LCCN 2015040782 | ISBN 9780199895625 (alk. paper)
Subjects: | MESH: Nervous System Diseases—Examination Questions. |
Neurology—Examination Questions. | Specialty Boards—Examination Questions.
Classification: LCC RC343.5 | NLM WL 18.2 | DDC 616.80076—dc23 LC record available at
http://lccn.loc.gov/2015040782

For my husband and my mother

NOTE FROM THE AUTHOR

This book was designed to prepare the reader for the American Board of Psychiatry and Neurology (ABPN) board certification and recertification examinations. It covers the topics listed on the content outline provided by the ABPN. I recommend that you personally review this document prior to your test. This book is not a clinical manual and is not intended to guide clinical decision making or treatment; it is designed for test preparation. In order to convey important information, I have used some question formats that will not be on the actual ABPN board examination. I strongly recommend that you check the ABPN website for the format of your test and review the information provided by the testing site, including any practice questions. This test is very different from the resident in-service training (RITE) examination. I also suggest that you take advantage of the excellent resources provided by the American Academy of Neurology. Best of luck on your exam!

AM

ACKNOWLEDGMENTS

First, I need to acknowledge my husband, who supported me during the writing of this book.

I am grateful to all those who proofread chapters: David McGregor, Jim Wheless, Joshua Lennon, Masanori Igarashi, Stephen Fulton, Namrata Shah, Marc Malkoff, Lisa Armitige, Bola Adamolekun, Abigail Adamson, Sandy Arnold, Asim Choudhri, Anne Cross, Michael Jacewicz, Swati Karmarkar, Thomas O'Donnell, Brent Orr, Linda Buckleair, Jyotsna Ranga, Zsila Sadighi, Elizabeth Vannucci, and Aparajitha Verma. Any mistakes contained in this book are mine.

I would also like to thank Craig Panner at Oxford University Press for his patience and encouragement and Emily Samulski for her assistance.

I have too many friends, family members, and colleagues to thank to list them all, but I greatly appreciate all of you!

Thank you also to my residents, past and present, who helped inspire me to write this. This book is for you!

CONTENTS

1.

AUTONOMIC NERVOUS SYSTEM

QUESTIONS

1. State whether each of the following is a sympathetic or a parasympathetic response.
   1) Pupil constriction
   2) Inhibition of digestion
   3) Stimulation of glucose release
   4) Systemic vasoconstriction
   5) Salivation
   6) Bronchodilation
   7) Lacrimation
   8) Intestinal vasodilation

2. Which of the following is *not* involved in the parasympathetic nervous system?
   A. Oculomotor nerve
   B. Facial nerve
   C. Trigeminal nerve
   D. Glossopharyngeal nerve

3. Which of the following is a part of the sympathetic nervous system?
   A. Superior cervical ganglia
   B. Otic ganglia
   C. Pterygopalatine ganglia
   D. Submandibular ganglia

4. Which cranial nerve innervates the chemoreceptors and baroreceptors of the carotid body?
   A. Trigeminal
   B. Facial
   C. Glossopharyngeal
   D. Vagus

5. Parasympathetic preganglionic fibers for the heart, lungs, and gastrointestinal tract arise from which of these structures?
   A. Dorsal motor nucleus of the vagus
   B. Nucleus tractus solitarius
   C. Nucleus ambiguus
   D. Trigeminal nucleus

6. Which neurotransmitter is released by parasympathetic preganglionic neurons?
   A. Acetylcholine
   B. Norepinephrine
   C. Epinephrine
   D. Glycine

7. Which neurotransmitter is released by sympathetic preganglionic neurons?

   A. Acetylcholine
   B. Norepinephrine
   C. Epinephrine
   D. Glutamate

8. Which neurotransmitter is released by *most* sympathetic postganglionic neurons?
   A. Acetylcholine
   B. Norepinephrine
   C. Epinephrine
   D. Glutamate

9. **True or False?**
   During urination, the sympathetics are inhibited, causing relaxation of the bladder neck, and the parasympathetics are activated, causing contraction of the detrusor muscle.

10. **A patient has a suspected small-fiber neuropathy with autonomic dysfunction. Which of the following tests is the most sensitive?**
    A. Sudomotor testing
    B. Electromyography and nerve conduction studies (EMG/NCS)
    C. Holter test
    D. Tilt table test

11. **A 60-year-old man presents with fatigue and falls. On review of systems, he reports constipation and bruising. Neurologic examination identifies a peripheral neuropathy. General examination identifies macroglossia, hepatomegaly, and ecchymoses. Which test is most likely to confirm the diagnosis?**
    A. Immunofixation electrophoresis
    B. Kidney biopsy
    C. Liver biopsy
    D. Glucose tolerance test

12. **A 45-year-old woman presents with multiple falls. Which of the following would be most helpful in ruling out dysautonomia as the cause?**
    A. Denial of lightheadedness
    B. A history of constipation
    C. A history of urinary urgency
    D. A normal tilt table test

13. **A 15-year-old girl presents with lightheadedness, headaches, and fatigue that began after a viral illness. With minimal activity, she develops palpitations and sweating. When sitting, her heart rate is 80 beats per minute (bpm). Her heart rate increases to 120 bpm after she stands. Her blood pressure does not change significantly. What is the most likely diagnosis?**

A. Diabetes
B. Orthostatic hypotension
C. Postural orthostatic tachycardia syndrome (POTS)
D. Rapid-onset obesity with hypothalamic dysfunction, hypoventilation, and autonomic dysregulation (ROHHAD) syndrome

14. **A patient with suspected autonomic dysfunction performing the Valsalva maneuver does not demonstrate the normal increase in blood pressure during phase 4. What does this finding suggest?**
A. Orthostatic hypotension
B. Parkinson disease
C. Parasympathetic dysfunction
D. Sympathetic dysfunction

15. **True or False?**
A patient with anhidrosis on thermoregulatory sweat testing and a normal result on quantitative sudomotor autonomic reflex testing has a preganglionic sudomotor abnormality.

16. **Which of the following is associated with autonomic neuropathy?**
A. Anti-Hu antibodies (also known as antineuronal nuclear antibody type 1 [ANNA-1])
B. Nicotinic ganglionic acetylcholine receptor (α3-AChR) antibodies
C. P/Q-type calcium channel antibodies
D. All of the above

17. **Which of the following can cause autonomic neuropathy?**
A. Chagas disease
B. Diphtheria
C. Leprosy
D. All of the above

AUTONOMIC NERVOUS SYSTEM

ANSWERS

1. Sympathetic or parasympathetic responses

1) Pupil constriction—Parasympathetic
2) Inhibition of digestion—Sympathetic
3) Stimulation of glucose release—Sympathetic
4) Systemic vasoconstriction—Sympathetic
5) Salivation—Parasympathetic
6) Bronchodilation—Sympathetic
7) Lacrimation—Parasympathetic
8) Intestinal vasodilation—Parasympathetic

(See Table 1.1.)

Table 1.1 FUNCTIONS OF THE SYMPATHETIC AND PARASYMPATHETIC NERVOUS SYSTEMS

SYMPATHETIC	PARASYMPATHETIC
Pupil dilation	Pupil constriction
Increased heart rate and contraction	Decreased heart rate
Inhibition of digestion	Stimulation of digestion
Bronchodilation	Bronchoconstriction
Ejaculation	Erection

The parasympathetic nervous system is also known as the craniosacral division of the autonomic nervous system.

The preganglionic neurons of the sympathetic nervous system are in the intermediolateral nucleus (T1–L2) of the spinal cord.

2. C

The oculomotor, facial, glossopharyngeal, and vagus nerves are part of the parasympathetic nervous system; the trigeminal nerve is not.

The oculomotor nerve causes constriction of the pupil and ciliary body.

The facial nerve causes lacrimation and salivation.

The glossopharyngeal nerve causes salivation.

The vagus nerve causes heart deceleration, bronchoconstriction, stimulation of digestion by the stomach and release of bile from the gallbladder, and vasodilation of intestinal blood vessels.

3. A

The superior cervical ganglia is a part of the sympathetic nervous system. It is involved in pupil dilation.

4. C

The glossopharyngeal nerve innervates the chemoreceptors and baroreceptors of the carotid body. Information regarding blood volume and blood pressure from mechanoreceptors in the carotid arteries is relayed to the nucleus tractus solitarius (NTS). Similar information is carried from the aorta to the NTS through the vagus nerve.

Glossopharyngeal neuralgia causes pharyngeal pain. It can also result in reflex bradycardia and syncope.

5. A

Parasympathetic preganglionic fibers for the heart, lungs, and gastrointestinal tract arise from the dorsal motor nucleus of the vagus. This nucleus receives information from the nucleus tractus solitarius.

6. A

Acetylcholine is released by parasympathetic preganglionic neurons.

7. A

Acetylcholine is released by sympathetic preganglionic neurons.

8. B

Norepinephrine is released by most sympathetic postganglionic neurons. Sweat glands are an exception. Postganglionic neurons of sweat glands release acetylcholine; postganglionic sympathetic sweat glands have muscarinic receptors.

9. True

The overall effect of sympathetic autonomic innervation of the bladder is inhibition of micturition via urethral smooth muscle.

10. A

Sudomotor testing is sensitive to autonomic dysfunction associated with small-fiber neuropathy. EMG/NCS do not assess the appropriate nerve fibers and therefore miss small-fiber neuropathies. Skin biopsy is the gold standard for diagnosing small-fiber neuropathy.

11. A

This is primary amyloidosis, which causes autonomic neuropathy. Immunofixation electrophoresis can confirm the diagnosis.

The most common types of amyloidosis are primary amyloidosis, which is caused by a monoclonal gammopathy, and familial amyloidosis, which is caused by mutations in transthyretin.[1]

12. D

A normal tilt table test result would be the most helpful finding in ruling out dysautonomia. Patients with autonomic disorders do not always complain of lightheadedness. Constipation and urinary urgency can occur with dysautonomia.

13. C

Diabetes is the most common cause of autonomic neuropathy, but this case is most consistent with POTS.

POTS is a type of orthostatic intolerance. Orthostatic hypotension is defined by a decrease in systolic blood pressure of at least 20 mm Hg and/or a decrease in diastolic blood pressure of at least 10 mm Hg in the first 3 minutes of standing. If this decrease is not present but the patient has tachycardia and is symptomatic, then the patient has orthostatic intolerance. In adults with POTS, the heart rate increases by at least 30 bpm when standing. In children with POTS, it can increase by 40 bpm. POTS symptoms may manifest after an illness. Treatment involves hydration, increased salt intake, conditioning and strengthening, and sometimes support stockings. Medications used to treat POTS include beta-blockers, midodrine, and fludrocortisone. Midodrine is a sympathomimetic that can cause supine hypertension.

ROHHAD syndrome manifests in early childhood with rapid weight gain in a previously normal child. Autonomic dysfunction then occurs, followed by hypoventilation, which can be fatal. In addition to weight gain, polydipsia and hypernatremia are other common manifestations of hypothalamic dysfunction in patients with ROHHAD syndrome. Autonomic dysfunction causes ophthalmologic abnormalities such as pupillary dysfunction; thermal dysregulation; and gastrointestinal dysmotility. Some patients with ROHHAD syndrome develop neural crest tumors. ROHHAD syndrome shares some features with congenital central hypoventilation syndrome (CCHS), but CCHS is associated with mutations in *PHOX2B*.[2]

14. D

A lack of increase in blood pressure during phase 4 is consistent with sympathetic dysfunction.

15. True

Quantitative sudomotor autonomic reflex testing (QSART) assesses the postganglionic sympathetic sudomotor axon. If the patient has anhidrosis during thermoregulatory sweat testing and the QSART is normal, the lesion is preganglionic.

16. D

Anti-Hu antibodies can be seen in small-cell lung cancer.

Nicotinic ganglionic acetylcholine receptor (α3-AChR) antibodies are seen in autoimmune autonomic ganglionopathy, which causes pandysautonomia.

P/Q-type calcium channel antibodies occur in Lambert-Eaton syndrome (see Box 1.1).

Box 1.1 ANTIBODIES ASSOCIATED WITH AUTONOMIC NEUROPATHY

- Nicotinic ganglionic acetylcholine receptor (α3-AChR) antibodies
- Anti-Hu antibodies
- Purkinje cell antibodies type 2
- Collapsing response mediator protein-5 (anti-CV2)
- P/Q-type calcium channel antibodies
- *N*-Methyl-D-aspartate (NMDA) receptor antibodies

---

17. D

Chagas disease (due to the parasite *Trypanosoma cruzi*) causes megaesophagus and megacolon. It can also cause orthostatic hypotension, syncope, palpitations, and sudden death.

Leprosy causes asymmetric sensory loss. Sensitivity to pain and temperature are affected first. Leprosy also can affect autonomic skin fibers, resulting in loss of sweating. Cardiac autonomic neuropathy can be seen. Nerve enlargement occurs in leprosy; nerves may be palpable.

Diphtheria causes a distal polyneuropathy involving the limbs (a symmetric sensorimotor peripheral neuropathy) and a palatal neuropathy. In addition to palatal paralysis, other cranial nerves may become involved. Patients may have lack of accommodation with preservation of the light reflex. Involvement of the nodose ganglion of the vagus nerve can result in tachycardia. Hypotension can also occur.

Human immunodeficiency virus infection and botulism can also cause autonomic neuropathy.[1]

REFERENCES

1. Iodice V, Sandroni P. Autonomic neuropathies. *Continuum (Minneap Minn)* 2014;20:1373–1397.
2. Ize-Ludlow D, Gray JA, Sperling MA, et al. Rapid-onset obesity with hypothalamic dysfunction, hypoventilation, and autonomic dysregulation presenting in childhood. *Pediatrics* 2007;120:e179–e188.

2.

BEHAVIORAL NEUROLOGY

QUESTIONS

1. Which of the following is the most consistent finding in delirium?
   A. Auditory hallucinations
   B. Distractibility
   C. Aggression
   D. Seizures

2. A patient with renal failure develops confusion. He has asterixis on examination. Head computed tomography (CT) findings are normal. Besides diffuse background slowing, what is the most likely electroencephalography (EEG) finding?
   A. Focal slowing over the temporal lobes
   B. Focal slowing over the frontal lobes
   C. Intrusion of rapid eye movement sleep
   D. Triphasic waves

3. A 52-year-old man with a history of migraines is brought to the emergency department because of altered mental status. On examination, he is alert and oriented to self but repeats the same questions over and over. He has anterograde amnesia, but remote memory, speech, and attention are intact. Physical examination is normal. CT and EEG are normal. Routine laboratory test results are unremarkable. Seven hours later, he recovers. What is the most likely diagnosis?
   A. Transient global amnesia
   B. Basilar migraine
   C. Acute confusional state
   D. Postictal psychosis

4. True or False?
   The majority of left-handed people are left hemisphere dominant for language.

5. Motor impersistence is suggestive of a lesion in which part of the brain?
   A. Nondominant frontal lobe
   B. Nondominant parietal lobe
   C. Nondominant temporal lobe

6. A right-handed patient eats food only from the right side of his plate and denies that his left arm is his. Where is the lesion?
   A. Right frontal lobe
   B. Right parietal lobe
   C. Right temporal lobe
   D. Left frontal lobe

7. Which lobe is responsible for identification of problems, formulations of strategies, execution of plans, and evaluation of outcomes?
   A. Frontal
   B. Occipital
   C. Parietal
   D. Temporal

8. Which type of memory is most likely to be affected by normal aging?
   A. Episodic
   B. Implicit
   C. Semantic

9. What is the most common cause of episodic memory impairment?
   A. Alzheimer disease
   B. Parkinson disease
   C. Frontotemporal dementia
   D. Vascular cognitive impairment

10. What is the most common cause of semantic memory impairment?
    A. Alzheimer disease
    B. Parkinson disease
    C. Frontotemporal dementia
    D. Vascular cognitive impairment

11. The supplementary motor area, cerebellum, and basal ganglia are critical for which type of memory?
    A. Episodic
    B. Procedural
    C. Semantic
    D. Working

12. Which of the following is the most common cause of procedural memory impairment?
    A. Alzheimer disease
    B. Parkinson disease
    C. Frontotemporal dementia
    D. Vascular cognitive impairment

13. Which lobe of the brain is primarily responsible for working memory?
    A. Frontal
    B. Occipital
    C. Parietal
    D. Temporal

14. A patient has impaired immediate memory, free recall, and recollection but normal item memory and cued recall. He has false memories. His memory improves

significantly with environment support. Where is his lesion?
- A. Frontal lobe
- B. Lateral temporal lobe
- C. Medial temporal lobe
- D. Parietal lobe

15. Which of the following is *least* likely to be seen with a lesion of the orbitofrontal cortex?
- A. Insensitive remarks
- B. Akinetic mutism
- C. Perseveration
- D. Impulsivity

16. Which of the following is *not* part of Balint syndrome?
- A. Simultagnosia
- B. Optic ataxia
- C. Optic apraxia
- D. Inability to identify an object unless it moves

17. A lesion of the left occipital lobe and adjacent corpus callosum causes which of the following?
- A. Alexia with agraphia
- B. Alexia without agraphia
- C. Ideomotor apraxia
- D. Pure word deafness

18. A 60-year-old woman presents with difficulties writing and performing calculations. On examination, she is confused as to her left and right and has difficulty identifying fingers. Where is her lesion?
- A. Dominant inferior parietal lobe
- B. Dominant superior temporal lobe
- C. Nondominant inferior frontal lobe
- D. Nondominant parietal lobe

19. What is the term used when a patient believes that his friends and family have been replaced by imposters?
- A. Capgras syndrome
- B. Fregoli syndrome
- C. Reduplicative paramnesia
- D. Simultagnosia

20. A patient with bilateral posterior cerebral artery strokes cannot see, but he denies it. What is the name of this syndrome?
- A. Anton syndrome
- B. Charles Bonnet syndrome
- C. Ganser syndrome
- D. Geschwind syndrome

21. Where is the lesion that causes prosopagnosia?
- A. Right parietal lobe
- B. Left parietal lobe
- C. Right frontal lobe
- D. Bilateral occipitotemporal cortex

22. Which lobe of the brain is tested by the Wisconsin Card Sorting Test, the Stroop color word task, trail-making, and category fluency?
- A. Frontal
- B. Occipital
- C. Parietal
- D. Temporal

23. Which lobe is tested with go/no-go and sequencing tasks, such as the written alternating sequencing task or the manual sequencing task?
- A. Frontal
- B. Occipital
- C. Parietal
- D. Temporal

24. A 70-year-old woman is brought by her family to the emergency department because she is unable to speak. She obeys commands, except that she is unable to repeat when asked to do so and she cannot write. Where is the lesion?
- A. Dominant inferior frontal gyrus
- B. Dominant middle frontal gyrus
- C. Dominant superior frontal gyrus
- D. Dominant superior temporal gyrus

25. A patient has fluent but nonsensical speech. He also has impairments in comprehension, repetition, naming, reading, and writing. Where is the lesion?
- A. Inferior frontal gyrus
- B. Superior temporal gyrus
- C. Middle temporal gyrus
- D. Inferior temporal gyrus

26. A patient who has fluent speech and comprehends but cannot repeat has which of the following?
- A. Aphemia
- B. Conduction aphasia
- C. Transcortical motor aphasia
- D. Transcortical sensory aphasia
- E. Mixed transcortical aphasia

27. A patient with global aphasia, right hemiplegia, and right hemianesthesia most likely has a stroke in which territory?
- A. Left anterior cerebral artery
- B. Left middle cerebral artery
- C. Inferior division of the left middle cerebral artery
- D. Superior division of the left middle cerebral artery

28. A patient has a stroke resulting in aphasia and right arm and facial weakness without sensory deficits. Which type of aphasia is most likely in this patient?
- A. Broca aphasia
- B. Transcortial sensory aphasia
- C. Wernicke aphasia
- D. Mixed transcortical aphasia

29. **Anomic aphasia is most likely to occur with a lesion in which region?**
    A. Frontal operculum
    B. Supplementary motor area
    C. Angular gyrus
    D. Inferior temporal gyrus

30. **True or False?**
    Loss of emotional content of speech can occur with non-dominant hemisphere lesions.

31. **Which of the following differentiates aphemia (pure word mutism) from Broca aphasia and transcortical motor aphasia?**
    A. The ability to comprehend
    B. The ability to repeat
    C. The ability to write
    D. The ability to do calculations

BEHAVIORAL NEUROLOGY

ANSWERS

1. B

Attention difficulties are characteristic of delirium. Patients with delirium are distractible and have difficulty performing goal-directed tasks. Working memory is impaired, and patients have difficulty with digit span testing.

Risk factors include advanced age, multiple medications, underlying medical and neurologic conditions, vision or auditory impairment, and sleep deprivation. Environmental conditions such as isolation and lack of daylight also contribute.

Medications are a common cause of delirium.

2. D

Triphasic waves are seen in the setting of metabolic encephalopathy. Focal slowing indicates local dysfunction.

3. A

This patient has transient global amnesia (TGA), which is characterized by repetitive questioning and anterograde amnesia for several hours with normal findings on neurologic examination. Cognition is normal apart from the amnesia, and the patient remains oriented to self. Immediate memory and remote memories are intact, but there may be retrograde amnesia for the past weeks or years. Unlike patients with an acute confusional state, patients with TGA are able to maintain attention. Age greater than 50 years is a risk factor. Some patients have a history of migraine. On magnetic resonance imaging (MRI), an abnormality in the hippocampus has been found in some patients.

4. True

The Wada test (intracarotid sodium amobarbital test) is the gold-standard for determining hemispheric dominance for speech and memory.

5. A

Motor impersistence, in which a patient has difficulty maintaining a motor task, may occur with nondominant frontal lobe lesions.

6. B

The patient has neglect of the left side, consistent with a right parietal lobe lesion. The patient also has asomatognosia (i.e., he denies ownership of a limb). This is usually caused by a contralateral parietal lobe lesion. The term *asomatognosia* may also be used when a patient lacks awareness of sensation from part of the body (e.g., due to posterior column or peripheral nerve disease).

The term *anosognosia* also applies in this case. This term refers to denial of deficits, which is typically a result of right parietal lesions. This denial may include denial of ownership of a limb.

Anosodiaphoria is the term for lack of concern about one's illness.

7. A

The frontal lobe is responsible for identification of problems, formulations of strategies, execution of plans, and evaluation of outcomes.

8. A

Episodic memory is most likely to be affected by normal aging. Episodic memory refers to memory of an event. Impaired episodic memory may cause patients to lose objects or ask questions repetitively.

9. A

Alzheimer disease is the most common cause of episodic memory impairment. Normal episodic memory relies on the hippocampus and medial temporal lobe structures.

10. A

Semantic memory is declarative memory—knowledge of facts rather than memories about personal experience. It may manifest with anomia for words used infrequently.

Alzheimer disease affects the inferolateral temporal lobes, which are critical for semantic memory.

11. B

Procedural memory refers to skills that are usually performed automatically, such as riding a bike. The supplementary motor area, cerebellum, and basal ganglia are crucial for procedural memory.

12. B

Parkinson disease is the most common cause of impaired procedural memory.

13. A

Working memory allows one to temporarily store and manipulate information, for instance to perform calculations "in one's head." It allows short-term recall and is necessary for multitasking. The frontal lobe is primarily responsible.

14. A

Patients with memory deficits due to a frontal lobe lesion have impaired immediate memory, free recall, and recollection. Cued recall (recall after clues are given) and item memory tend to be normal. Patients may have false memories or confabulate. Environmental support improves memory performance.

Patients with medial temporal lobe lesions have impaired free recall, cued recall, recollection, and item memory. Environmental support is less likely to improve memory performance in these patients.

15. B

The orbitofrontal cortex is connected to the limbic system. Lesions of the orbitofrontal cortex cause disinhibition, impulsivity, and inappropriate jocularity (witzelsucht). Bilateral orbitofrontal lesions can cause imitation of gestures (echopraxia) and utilization behavior (manipulation of objects in the environment).

Lesions of the lateral frontal cortex cause apathy with intermittent bursts of anger/aggression. Patients have poor word list generation and psychomotor retardation.

Lesions of the medial frontal lobe cause akinetic mutism, lower extremity weakness, and incontinence.

Perseveration is the tendency to repeat a behavior excessively. It is seen with certain frontal lobe lesions, including orbitofrontal lobe lesions. Also, motor perseveration can be seen with medial frontal lesions.

16. D

In Balint syndrome, the patient has difficulty identifying moving objects. Patients who can identify an object *only* when it is moving have visual static agnosia. Balint syndrome occurs with bilateral parieto-occipital lesions. It is a type of disconnection syndrome. Other disconnection syndromes include alexia without agraphia, pure word deafness, and ideomotor apraxia.

17. B

A lesion of the left occipital lobe and adjacent corpus callosum causes alexia *without* agraphia. The patient may also have a right homonymous hemianopsia and difficulty naming colors.

Alexia *with* agraphia occurs with angular gyrus lesions.

Patients with pure word deafness (auditory verbal agnosia) have intact hearing but are unable to understand spoken language. Reading and writing are intact. Bilateral superior temporal gyrus lesions and certain dominant temporal lobe lesions can cause this pattern.

Ideomotor apraxia is difficulty acting out an action when instructed to do so. When given an object with which to act out the action, the patient is better able to perform the action.

Patients with *ideational* apraxia have difficulty knowing which action to perform and have difficulty performing a series of actions in the correct sequence. There is a loss of plan for performing a task (see Table 2.1).

Table 2.1 NEUROANATOMY OF BEHAVIORAL NEUROLOGY CONDITIONS

CONDITION	LESION(S)
Alexia without agraphia	Left occipital region and adjacent corpus callosum
Balint syndrome	Bilateral parieto-occipital
Ideomotor apraxia	Dominant inferior parietal lobe, supplementary motor area, or frontal cortex and adjacent corpus callosum
Ideational apraxia	Dominant parietal lobe

18. A

The condition described is Gerstmann syndrome. It is characterized by four primary symptoms: a writing disability (agraphia or dysgraphia), a lack of understanding of the rules for calculation or arithmetic (acalculia or dyscalculia), an inability to distinguish right from left, and an inability to identify fingers (finger agnosia). It is caused by a lesion in the dominant inferior parietal lobe.

19. A

Capgras syndrome is the term used when a patient believes his friends and family are duplicate imposters. It is a misidentification syndrome.

Fregoli syndrome is another misidentification syndrome. It is the belief that a stranger is actually a friend in disguise.

Reduplicative paramnesia is the belief that locations have been duplicated.

Simultagnosia is the inability to see two objects at the same time. Only portions of the visual field are perceived, not the whole scene. This occurs in Balint syndrome.

20. A

Anton syndrome is the term for patients who deny their blindness. It can occur with bilateral posterior cerebral artery strokes.

A patient with impaired vision who has visual hallucinations has Charles Bonnet syndrome.

Patients with Ganser syndrome respond to questions with inaccurate, approximate answers.

21. D

Prosopagnosia is the term for difficulty recognizing faces. It is caused by bilateral occipitotemporal cortex lesions.

22. A

The Wisconsin Card Sorting Test, the Stroop color word test, trail-making, and category fluency assess the frontal lobe.

The Stroop color word test evaluates attention and executive function, specifically response inhibition. During the task, the patient is asked to report the font color of a word when the word actually names a different color. For instance, if the word "yellow" is written in green ink, The correct response is green.

23. A

Go/no-go and sequencing tasks test the frontal lobe.

24. A

This patient's speech is not fluent, she comprehends, and she cannot repeat. This is Broca aphasia, which occurs with lesions of the dominant inferior frontal cortex, specifically the opercular and triangular parts of this gyrus.

If she could repeat, this would be transcortical motor aphasia, which is caused by a lesion anterior or superior to Broca's area. For instance, transcortical motor aphasia can occur with a stroke in the anterior cerebral artery (ACA) distribution or in the watershed area between the ACA and middle cerebral artery (MCA) territories.

25. B

This patient has Wernicke aphasia, which is caused by lesions of the dominant superior temporal gyrus. A visual field defect (homonymous hemianopia or quadrantanopia) may accompany Wernicke aphasia if the optic radiations are affected by the lesion. Anosognosia may also occur in patients with Wernicke aphasia.

26. B

This patient has conduction aphasia. Patients with conduction aphasia have fluent speech and are able to comprehend but cannot repeat. It can result from lesions in the insula, the posterior part of the superior temporal gyrus, or the supramarginal gyrus. Historically, it was thought to be caused by lesions of the arcuate fasciculus, which was thought to connect Broca's and Wernicke's areas; however, modern neuroimaging suggests that the connections between these areas are more complex than that.[1]

Aphemia is a nonfluent aphasia.

Repetition is intact in transcortical aphasias.

27. B

This patient has a stroke in the left middle cerebral artery (MCA) territory. The lesion is at the stem of the MCA. A right homonymous hemianopsia is also seen with this lesion. A left gaze preference may be seen at the onset of symptoms.

A stroke in the territory of the superior division of the left MCA can cause Broca aphasia.

A stroke in the territory of the inferior division of the left MCA can cause Wernicke aphasia.

A lesion of the left anterior cerebral artery (ACA) could cause weakness and sensory loss in the right leg and a transcortical motor aphasia.

28. A

This patient is most likely to have Broca aphasia. Broca's area is adjacent to primary motor cortex for the face, so a single lesion could cause Broca aphasia and facial weakness.

A stroke in the superior division of the left middle cerebral artery (MCA) could cause the clinical picture described in this case.

Transcortical sensory aphasia occurs with lesions near Wernicke's area.

Mixed transcortical aphasia can occur with strokes that affect the watershed region between the anterior cerebral artery (ACA) and the MCA or the watershed region between the MCA and posterior cerebral artery (PCA) in the dominant hemisphere, for instance due to occlusion of the internal carotid artery.

29. C

Anomic aphasia is more difficult to localize than other aphasias. Some cases are caused by lesions of the dominant angular gyrus. Anomic aphasia is characterized by

---

Box 2.1 OVERVIEW OF THE APHASIAS

Fluent aphasias:
- Anomic
- Wernicke
- Conduction
- Transcortical sensory

Non-fluent aphasias:
- Global
- Broca
- Transcortical motor
- Mixed transcortical
- Aphemia

Problems with naming:
- Global
- Broca
- Wernicke
- Transcortical (motor, sensory, and mixed)
- Anomia
- Aphemia

Problems with repetition:
- Global
- Broca
- Wernicke
- Conduction
- Aphemia

Problems with comprehension:
- Global
- Wernicke
- Transcortical sensory
- Mixed transcortical

word-finding difficulties, specifically difficulty naming. Otherwise, speech is fluent. Repetition and comprehension are intact. Anomia can occur in patients with Alzheimer disease or the semantic variant of primary progressive aphasia. It can also be seen in patients who are recovering from a more severe aphasia.

Lesions of the dominant angular gyrus can also cause Gerstmann syndrome and alexia.

Lesions to the frontal operculum are more likely to cause Broca aphasia.

30. True

Loss of emotional content of speech can occur with nondominant hemisphere lesions.

31. C

Aphemia is also referred to as pure word mutism. It is caused by small lesions in Broca's area or the adjacent subcortical white matter. Speech is difficult/effortful for patients with aphemia. However, comprehension, grammar, and writing are intact. Patients with Broca aphasia or transcortical motor aphasia are unable to write (see Box 2.1).

REFERENCE

1. Bernal B, Ardila A. The role of the arcuate fasciculus in conduction aphasia. *Brain* 2009;132:2309–2316.

3.

CEREBROVASCULAR DISEASE

QUESTIONS

1. A 60-year-old man presents with recent onset of right facial weakness. He cannot lift his right eyebrow or close his right eye. He has a depressed right nasolabial fold. He also reports decreased taste. What is the best treatment?
   A. Aspirin
   B. Heparin drip
   C. Prednisone
   D. Intravenous recombinant tissue plasminogen activator (rtPA) if he presents within 4.5 hours of symptom onset.

2. What is the most common cause of amaurosis fugax (transient monocular blindness)?
   A. Hypotension
   B. Ipsilateral internal carotid artery atherosclerosis
   C. Migraine
   D. Ophthalmic artery vasospasm
   E. Temporal arteritis

3. Which of the following is *least* likely to be due to a lacunar stroke in a left hemisphere dominant person?
   A. Left-sided weakness involving the face, arm, and leg
   B. Left-sided numbness involving the face, arm, and leg
   C. Dysarthria and a clumsy left arm
   D. Left face and arm weakness and left hemineglect

4. A 42-year-old man presents with ptosis on the left, numbness of his left face and right arm and leg, vomiting, vertigo, and falling to the right. Occlusion of which artery is most likely responsible?
   A. Vertebral artery
   B. Anterior inferior cerebellar artery
   C. Superior cerebellar artery
   D. Posterior cerebral artery

5. A stroke in which of these territories causes the lateral pontine syndrome (ipsilateral facial paralysis, unilateral deafness, vertigo, facial hemianesthesia, contralateral loss of pain and temperature, ataxia, and ipsilateral Horner syndrome).
   A. Anterior inferior cerebellar artery (AICA)
   B. Anterior spinal artery
   C. Paramedian branches of the basilar artery
   D. Posterior inferior cerebellar artery (PICA)

6. A 60-year-old man presents with left face and arm weakness. Sensation is normal. What artery is most likely involved?
   A. The right recurrent artery of Huebner
   B. The right anterior cerebral artery

   C. The right lateral lenticulostriate arteries
   D. The right anterior choroidal artery

7. A 70-year-old woman presents with a stroke of the medial thalami bilaterally. Where is the lesion?
   A. The artery of Percheron
   B. Posterior choroidal artery
   C. Polar/thalamotuberal artery
   D. Thalamogeniculate artery

8. A 55-year-old man taking no medications presents with acute stroke. His oxygen saturation is 96% on room air. Which of the following is *false*?
   A. Supplemental oxygen should be given.
   B. Cardiac monitoring should be performed for the first 24 hours after the stroke to rule out atrial fibrillation.
   C. Since there is no history of anticoagulant use, the only blood test required before administration of recombinant tissue plasminogen activator (rtPA), if there is no reason to suspect a bleeding abnormality, is a blood glucose measurement.
   D. Baseline troponins should not delay administration of rtPA.

9. Which of the following statements is *false*?
   A. If a patient clinically has a transient ischemic attack, the findings on diffusion-weighted imaging (DWI) will be negative.
   B. Some patients with stroke have negative diffusion-weighted imaging findings.
   C. Recombinant tissue plasminogen activator (rtPA) can be given to a stroke patient who is improving clinically if the remaining deficit is not minor.
   D. The guidelines now state that rtPA can be given to patients up to 4.5 hours after the onset of stroke, but there are additional exclusion criteria after 3 hours.

10. A 60-year-old patient presents with stroke. Symptoms began 30 minutes ago. No contraindications to recombinant tissue plasminogen activator are found in the history or laboratory studies. Computed tomography (CT) shows blurring of the gray-white junction involving more than one third of the middle cerebral artery territory. Which of the following is the most appropriate treatment?
    A. Aspirin
    B. Clopidogrel
    C. Heparin drip
    D. Recombinant tissue plasminogen activator

11. True or False?
    According to the 2015 American Heart Association/ American Stroke Association (AHA/ASA) endovascular

therapy guideline, a patient may receive recombinant tissue plasminogen activator (rtPA) and endovascular therapy.

12. Which of the following statements is *false*?
    A. In addition to being invasive, conventional angiography does not provide good visualization of intramural hematomas.
    B. Intravenous tissue plasminogen activator is contraindicated in cases of stroke from carotid dissection.
    C. Infection, hypoglycemia, and other metabolic disturbances can reactivate old stroke symptoms.
    D. Hemiparesis is the most common presentation of acute stroke in children.

13. What is the mechanism of action of recombinant tissue plasminogen activator?
    A. It converts plasminogen to plasmin, which initiates fibrinolysis.
    B. It inhibits platelet cyclooxygenase.
    C. It inhibits platelet aggregation.
    D. It is a thrombin inhibitor.

14. A 55-year-old man has a right middle cerebral artery infarct. Thirty six hours after the stroke, he is difficult to arouse. CT shows mass effect and slight midline herniation. Which treatment should be considered?
    A. Corticosteroids
    B. Hemicraniectomy
    C. Hypothermia
    D. Suboccipital decompression

15. A patient with hypertension is found to have asymptomatic carotid stenosis. Which of the following is recommended to prevent stroke?
    A. Initiation of aspirin and a statin
    B. Self-measured blood pressure at home to try to improve blood pressure measurements
    C. A diet that is low in sodium and high in potassium
    D. All of the above

16. A 70-year-old man presents with right middle cerebral artery stroke. Investigations reveal 90% stenosis of his right middle cerebral artery. Which of the following treatments is recommended?
    A. Aspirin 325 mg daily
    B. Warfarin
    C. Angioplasty of the right middle cerebral artery
    D. Stenting of the right middle cerebral artery

17. A 60-year-old man presents the day after a stroke. A patent foramen ovale (PFO) is found. The rest of his workup is unremarkable. He has never had a deep vein thrombosis. What treatment is recommended?
    A. Aspirin
    B. PFO closure in 1 month
    C. PFO closure as soon as possible
    D. Warfarin

18. A 40-year-old woman presents with a stroke. She has a history of three spontaneous abortions. Her partial thromboplastin time (PTT) is prolonged. Which of the following tests is most likely to confirm her diagnosis?
    A. Quantitative von Willebrand factor testing
    B. Antithrombin III level
    C. Testing for antiphospholipid antibodies
    D. Testing for protein S deficiency

19. In which stroke patients may carotid endarterectomy (CEA) be associated with an improved outcome compared with carotid artery stenting (CAS)?
    A. Age greater than 70 years
    B. Patients with hyperlipidemia
    C. Patients with mild diabetes
    D. Patients taking aspirin

20. Which of the following is *least* likely to increase the risk for stroke due to atrial fibrillation?
    A. Congestive heart failure
    B. Hypertension
    C. Diabetes
    D. Age 60 years

21. What is an advantage of warfarin compared with other oral anticoagulants such as apixaban and dabigatran?
    A. It is reversible with vitamin K and fresh frozen plasma.
    B. It is shorter acting.
    C. Less risk for intracranial hemorrhage
    D. Less risk for gastrointestinal hemorrhage

22. What is the mechanism of action for clopidogrel?
    A. It antagonizes the vitamin K–dependent clotting pathway.
    B. It prevents binding of adenosine diphosphate (ADP) to its receptor on platelets.
    C. It is a factor Xa inhibitor.
    D. It is a thrombin inhibitor.

23. What is the mechanism of action for dabigatran?
    A. It antagonizes the vitamin K–dependent clotting pathway.
    B. It is a factor Xa inhibitor.
    C. It inhibits platelet aggregation.
    D. It is a thrombin inhibitor.

24. A 30-year-old woman with a history of migraines presents with stroke. Her father had a history of recurrent strokes beginning at age 40. Her paternal grandmother had early dementia. Magnetic resonance imaging (MRI) shows extensive white matter disease. Which of the following is expected?
    A. Mutation in the *GLA* gene
    B. Mutation in the *HTRA1* gene
    C. Mutation in the *KRIT1* gene
    D. Mutation in the *NOTCH3* gene

25. A 20-year-old man with a history of intellectual disability and myopia presents with stroke. On examination, he is tall and thin. Serum and urine amino acids confirm his diagnosis. A trial of which medication is recommended to treat the underlying condition?
    A. Carnitine
    B. Coenzyme Q10
    C. Pyridoxine
    D. Warfarin

26. In a patient with sickle cell disease and high-velocity flow in the middle cerebral artery demonstrated on transcranial Doppler ultrasonography, what is the best method to prevent stroke?
    A. Avoid iron deficiency anemia.
    B. Transfuse the patient to maintain a hemoglobin S concentration at less than 30% of the total hemoglobin concentration.
    C. Transfuse the patient when symptoms occur.
    D. Transfuse the patient if symptoms persist after hydration.

27. Fill in the blank.

    Oxygen delivery is the product of cerebral blood flow and _____.
    A. Blood oxygen content
    B. Percentage of hemoglobin A
    C. Oxygen saturation measured by pulse oximeter
    D. Hematocrit

28. Which of the following is *least* susceptible to hypoxic injury?
    A. Pyramidal cells in area CA1 (Sommer's sector) of the hippocampus
    B. Purkinje cells in the cerebellum
    C. Neurons of layers III, V, and VI of the cortex
    D. Granule cells of the cerebellum

29. Which of the following causes acquired antithrombin deficiency?
    A. Asparaginase
    B. Cyclophosphamide
    C. 5-Fluorouracil
    D. Methotrexate

30. Which of the following is the most common inherited risk factor for thrombophilia?
    A. Factor V Leiden
    B. Prothrombin gene mutation
    C. Protein C deficiency
    D. Protein S deficiency

31. A 58-year-old woman presents with a small subcortical intracerebral hemorrhage. Her blood pressure is 185/115 mm Hg. Which of the following is recommended at this time?
    A. Mannitol
    B. 3% hypertonic saline
    C. Nicardipine
    D. Intravenous fosphenytoin

32. A 50-year-old man presents with a lobar intracerebral hemorrhage. Which of the following is *not* recommended?
    A. Screen for a myocardial infarction.
    B. Screen for dysphagia.
    C. Administer corticosteroids to decrease intracranial pressure.
    D. Consider continuous electroencephalographic (EEG) monitoring if his mental status is worse than expected.

33. A 55-year-old man with cerebellar hemorrhage begins to worsen neurologically. Which of the following is most likely to be effective?
    A. Ventricular drainage
    B. Mannitol
    C. Hypertonic saline
    D. Surgery

34. What is the most common site of intracerebral hemorrhage due to hypertension?
    A. Cerebellum
    B. Putamen
    C. Pons
    D. Thalamus

35. A 24-year-old man presents with severe headache that started when he was moving his couch. He reports even more pain with neck movement. CT of the head is normal. What is the next step?
    A. Administer intravenous ketorolac.
    B. Administer subcutaneous sumatriptan.
    C. Administer intravenous valproic acid.
    D. Lumbar puncture

36. A 55-year-old man develops a severe headache while straining. He is found to have subarachnoid hemorrhage. His angiogram is negative. Subarachnoid hemorrhage with a negative angiogram is most likely to be associated with which of the following?
    A. An anterior cerebral artery aneurysm
    B. An anterior communicating artery aneurysm
    C. A middle cerebral artery aneurysm
    D. Perimesencephalic hemorrhage

37. Which of the following is *not* a risk factor for aneurysmal subarachnoid hemorrhage?
    A. Aneurysm more than 7 mm in size
    B. Pregnancy and delivery
    C. Significant life event in the past month
    D. Smoking

38. A 71-year-old patient presents with aneurysmal subarachnoid hemorrhage. Which of the following statements is *false*?
    A. Myocardial infarction and arrhythmias can occur after subarachnoid hemorrhage.
    B. Coiling of the aneurysm is preferred because of the patient's age.
    C. Treatment of the aneurysm by coiling or clipping should be postponed for 1 week to allow for the patient's condition to stabilize.
    D. After treatment of the aneurysm, repeat imaging should be performed.

39. Which of the following is the most effective therapy to prevent delayed cerebral ischemia in a patient with subarachnoid hemorrhage?
    A. Hypertension, hypervolemia, and hemodilution (HHH) therapy
    B. Labetalol

C. Oral nimodipine

D. Nitroprusside

40. A 16-year-old presents with a seizure and is found to have an aneurysm. On review of systems, the mother mentions academic difficulties and nose bleeds. There is a family history of arteriovenous malformation and hearing loss. The mother has telangiectasias on her face. A defect in the gene encoding which of the following proteins needs to be considered?

A. Endoglin

B. Tuberin

C. Hamartin

D. Merlin

41. A 30-year-old woman suffers a carotid dissection. An angiogram shows a "string of beads" formation. Which of the following is the most likely diagnosis?

A. Ehlers-Danlos syndrome

B. Fibromuscular dysplasia

C. Marfan syndrome

D. Moyamoya disease

42. A child with a history of narrowing of the internal carotid arteries develops left-sided weakness when she is running on the playground and when crying. What diagnosis should be suspected?

A. Hemiplegic migraine

B. Dissection

C. Moyamoya syndrome

D. Transient cerebral arteriopathy

43. Which of the following is *least* likely to be present if a patient has dissection of the internal carotid artery?

A. Ptosis

B. Miosis

C. Anhidrosis

44. A 20-year-old woman who gave birth 3 days earlier presents with a seizure, severe headache, and vomiting. She has papilledema on examination. Which of the following would most likely provide the diagnosis?

A. Magnetic resonance angiogram (MRA)

B. Magnetic resonance venography (MRV)

C. Carotid ultrasound

D. Ophthalmology consult

45. A patient is diagnosed with sagittal sinus thrombosis. Which of the following statements is *false*?

A. On a contrast CT study, the empty delta sign may be seen.

B. Anti-epileptic medication should be started to prevent seizures.

C. Steroids are not recommended.

D. Tests for protein C and protein S deficiency should be done 2 to 4 weeks after anticoagulation is completed.

46. What is the best way to diagnose small-vessel vasculitis?

A. Magnetic resonance angiography (MRA)

B. Computed tomography angiography (CTA)

C. Conventional angiography

D. Brain biopsy

CEREBROVASCULAR DISEASE

ANSWERS

1. C

This patient has facial weakness involving the upper and lower face. This is consistent with a *peripheral* cranial nerve 7 palsy, *not* a central cranial nerve 7 palsy. Also, his taste sensation is decreased. This patient has Bell palsy. Bell palsy is in the differential diagnosis for facial weakness. Non-neurologists may mistake facial weakness due to Bell palsy for a stroke. A patient with Bell palsy could have also have hyperacusis. New-onset Bell palsy is treated with prednisone. Antivirals may be offered, but the patient should be counseled that there is no evidence of significant improvement with antivirals.[1]

2. B

Ipsilateral internal carotid artery atherosclerosis is the most common cause of amaurosis fugax.

3. D

A stroke in the superior division of the right middle cerebral artery (MCA) causes left face and arm weakness and left hemineglect in a left hemisphere dominant person. There may also be sensory loss in the face and arm. This is not a lacunar stroke syndrome. The other clinical scenarios are consistent with lacunar stroke.

Pure motor hemiparesis results from lesions in the internal capsule, basis pontis, or corona radiata.

A lesion in the ventroposterolateral nucleus of the thalamus can cause a pure hemisensory stroke.

Dysarthria–clumsy hand syndrome occurs with lesions involving the basis pontis, internal capsule, or cerebral peduncle.

Ataxic hemiparesis is another lacunar stroke syndrome. It can occur with lesions of the posterior limb of the internal capsule or the basis pontis.

A lacune involving the internal capsule and thalamus can cause a sensorimotor stroke characterized by hemisensory loss and hemiparesis contralateral to the lesion.

4. A

This is Wallenberg syndrome (lateral medullary syndrome), which most often is caused by occlusion of the vertebral artery but also can be caused by occlusion of the posterior inferior cerebellar artery. Patients with Wallenberg syndrome have ipsilateral ataxia due to involvement of the

inferior cerebellar peduncle; vertigo due to involvement of the vestibular nuclei; decreased pain and temperature in the ipsilateral face due to involvement of the trigeminal nucleus and tract; decreased pain and temperature in the contralateral body due to involvement of the spinothalamic tract; an ipsilateral Horner syndrome due to involvement of descending sympathetic fibers; hoarseness and dysphagia due to involvement of the nucleus ambiguus; and decreased taste due to involvement of the nucleus solitarius (see Figure 3.1).

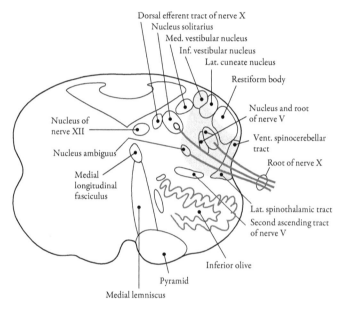

Figure 3.1 Cross-section of the medulla illustrating the zone of infarction with Wallenberg syndrome. Inf. = inferior; Lat. = lateral; Med. = medial. (From Baloh RW, Honrubia V, Kerber K, eds. *Baloh and Honrubia's Clinical Neurophysiology of the Vestibular System,* 4th edition, Fig. 14-1. New York, Oxford University Press, 2011.)

5. A

A stroke in the AICA distribution causes the lateral pontine syndrome.

Medial medullary syndrome may be caused by an anterior spinal artery stroke or a stroke involving branches of the vertebral artery. The medial medullary syndrome affects the pyramid, medial lemniscus, and hypoglossal nerve. Patients have contralateral weakness, usually sparing the face, ipsilateral tongue weakness, and contralateral loss of position and vibration sense.

A stroke in the PICA territory can cause a cerebellar stroke or a lateral medullary syndrome.

A stroke in the distribution of the paramedian branches of the basilar artery causes medial inferior pontine syndrome. The medial lemniscus, corticospinal tract, and abducens nerve roots are affected.

6. A

This patient had a stroke in the distribution of the right recurrent artery of Huebner. This is a branch of the anterior cerebral artery. A stroke in this territory causes contralateral face and arm weakness.

A stroke in the distribution of the right anterior cerebral artery would cause contralateral lower extremity weakness and sensory loss with less involvement of the arm.

A stroke in the distribution of the right lateral lenticulostriate arteries would cause a contralateral pure motor hemiparesis. This usually affects the face, arm, and leg; strokes affecting two of these three areas are possible but rare. The lateral lenticulostriate arteries are a branch of the middle cerebral artery and help to supply the internal capsule.

A stroke in the distribution of the right anterior choroidal artery would cause contralateral hemiplegia due to injury to the posterior limb of the internal capsule. Contralateral hemianesthesia occurs with thalamic injury. Involvement of the lateral geniculate body causes a sectoranopia with sparing in the horizontal meridian.

7. A

The artery of Percheron is an anatomic variant of the posterior circulation. Typically, the paramedian thalamus is supplied by ipsilateral paramedian/thalamoperforating arteries, which are branches of the P1 segment of the posterior cerebral artery (PCA). The artery of Percheron is a single dominant thalamoperforating artery that arises from one P1 segment and supplies both paramedian thalami. It may also supply the midbrain.

The anterior thalamus is supplied by the polar/thalamotuberal arteries, which are branches of the posterior communicating artery. The inferolateral thalamus is supplied by the thalamogeniculate arteries, which are branches from the P2 segment of the PCA. The posterior thalamus is supplied by the posterior choroidal arteries, which also are branches from the P2 segment of the PCA.

Other causes of bilateral thalamic lesions are cerebral venous thrombosis, Wernicke encephalopathy, extrapontine myelinolysis, Wilson disease, Creutzfeldt-Jakob disease, neurofibromatosis type 1, Leigh disease, and bilateral thalamic glioma.

8. A

Oxygen does not need to be given to all acute stroke patients. The goal is for the oxygen saturation to be greater than 94%.

Obtaining an electrocardiogram and a chest radiograph should not delay administration of recombinant tissue plasminogen activator.[2]

9. A

Some patients with transient ischemic attack (TIA) have been found to have a positive DWI study, and some patients with stroke have a negative DWI. A false-negative DWI is more likely if the stroke is mild, in the brainstem, or very early.

Intravenous rtPA can be given to patients up to 4.5 hours after the onset of stroke, but there are additional exclusion criteria after 3 hours (see Box 3.1).[2]

Box 3.1 EXCLUSION CRITERIA
FOR ADMINISTRATION OF RTPA BETWEEN 3 AND
4.5 HOURS AFTER THE ONSET OF A STROKE

- Age greater than 80 years
- Patient is taking anticoagulants (regardless of the international normalized ratio)
- National Institutes of Health Stroke Scale (NIHSS) score greater than 25
- Ischemic injury involves more than one third of the middle cerebral artery territory
- History of both stroke and diabetes mellitus

10. D

Obvious hypodensity would be a contraindication to recombinant tissue plasminogen activator, but early ischemic changes indicating involvement of more than one third of the middle cerebral artery (MCA) territory is not a contraindication according to the latest guidelines.

Loss of gray-white differentiation is an early sign of ischemia on CT. This may be seen in the basal ganglia (lenticular obscuration), over the convexities (cortical ribbon sign), and at the junction of the cortex and insula (insular ribbon sign). Also, the gyri may swell, producing sulcal effacement. A hyperdense MCA suggests occlusion of this artery. A clot in the branch of the MCA may be seen as a dot (MCA dot sign) (see Box 3.2).[2]

Box 3.2 EARLY SIGNS OF ISCHEMIA
ON COMPUTED TOMOGRAPHY

- Loss of gray-white differentiation
  - Lenticular obscuration
  - Cortical ribbon sign
  - Insular ribbon sign
- Sulcal effacement
- Hyperdense MCA or MCA dot sign

11. True

According to the 2015 American Heart Association/American Stroke Association endovascular therapy guideline, if a patient is eligible for rtPA, it should be administered even if endovascular treatment is being considered. There is no need to monitor the patient for response to intravenous rtPA before proceeding with endovascular therapy. The guideline also states that endovascular therapy with a stent retriever is preferred over intra-arterial rtPA, because rtPA has not been approved for intra-arterial use. According to the guideline, intra-arterial fibrinolysis may be performed within 6 hours of stroke onset in selected patients who have contraindications to intravenous rtPA; however, the consequences are unknown.[3]

12. B

Conventional angiography does not provide good visualization of intramural hematomas. MRI with magnetic resonance angiography (MRA) can be used to identify intramural hematomas. Computed tomography angiography (CTA) is helpful for identifying intimal flaps, pseudoaneurysms, high-grade stenosis, and vertebral dissections.

Carotid dissection is *not* a contraindication to rtPA.

13. A

Recombinant tissue plasminogen activator converts plasminogen to plasmin, which initiates fibrinolysis.

14. B

Fever, seizures, and hypercapnia contribute to increased intracranial pressure and should be avoided in patients with ischemia. Hyperglycemia can contribute to edema and should also be avoided. Hypoglycemia can increase the size of infarction.

Osmotic therapy may be used in patients with cerebral edema who deteriorate. Current guidelines state that hypothermia, barbiturates, and corticosteroids are not recommended to treat swelling in patients with edema following ischemia.

This patient is a candidate for hemicraniectomy. Guidelines from the AHA/ASA state that decompressive craniectomy with dural expansion is effective in patients with unilateral middle cerebral artery (MCA) infarctions who are younger than 60 years of age and whose condition deteriorates within 48 hours despite medical therapy.

Suboccipital craniectomy with dural expansion is indicated in patients with cerebellar infarctions who deteriorate despite medical therapy.[4]

15. D

The patient's stroke risk should be assessed, and risk factors should be addressed. The patient's hypertension should be treated. The goal is a blood pressure less than 140/90 mm Hg. The patient should be placed on aspirin and a statin given his asymptomatic carotid stenosis. A diet that is low in sodium and high in potassium has been recommended. Other dietary recommendations include a DASH-style diet (fruits, vegetables, low-fat dairy products, reduced saturated fat); a Mediterranean diet with addition of nuts; or a diet rich in fruits and vegetables. The 2014 AHA/ASA guidelines for primary stroke prevention state that carotid endarterectomy may be considered in asymptomatic patients who have greater than 70% stenosis of the internal carotid artery if the operative risks are low.[5]

16. A

According to the AHA/ASA guidelines for secondary stroke prevention, aspirin 325 mg daily is recommended for this patient. Clopidogrel 75 mg daily may be added for 90 days if it is initiated within 1 month after a stroke (or a transient ischemic attack). Stenting and angioplasty are considered investigational in this setting. Stenting with the Wingspan stent system is not recommended.

Since the patient has more than 50% stenosis of a major intracranial artery, it is also recommended that his systolic blood pressure be less than 140 mm Hg and that he be placed on high-intensity statin therapy.[6]

17. A

There is no indication for anticoagulation. Antiplatelet therapy is recommended. Closure of the PFO is *not* indicated in a patient with cryptogenic ischemic stroke who does not have a deep vein thrombosis (DVT). It may be considered if the patient has a DVT and a risk for recurrence of DVT.[6]

18. C

This patient most likely has antiphospholipid antibodies. Antiphospholipid antibodies increase one's risk for venous and arterial thromboses. Examples of antiphospholipid antibodies are lupus anticoagulant, anticardiolipin, and anti-β_2-glycoprotein I antibodies. Livedo reticularis, unexplained thrombocytopenia, a prolonged PTT, and fetal loss raise concern for antiphospholipid antibody syndrome.

According to the 2015 AHA/ASA guidelines for secondary stroke prevention, routine testing for antiphospholipid antibodies is not required in a patient with ischemic stroke or a transient ischemic attack (TIA) if another explanation is found. Patients who have had an ischemic stroke or TIA and meet criteria for antiphospholipid antibody syndrome may be placed on anticoagulation depending on the risk for recurrent thrombotic events and the risk for bleeding. If anticoagulation is not initiated, antiplatelet therapy is recommended. If a patient has antiphospholipid antibodies but does not meet full criteria for the antiphospholipid antibody syndrome, antiplatelet therapy is recommended.[6]

19. A

According to the 2015 AHA/ASA guidelines for secondary stroke prevention, age may be considered when choosing between CEA and CAS. Patients older than 70 years of age may have improved outcome with CEA. In younger patients, the risks of CEA and CAS are equivalent.

CEA is recommended for patients with severe stenosis (70–99%) and a history of stroke or TIA within the past 6 months if the risks of surgery are low. It is recommended for patients with moderate (50–69%) stenosis and a history of stroke or TIA depending on patient-specific factors, if the risk of surgery is low. Neither CEA nor CAS is recommended for patients with less than 50% stenosis.

CAS is an alternative to CEA in symptomatic individuals if the lumen is shown to be more than 70% reduced by noninvasive imaging or more than 50% by angiography, if the patient is at low risk for complications. Likewise, if the patient is at increased risk from CEA surgery or had a restenosis after CEA, CAS may be considered if the patient has stenosis greater than 70% and is symptomatic.[6]

20. D

To estimate the risk for stroke in a patient with atrial fibrillation, the $CHADS_2$ score or the CHA_2DS_2-VASc score can be used (see Boxes 3.3 and 3.4).

Box 3.3 CHADS₂

The $CHADS_2$ score is used to estimate the risk for stroke in a patient with atrial fibrillation. The acronym $CHADS_2$ stands for

- Congestive heart failure
- Hypertension
- Age ≥75 years
- Diabetes mellitus
- Stroke or TIA previously

In scoring, a previous stroke or TIA gives 2 points, and the others give 1 point each. The maximum score is 6.

Box 3.4 CHA₂DS₂-VASC

The CHA_2DS_2-VASc score has been used since 2010 to estimate the risk for stroke in a patient with atrial fibrillation. It provides a better stratification of low-risk patients than the $CHADS_2$ score. The acronym CHA_2DS_2-VASc stands for

- Congestive heart failure
- Hypertension
- Age ≥75 years
- Diabetes mellitus
- Stroke or TIA previously
- Vascular disease
- Age 65–74 years
- Sex category (i.e., female sex)

In scoring, age ≥75 years or a previous stroke or TIA gives 2 points; age 65–74 and the others give 1 point each. The maximum score is 9.

The risk for bleeding from anticoagulation in a patient with atrial fibrillation is determined by the HAS-BLED score (see Box 3.5).

Box 3.5 HAS-BLED

The HAS-BLED score is used to determine the 1-year risk for major bleeding from anticoagulation in a patient with atrial fibrillation. The acronym HAS-BLED stands for

- Hypertension
- Abnormal liver or renal function
- Stroke
- Bleeding previously or predisposition to bleeding
- Labile international normalized ratio (INR)
- Elderly (age >65 years)
- Drug or alcohol use

Vitamin K antagonists (e.g., warfarin), apixaban, or dabigatran can be used to prevent recurrent stroke or TIA in patients with nonvalvular atrial fibrillation. Rivaroxaban can also be used.

If treating with a vitamin K antagonist, the target INR for a patient with atrial fibrillation and a history of stroke or TIA is 2.5.

If a patient with a stroke or TIA also has significant coronary artery disease, such as an acute coronary syndrome or stent placement, then the patient may be given both oral anticoagulation and antiplatelet therapy (if there are no contraindications).

In most patients who have atrial fibrillation and have had a stroke, oral anticoagulation can be started within 2 weeks of the stroke. However, if there is a high risk of hemorrhagic conversion, one can delay initiation of treatment.[6]

21. A

One advantage of warfarin over the newer anticoagulants is that it is reversible with vitamin K and fresh frozen plasma. Prothrombin complex concentrates are also being investigated. Specific antibodies exist for reversal of the novel oral anticoagulants (NOACs), especially the factor Xa inhibitors, but they may not be readily available.

The newer agents do have a short half-life.

Warfarin antagonizes the vitamin K–dependent clotting pathway. Activated vitamin K is needed to activate factors II (prothrombin), VII, IX, and X; protein C; and protein S. Vitamin K deficiency causes a prolonged prothrombin time (PT).

The ARISTOTLE (Apixaban for Reduction in Stroke and Other Thromboembolic Events in Atrial Fibrillation) trial found decreased risk for intracranial hemorrhage in patients taking apixaban compared with those taking warfarin. There was no significant difference in the rate of gastrointestinal hemorrhage.[6,7,8]

22. B

Clopidogrel prevents platelet aggregation. An active metabolite of clopidogrel prevents binding of ADP to its receptor on platelets (the $P2Y_{12}$ receptor). This prevents ADP-mediated activation of the glycoprotein IIb/IIIa complex, which is needed for platelet aggregation.

Patients with a reduced-function *CYP2C19* allele have a reduced response to clopidogrel and worse cardiovascular outcomes. There is also a variant that leads to an enhanced response and an increased risk for bleeding.

23. D

Dabigatran is a thrombin inhibitor (see Table 3.1).

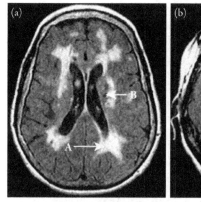
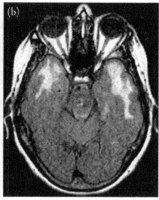
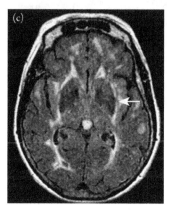

Table 3.1 MECHANISM OF ACTION OF ANTICOAGULANTS AND ANTIPLATELET AGENTS

MEDICATION	MECHANISM OF ACTION
Apixaban	Factor Xa inhibitor
Clopidogrel	Prevents binding of ADP to the $P2Y_{12}$ receptor on platelets. This prevents ADP-mediated activation of the GPIIb/IIIa complex.
Dabigatran	Thrombin inhibitor
Rivaroxaban	Factor Xa inhibitor
Warfarin	Antagonizes the vitamin K–dependent clotting pathway

Figure 3.2 Appearances of CADASIL on fluid-attenuated inversion recovery (FLAIR) magnetic resonance imaging. a: Leukoaraiosis (arrow A) and focal lacunar infarction (arrow B) b: Involvement of the anterior temporal pole c: Involvement of the external capsule (arrow) (From Markus H, Pereira A, Cloud G. *OSH Stroke Medicine*, Fig. 11.4. New York, Oxford University Press, 2010.)

24. D

This patient has cerebral autosomal dominant arteriopathy with subcortical infarcts and leukoencephalopathy (CADASIL), which causes fibrosis of small arteries and arterioles.

CADASIL causes migraine headaches (often with a visual aura), early stroke, recurrent stroke, seizures, and early dementia. Patients with CADASIL may also have mood disturbance and cognitive impairment. Hyperintensities in the white matter of the anterior temporal poles on T2-weighted MRI are characteristic. As the disease progresses, the white matter becomes more abnormal. Symmetric white matter lesions are seen in the periventricular regions and in the deep white matter (see Figure 3.2). Dilated perivascular spaces and cerebral microbleeds can also been seen. CADASIL is caused by a missense mutation of the *NOTCH3* gene on chromosome 19q12. If gene testing is negative but the diagnosis is still suspected, then skin biopsy can be performed. In CADASIL, there is deposition of eosinophilic granular material in the media of small arteries and arterioles. It is positive on periodic acid–Schiff (PAS) staining and stains with Congo red. Electron microscopy shows granular osmophilic material.

Mutations in *HTRA1* cause cerebral autosomal *recessive* arteriopathy with subcortical infarcts and leukoencephalopathy (CARASIL). The first symptom is often gait disturbance and spasticity, which manifest in early adulthood and are caused by white matter lesions. Similar to patients with CADASIL, patients with CARASIL may have early stroke, mood changes, and cognitive decline. Premature alopecia

and back pain are more characteristic of CARASIL than CADASIL.

Mitochondrial encephalomyopathy, lactic acidosis, and stroke-like episodes (MELAS) can also cause migraine-type headaches, early dementia, seizures, and stroke. Most cases of MELAS are caused by mutations in the *MT-TL1* (transfer RNA mitochondrial, leucine 1) gene.

Mutations in the gene *TREX1* cause retinal vasculopathy with cerebral leukodystrophy, which is also associated with small-vessel disease, migraine-like headaches, stroke, and dementia.

Mutations in the *GLA* gene lead to Fabry disease, which is a metabolic cause of early stroke. Fabry disease is a lysosomal storage disorder that results from deficiency of α-galactosidase A. It is X-linked recessive. In this condition, globotriaosylceramide accumulates in cells. Patients can have white matter abnormalities and dolichoectasia of cerebral vessels in addition to stroke. Patients can also have cardiomyopathy, cardiac conduction defects, autonomic dysfunction, and renal failure. Fabry disease produces a small-fiber neuropathy. Angiokeratoma in a bathing suit distribution and painful acroparesthesias are characteristic. Enzyme replacement therapy is available.

Familial cerebral amyloid angiopathy, which is caused by mutations in *APP*, also leads to white matter abnormalities, as well as lobar hemorrhage and microbleeds.

Mutations in *COL4A1* (collagen type IV, alpha 1) also cause small-vessel disease. A syndrome of hereditary angiopathy with nephropathy, aneurysms, and muscle cramps is caused by mutations in this gene.

Mutations in the *KRIT1* (or *CCM1*) gene are one cause of familial cerebral cavernous malformations.

25. C

This patient has homocystinuria, which is associated with thromboembolism, eye abnormalities (myopia or lens dislocation), and Marfanoid habitus. Homocystine is elevated in the blood and urine. Methionine is also elevated in the blood.

The most common cause of homocystinuria is cystathionine β-synthase (CBS) deficiency. Some patients with this condition respond to pyridoxine. Patients with homocystinuria due to CBS deficiency are at risk for other conditions such as dystonia, livedo reticularis, and pancreatitis.

Patients with homocystinuria who do not respond to pyridoxine can be treated with vitamin B12 and folate, which help convert homocystine to methionine. The medication betaine has the same effect.

Some forms of homocystinuria are associated with megaloblastic anemia. Homocystinuria can be found in some patients with methylmalonic acidemia.

26. B

The Stroke Prevention Trial in Sickle Cell Anemia (STOP) determined that maintaining a hemoglobin S concentration less than 30% of the total hemoglobin concentration reduced the risk for first stroke in patients with sickle cell disease who had rapid flow in the internal or middle cerebral artery on transcranial Doppler ultrasonography. Iron overload is a possible complication.[9]

27. A

Oxygen delivery is the product of cerebral blood flow and blood oxygen content.

28. D

The granule cells of the cerebellum are less susceptible to hypoxic injury than the other cell types listed.

The following cells are particularly susceptible to hypoxia: pyramidal cells in Sommer's sector of the hippocampus; Purkinje cells in the cerebellar cortex; and neurons of layers III, V, and VI of the cerebral cortex.

29. A

L-Asparaginase causes decreased fibrinogen, antithrombin III, protein C, and protein S. It can cause sinus venous thrombosis.

Cyclophosphamide, 5-fluorouracil, and methotrexate cause acquired protein C deficiency. Acquired protein C deficiency can also occur in the setting of severe infection, such as meningococcemia, liver disease, disseminated intravascular coagulation, and acute respiratory distress syndrome.

30. A

Factor V Leiden is the most common inherited risk factor for thrombophilia.

Factor V is involved in clot formation, specifically formation of fibrin. In a normal individual, activated protein C (APC) inactivates factor V. Patients with factor V Leiden have resistance to APC; in these patients, APC is not able to inactivate factor V as usual, and clotting continues. Patients with factor V Leiden are at risk for venous thromboembolism, especially deep vein thromboses in the leg.

31. C

If there is no contraindication, a patient with intracerebral hemorrhage and a systolic blood pressure between 150 and 220 mm Hg can be treated to lower the systolic blood pressure to 140 mm Hg. This can improve outcome. Blood pressure should be controlled as soon as possible to prevent recurrence of hemorrhage.[7]

32. C

Corticosteroids should *not* be used to treat intracranial pressure in cases of intracerebral hemorrhage.

Continuous EEG monitoring should be considered if the patient's mental status is worse than expected. Prophylactic anti-epileptic medication is *not* recommended.

Normoglycemia is recommended.

Graduated compression stockings are *not* helpful for prevention of deep vein thrombosis.

Intermittent pneumatic compression is recommended.

Multidisciplinary rehabilitation is recommended for patients with intracerebral hemorrhage.

Protamine sulfate may be given to reverse heparin in a patient with intracerebral hemorrhage. Activated charcoal may be administered if the patient recently took dabigatran, apixaban, or rivaroxaban. Hemodialysis has also been used for patients taking dabigatran.

Risk factors for intracerebral hemorrhage should be addressed, including treatment of obstructive sleep apnea, if present. Risk factors for recurrence include older age, microbleeds on gradient echo MRI, a prior history of intracerebral hemorrhage, anticoagulation, and apolipoprotein E ε2 or ε4. Cerebral amyloid angiopathy increases the risk for recurrence of lobar hemorrhage.[7]

33. D

Surgery is recommended as soon as possible for patients with cerebellar hemorrhage and worsening neurologic status, hydrocephalus, or brainstem compression. Studies have recommended surgery if a cerebellar hemorrhage is more than 3 cm in diameter.

Suboccipital craniectomy with dural expansion is indicated for patients with cerebellar ischemic stroke who deteriorate despite medical therapy. External ventricular drainage alone may not rescue all patients and is less effective overall than surgery. It may be used to temporize as surgery is arranged.[4,7]

34. B

The most common site of intracranial hemorrhage due to hypertension is the putamen.

35. D

This patient's story is concerning for subarachnoid hemorrhage. CT can miss some cases. Lumbar puncture should be performed to rule out subarachnoid hemorrhage in this patient. However, negative CT and cerebrospinal fluid analysis do not completely rule out a symptomatic unruptured aneurysm.

Reversible cerebral vasoconstriction syndrome (RCVS) is another cause of thunderclap headaches.

36. D

Patients with perimesencephalic hemorrhage often have nonaneurysmal subarachnoid hemorrhage; they usually have a negative angiogram. These patients tend to have a better prognosis than patients with subarachnoid hemorrhage (SAH) caused by an aneurysm.

Saccular aneurysmal rupture is the most common cause of nontraumatic SAH. Most aneurysms are present at the origin of the anterior communication artery. Mycotic aneurysms are typically more distal than saccular aneurysms.

37. B

The risk for aneurysmal subarachnoid hemorrhage (aSAH) is greater for women than for men, but pregnancy and delivery do not increase one's risk.

An aneurysm is more prone to rupture if it is large or symptomatic. Risk factors for aSAH include an aneurysm more than 7 mm in size, a significant life event in the past month, and tobacco use. Also, hypertension, excessive alcohol, sympathomimetic drugs, a positive family history, and particular genetic conditions (e.g., autosomal dominant polycystic kidney disease, Ehlers-Danlos type IV) are risk factors. A daughter sac may also suggest an increased risk for rupture. A diet with plenty of vegetables may decrease the risk of aSAH.

38. C

According to the 2012 AHA/ASA guidelines for the management of aneurysmal subarachnoid hemorrhage (aSAH), patients with aSAH should be assessed with the Hunt and Hess Grading Scale or the World Federation of Neurological Surgeons Scale (see Boxes 3.6 and 3.7).

The 2012 AHA/ASA guidelines also state that the patient should quickly be transferred to a hospital that has experience treating patients with aSAH. The systolic blood pressure should be lowered to less than 160 mm Hg using a medication that can be titrated. Tranexamic acid or aminocaproic acid can be used in the short term

---

Box 3.6 HUNT AND HESS GRADING SCALE

Grade 0 = Unruptured aneurysm
Grade 1 = No symptoms or mild headache and minimal neck stiffness
Grade 2 = Moderate to severe headache, neck rigidity; no neurologic deficits (apart from cranial nerve palsy)
Grade 3 = Drowsy, confused, or mild focal deficit
Grade 4 = Stupor, hemiparesis
Grade 5 = Coma, decerebrate posturing

Box 3.7 WORLD FEDERATION OF NEUROLOGICAL SURGEONS SCALE

Grade 1 = Glasgow coma score of 15 and no focal deficit.
Grade 2 = Glasgow coma score of 13 or 14 and no focal deficit.
Grade 3 = Glasgow coma score of 13 or 14 with a focal deficit.
Grade 4 = Glasgow coma score of 7 to 12.
Grade 5 = Glasgow coma score of 3 to 6.

---

if obliteration of the aneurysm is delayed, there is a significant risk of rebleeding, and there are no contraindications. The guidelines recommend surgical clipping or endovascular coiling as soon as possible after aSAH to prevent rebleeding. If a ruptured aneurysm can be coiled or clipped, coiling should be considered. Microsurgical clipping should be considered for large (>50 mL) intraparenchymal hematomas and middle cerebral artery aneurysms. Endovascular coiling should be considered for patients older than 70 years of age, those with a score of grade or 4 or 5 on the World Federation of Neurosurgical Surgeons classification, and those with aneurysms at the basilar apex. After coiling or clipping, repeat imaging should be performed.[10]

39. C

Treatment of an aneurysmal subarachnoid hemorrhage (aSAH) involves stabilizing the patient; securing the aneurysm; avoiding rebleeding, hydrocephalus, cerebral vasospasm, and cerebral ischemia; and preventing systemic complications.

According to the 2012 AHA/ASA guidelines for management of aSAH, all patients with aSAH should be treated with oral nimodipine. Hypertension, hypervolemia, and hemodilution (HHH) therapy is no longer in favor. HHH therapy can cause pulmonary edema, myocardial ischemia, hyponatremia, and hemorrhage. In order to avoid delayed cerebral ischemia, euvolemia is currently recommended. Transcranial Doppler ultrasonography can monitor for vasospasm. Perfusion imaging can identify areas prone to ischemia. If patients have delayed cerebral ischemia, hypertension may be induced unless the patient has hypertension at baseline or it is contraindicated from a cardiac standpoint. Patients with symptomatic cerebral vasospasm after aSAH who do not respond to hypertensive therapy can be treated with cerebral angioplasty or selective intra-arterial vasodilator therapy or both.

Nitroprusside is a vasodilator; it can increase cerebral edema and intracranial pressure.

Prophylactic anti-epileptic medication may be given in the immediate period after aSAH. Routine long-term use of anti-epileptic medications is not recommended.

Fever and hypoglycemia should be avoided in patients with aSAH. Patients with aSAH are at risk for deep vein thrombosis and heparin-induced thrombocytopenia.[10]

40. A

This patient has hereditary hemorrhagic telangiectasia (HHT), which is also called Osler-Weber-Rendu disease. Most patients present with epistaxis. Patients with HHT can have arteriovenous malformations in multiple organs, such as the brain, lungs, or liver. Patients can have stroke due to a cerebral arteriovenous malformation, cerebral aneurysm, or paradoxical emboli. Some have gastrointestinal bleeding. Telangiectasias can be seen on the skin. Mutations in *ENG*, the gene that encodes endoglin, cause HHT type 1.

Defects in hamartin and tuberin occur in patients with tuberous sclerosis (TSC1 and TSC2, respectively). Defects in merlin occur in patients with neurofibromatosis type 2.

41. B

Fibromuscular dysplasia is an angiopathy that can cause aneurysms, dissection, or stenosis of arteries. It occurs more commonly in women than in men. It can affect the carotid or vertebral arteries. The renal arteries are also commonly affected. Fibromuscular dysplasia causes alternating narrowing and dilatation of the vessel wall, resulting in a "string of beads" appearance.

Connective tissue disorders, such as Ehlers-Danlos and Marfan syndromes, also increase the risk for dissection.

42. C

This patient has moyamoya syndrome. Narrowing of the intracranial internal carotid arteries causes formation of collaterals. These collaterals cause a "puff of smoke" appearance on angiography. Hyperventilation results in decreased carbon dioxide, which causes cerebral vasoconstriction, resulting in neurologic symptoms. When no known cause is found, the phenomenon is called moyamoya disease. When it is secondary to another condition, it is called moyamoya syndrome. Moyamoya disease can be familial. Multiple conditions can cause moyamoya syndrome including sickle cell disease, neurofibromatosis type 1, trisomy 21, and cranial radiation. Patients may require surgery to promote revascularization.

Transient cerebral arteriopathy (also known as focal arteriopathy) is a cause of stroke in childhood. It is a nonprogressive, typically unilateral arteriopathy that usually is reversible. When the cause is varicella zoster virus, the transient cerebral arteriopathy is called post-varicella angiopathy. This tends to affect the M1 segment of the middle cerebral artery.

43. C

Dissection of the internal carotid artery can cause Horner syndrome; however, anhidrosis typically is not present.

The oculosympathetic pathway that is responsible for the symptoms of Horner syndrome (ptosis, miosis, anhidrosis) is a three-neuron pathway. Sympathetic fibers travel from the first-order neuron in the hypothalamus through the brainstem and spinal cord to synapse at the ciliospinal center of Budge (C8–T2). Then, the second-order (preganglionic) fibers exit the spinal cord and travel through the cervical sympathetic chain. Next, they travel through the brachial plexus and over the apex of the lung. They synapse in the superior cervical ganglion, which is near the bifurcation of the common carotid artery. The third-order (postganglionic) fibers travel with the internal carotid artery into the cavernous sinus and then to the eye. The sympathetic fibers that affect sweating travel with the external carotid artery rather than the internal carotid artery. Therefore, anhidrosis is not expected with internal carotid artery dissection.

If a patient has headache, eye pain, or neck pain and a third-order Horner syndrome, internal carotid dissection should be considered (see Figure 3.3).

44. B

This patient has a sinus venous thrombosis. Pregnant women and women in the peripartum period are hypercoagulable and are at increased risk for sinus venous thrombosis.

45. B

The superior sagittal sinus is the sinus most often affected by thrombosis. The most common symptom in adults is headache. Other symptoms include intracranial hypertension, focal deficits, encephalopathy, and seizures.

Risk factors for cerebral venous thrombosis are blood stasis, changes to the wall of the vessel, and changes to blood composition. Dehydration is a risk factor. The use of oral contraceptives in women with the prothrombin G20210A mutation increases the risk for cerebral venous thrombosis. Hyperhomocysteinemia has not been proven to significantly increase one's risk. It is a risk factor for deep vein thrombosis and stroke.

Cerebral venous thrombosis is treated with anticoagulation if there is no contraindication. Endovascular therapy may be considered if anticoagulation is contraindicated or if the thrombosis progresses despite medical therapy.[11]

46. D

Small-vessel vasculitis affects vessels not seen on angiography. It affects venules, capillaries, and arterioles. The

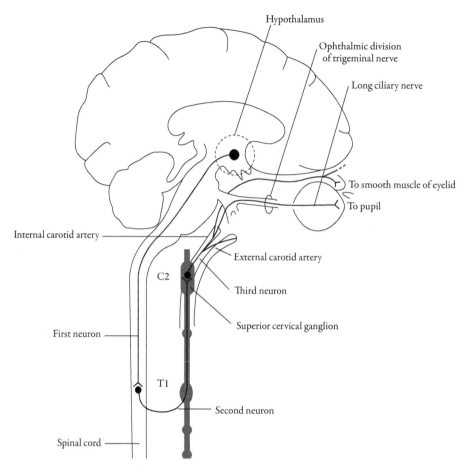

Hypothalamus

Ophthalmic division
of trigeminal nerve

Long ciliary nerve

To smooth muscle of eyelid

To pupil

Internal carotid artery

External carotid artery

C2

Third neuron

Superior cervical ganglion

First neuron

T1

Second neuron

Spinal cord

Figure 3.3 Sympathetic pupil pathway. C2 = second cervical vertebra; T1 = first thoracic vertebra. (From Sundaram V, Barsam A, Alwitry A, Khaw P. *Training in Ophthalmology*, Figures 9.1, 9.2, and 9.5. New York, Oxford University Press, 2009.)

best method for diagnosis of small-vessel vasculitis is brain biopsy.

REFERENCES

1. Gronseth GS, Paduga R. Evidence-based guideline update: Steroids and antivirals for Bell palsy. Report of the Guideline Development Subcommittee of the American Academy of Neurology. *Neurology* 2012;79:2209–2213.
2. Jauch EC, Saver JL, Adams HPJr, et al. Guidelines for the early management of patients with acute ischemic stroke: A guideline for healthcare professionals from the American Heart Association/ American Stroke Association. *Stroke* 2013;44:870–947.
3. Powers WJ, Derdeyn CP, Biller J, et al. 2015 AHA/ASA focused update of the 2013 guidelines for the early management of patients with acute ischemic stroke regarding endovascular treatment: A guideline for healthcare professionals from the American Heart Association/American Stroke Association. *Stroke*. Published online June 29, 2015.
4. Wijdicks EF, Sheth KN, Carter BS, et al. Recommendations for the management of cerebral and cerebellar infarction with swelling: A statement for healthcare professionals from the American Heart Association/American Stroke Association. *Stroke* 2014;45:1222–1238.
5. Meschia JF, Bushnell C, Boden-Albala B, et al. Guidelines for the primary prevention of stroke: A statement for healthcare professionals from the American Heart Association/American Stroke Association. *Stroke* 2014;45:3754–3832.
6. Kernan WN, Ovbiagele B, Black HR, et al. Guidelines for the prevention of stroke in patients with stroke and transient ischemic attack: A guideline for healthcare professionals from the American Heart Association/American Stroke Association. *Stroke* 2014;45:2160–2236.
7. Hemphill JCIII, Greenberg SM, Anderson CS, et al. Guidelines for the management of spontaneous intracerebral hemorrhage: A guideline for healthcare professionals from the American Heart Association/American Stroke Association. *Stroke* 2015;46:2032–2060.
8. Hylek EM, Held C, Alexander JH, et al. Major bleeding in patients with atrial fibrillation receiving apixaban or warfarin: The ARISTOTLE trial (Apixaban for Reduction in Stroke and Other Thromboembolic Events in Atrial Fibrillation)— Predictors, characteristics, and clinical outcomes. *J Am Coll Cardiol* 2014;27;63:2141–2147.
9. Adams RJ, McKie VC, Hsu L, et al. Prevention of a first stroke by transfusion in children with sickle cell anemia and abnormal results on transcranial Doppler ultrasonography. *N Engl J Med* 1998;339:5–11.
10. Connolly ESJr, Rabinstein AA, Carhuapoma JR, et al. Guidelines for the management of aneurysmal subarachnoid hemorrhage: A guideline for healthcare professionals from the American Heart Association/American Stroke Association. *Stroke* 2012;43:1711–1737.
11. Saposnik G, Barinagarrementeria F, Brown RD, et al. Diagnosis and management of cerebral venous thrombosis: A statement for healthcare professionals from the American Heart Association/American Stroke Association. *Stroke* 2011;42;1158–1192.

4.

CONGENITAL DISORDERS INCLUDING NEUROCUTANEOUS DISORDERS

1. Fill in the blank: The central nervous system is formed from _____.
   A. Ectoderm
   B. Endoderm
   C. Mesoderm

2. Failure of the anterior neural tube to close results in which of the following?
   A. Agenesis of the corpus callosum
   B. Alobar holoprosencephaly
   C. Anencephaly
   D. Atelencephaly

3. In which condition do encephaloceles occur?
   A. Meckel syndrome
   B. Pallister-Killian syndrome
   C. Rubenstein-Taybi syndrome
   D. Kallmann syndrome

4. Which of the following is most likely to be seen in a patient with cyclopia, anosmia, and a central tooth?
   A. A Chiari II malformation
   B. Holoprosencephaly
   C. Porencephaly
   D. Schizencephaly

5. Which of the following can cause polymicrogyria?
   A. In utero cytomegalovirus (CMV) infection
   B. Peroxisomal disorders
   C. Mutations in tubulin genes
   D. All of the above

6. A child with a history of infantile spasms is found to have chorioretinal lacunae. Which of the following is most likely to occur in this condition?
   A. Deafness
   B. Glaucoma
   C. Agenesis of the corpus callosum
   D. Periventricular nodular heterotopia

7. Which of the following is *least* likely to cause microcephaly?
   A. Achondroplasia
   B. Miller-Dieker syndrome
   C. Velo-cardio-facial syndrome
   D. Wolf-Hirschhorn syndrome

8. Mutation of which gene is *least* likely to cause lissencephaly?
   A. *ARX*
   B. *DCX*
   C. *PCDH19*
   D. *TUBA1A*

9. A 6-month-old child presents with infantile spasms. He has facial asymmetry and a whirled hypopigmented lesion on his trunk that follows Blaschko lines. Magnetic resonance imaging (MRI) shows hemimegalencephaly. What is the most likely diagnosis?
   A. Epidermal nevus syndrome
   B. Hypomelanosis of Ito
   C. Incontinentia pigmenti
   D. Proteus syndrome

10. Which of the following should be performed in a patient diagnosed with periventricular nodular heterotopia due to a filamin-A defect?
   A. Echocardiography
   B. Hearing screen
   C. Ophthalmology examination
   D. Renal ultrasound study

11. A child with a family history of spastic paraplegia is born with hydrocephalus and adducted thumbs. A mutation in which of the following genes is most likely to be responsible?
   A. *ARG1*
   B. *ASPM*
   C. *IKBKG*
   D. *L1CAM*

12. A child with Dandy-Walker syndrome presents with new-onset seizure. He has agenesis of the cerebellar vermis and cystic dilatation of the fourth ventricle. Which of the following is also expected to be present?
   A. Midbrain atrophy
   B. Pontocerebellar hypoplasia
   C. Optic nerve hypoplasia
   D. An enlarged posterior fossa with an elevated tentorium

13. A newborn has a lumbar myelomeningocele. Which of the following is most likely to occur with this condition?
   A. Chiari I malformation
   B. Chiari II malformation

C. Klippel-Feil syndrome

D. Diastematomyelia

14. A patient with a history of Chiari I malformation presents with decreased sensitivity to pain in her arms. On examination, she is noted to have decreased pain and temperature sensation in her upper extremities; however, vibration, position, and light touch sensation are intact. What is the most likely diagnosis?

A. Multiple sclerosis

B. Syrinx

C. Bilateral carpal tunnel syndrome

D. Vitamin B12 deficiency

15. Caudal regression is most likely to occur in patients born to mothers with which of the following conditions?

A. Diabetes

B. Hypothyroidism

C. Hyperthyroidism

D. Rickets

16. In which condition is a molar tooth seen on brain MRI?

A. Joubert syndrome

B. COACH syndrome

C. CORS syndrome

D. All of the above

17. Which of the following statements is *false*?

A. The most common cause of plagiocephaly is craniosynostosis.

B. Craniosynostosis is most often caused by premature closure of the sagittal suture.

C. Mutations in fibroblast growth factor receptors can cause craniosynostosis.

D. Hyperthyroidism can cause craniosynostosis.

18. A 9-year-old girl presents with attention deficit hyperactivity disorder. On examination, she has macrocephaly, ten hyperpigmented macules measuring more than 5 mm, and a tibia deformity. Which of the following is *least* likely to occur in this condition?

A. Renal artery stenosis

B. Pulmonary lymphangioleiomyomatosis

C. Optic nerve glioma

D. Iris hamartomas

19. A 20-year-old man presents with decreased hearing and unsteadiness. His father has a history of meningioma,

glioma, and posterior subcapsular lens opacities. Masses are seen in the cerebellopontine angle bilaterally on the patient's brain MRI. What are the lesions?

A. Neurofibromas

B. Vestibular schwannomas

C. Astrocytomas

D. Ependymomas

20. A newborn with hypopigmented lesions undergoes echocardiography for a heart murmur and is found to have cardiac rhabdomyomas. The electrocardiogram shows Wolff-Parkinson-White syndrome. Which of the following tests is most important to perform at this time?

A. Brain neuroimaging

B. Hearing test

C. Electroretinogram

D. MRI of the lungs

21. A patient with tuberous sclerosis complex develops infantile spasms. What is the best treatment?

A. Adrenocorticotropic hormone (ACTH)

B. The ketogenic diet

C. Topiramate

D. Vigabatrin

22. A patient with a port-wine stain involving the first division of the trigeminal nerve develops seizures. Head computed tomography shows dystrophic calcification. Which of the following is most likely to occur in this condition?

A. Cataract

B. Coloboma

C. Glaucoma

D. Optic nerve hypoplasia

23. A child presents with increased falls. He has a history of sinus infections and oculomotor apraxia. His mother says she thinks he has terrible allergies because his eyes seem irritated and red all the time. He is ataxic on examination. His alpha-fetoprotein (AFP) level is elevated, and immunoglobulin G (IgG), IgE, and IgA levels are low. Which of the following is most likely in this condition?

A. Increased risk for lymphoma

B. Lung cancer

C. Steatorrhea

D. Vitamin E deficiency

CONGENITAL DISORDERS INCLUDING NEUROCUTANEOUS DISORDERS

ANSWERS

1. A

The central nervous system is formed from ectoderm.

2. C

Failure of the anterior neural tube to close can cause anencephaly. This usually occurs between 18 and 24 days of embryonic development. (The anterior neuropore usually closes on day 25.) The lamina terminalis is where the anterior neuropore closes. It becomes a part of the wall of the third ventricle.

Folate helps prevent neural tube defects. Menstruating women who are taking an anti-epileptic drug should be placed on folate. Women with mutations in the *MTHFR* gene, which encodes methylenetetrahydrofolate reductase, may require higher doses of folate to prevent neural tube defects. Mutations in *MTHFR* can cause anencephaly, spina bifida, and homocystinuria.

Aprosencephaly and atelencephaly are disorders of prosencephalic development.

3. A

Encephaloceles represent a restricted defect in anterior neural tube closure that allows protrusion of brain and its coverings.

Meckel syndrome, also known as Meckel-Gruber syndrome, is characterized by an occipital encephalocele, cleft lip and palate, polycystic kidneys, and polydactyly. It is a ciliopathy (a disease with cilia dysfunction).

Encephaloceles also can occur in Walker-Warburg syndrome.

4. B

During development, the neural tube undergoes segmentation, which creates the prosencephalon, mesencephalon, and rhombencephalon. The prosencephalon gives rise to the forebrain; the mesencephalon gives rise to the midbrain; and the rhombencephalon gives rise to the hindbrain.

Prosencephalic development involves prosencephalic formation, prosencephalic cleavage, and midline prosencephalic development.

Normally, the prosencephalon is formed from the rostral end of the neural tube and divides into the telencephalon and diencephalon. The telencephalon becomes the cerebral hemispheres, and the diencephalon gives rise to the thalamus and hypothalamus. Aprosencephaly and atelencephaly are disorders of prosencephalic formation. In aprosencephaly, neither the telencephalon nor the diencephalon forms. In atelencephaly, the telencephalon does not form, but the diencephalon is present.

Failure of prosencephalic cleavage causes holoprosencephaly.

The most severe form of holoprosencephaly is alobar holoprosencephaly. There is no separation of the hemispheres, no interhemispheric fissure, and no corpus callosum. There is a single midline ventricle, and the basal ganglia and thalami are fused. The patient may have cyclopia, and the olfactory bulbs and tracts are absent. The septum pellucidum is absent in all types of holoprosencephaly.

Semilobar holoprosencephaly is the intermediate form of holoprosencephaly. There is some division of the cerebral hemispheres posteriorly. The anterior corpus callosum is absent.

Lobar holoprosencephaly is less severe. There is almost complete separation of the hemispheres except in the most ventral and rostral portion. The anterior corpus callosum may be underdeveloped.

A cleft lip/palate or a central tooth can be seen in holoprosencephaly. Diabetes insipidus, as well as other endocrinopathies, can occur in patients with holoprosencephaly.

There are multiple environmental and genetic causes of holoprosencephaly. Maternal diabetes is a risk factor. Holoprosencephaly is seen in trisomy 13 and 18 and in Smith-Lemli-Opitz, Pallister-Killian, Rubenstein-Taybi, and Kallmann syndromes. Mutations in *SHH* and *ZIC2* have been found in patients with holoprosencephaly.

Schizencephaly is characterized by a cleft in the cortical surface that is lined in gray matter and extends toward the ventricle. It is thought to be caused by vascular injury or infection.

Porencephaly refers to an intraparenchymal cyst that communicates with the ventricle. Mutations in *COL4A1* cause hereditary porencephaly. Mutations in this gene also cause the conditions brain small-vessel disease (with or without ocular anomalies) and hereditary angiopathy with nephropathy, aneurysms, and muscle cramps (HANAC).

5. D

There are multiple causes of polymicrogyria. In utero infection, for instance with CMV; in utero ischemia; and metabolic diseases such as Zellweger syndrome can cause polymicrogyria. There are also multiple genetic mutations that cause polymicrogyria. Mutations in tubulin, which is required for the formation of microtubules, can cause polymicrogyria as well as other brain malformations. Mutations in *GPR56* cause bilateral frontoparietal polymicrogyria. Mutations in the gene *SRPX2* on chromosome Xq22 can cause bilateral perisylvian polymicrogyria, which is a common form of polymicrogyria. It is associated with seizures and oromotor dyspraxia. Intellectual disability may also be present.

6. C

This patient has Aicardi syndrome. Aicardi syndrome is characterized by agenesis of the corpus callosum, infantile spasms, and chorioretinal lacunae. It is an X-linked dominant condition.

Agenesis of the corpus callosum, agenesis of the septum pellucidum, and septo-optic dysplasia are disorders of midline prosencephalic development. There are genetic, metabolic, and environmental causes of agenesis of the corpus callosum. Agenesis of the corpus callosum can occur as part of syndrome or independently. Other midline defects may also be present. For instance, agenesis of the corpus callosum, congenital heart defects, Hirschsprung disease, and genitourinary anomalies are seen in Mowat-Wilson syndrome, which is caused by mutations in *ZEB2*.

7. A

Achondroplasia causes megalencephaly and macrocephaly. It results from mutations in *FGFR3* and is autosomal dominant. It causes short stature with shortening of the proximal limbs, lumbar lordosis, hypotonia, and developmental delay. Cervicomedullary compression can result in early death. Hydrocephalus can occur due to stenosis of the jugular foramina.

Miller-Dieker syndrome is caused by mutations in chromosome 17p13.3 that include the *LIS1* gene (*PAFAH1B1*) and the gene *YWHAE*. Patients have microcephaly, lissencephaly, a furrowed brow, and cardiac defects.

Velo-cardio-facial syndrome is a chromosome 22q11.2 deletion syndrome. The term CATCH-22 has been used for the 22q11.2 deletion syndromes, which also include DiGeorge syndrome and Cayler cardiofacial syndrome. CATCH stands for cardiac abnormality, anomalous face, thymus hypoplasia, cleft palate, and hypocalcemia.

Wolf-Hirschhorn syndrome is caused by chromosome 4p monosomy. Patients with Wolf-Hirschhorn syndrome have "Greek warrior helmet" facies, microcephaly, seizures, hypotonia, and intellectual disability. Skeletal and cardiac anomalies may also be present.

8. C

Mutations in *LIS1 (PAFAH1B1)* on chromosome 17; *DCX* on the X chromosome; and *TUBA1A* can cause classic lissencephaly, which is characterized by a thick, four-layer cortex rather than a six-layer cortex. Specifically, mutations in *DCX*, which encodes doublecortin, cause lissencephaly in males and subcortical band heterotopia in girls. *LIS1 (PAFAH1B1)* and *DCX* regulate the function of microtubules, which are required for cell division.

Mutations in *TUBA1A* and *TUBG1*, which result in tubulinopathies, cause lissencephaly and microlissencephaly (i.e., lissencephaly plus a head circumference <3 standard deviations below the mean). Dysmorphic basal ganglia are typical of tubulinopathies. Cerebellar anomalies are also common. Agenesis of the corpus callosum can occur.

Mutations in *TUBA1A* can cause lissencephaly with cerebellar hypoplasia. Mutations in *RELN* can also cause this condition.

In classic lissencephaly, which is also known as type 1 lissencephaly, there is undermigration of neurons. Overmigration of neurons causes cobblestone cortical malformation (CCM), which is also known cobblestone lissencephaly or type 2 lissencephaly. This is seen in Fukuyama congenital muscular dystrophy, Walker-Warburg syndrome, and muscle-eye-brain disease. CCM is caused by defects in the O-linked glycosylation of α-dystroglycan.

Mutations in the gene *ARX*, which is a homeobox gene, cause X-linked lissencephaly-2. X-linked lissencephaly-2 is associated with a three-layer cortex. Ambiguous genitalia and agenesis of the corpus callosum can also occur in this condition. X-linked lissencephaly-2 has also been called X-linked lissencephaly with ambiguous genitalia, or XLAG. Mutations in *ARX* can also cause X-linked intellectual disability and X-linked early infantile epileptic encephalopathy-1 (EIEE1), which has also been known as X-linked infantile spasm syndrome-1. [1,2]

Mutations in *PCDH19*, which encodes protocadherin, cause an early-onset X-linked epileptic encephalopathy in females that can be associated with autism and intellectual disability.

9. B

This patient has hypomelanosis of Ito, which is a neurocutaneous disorder caused by chromosomal mosaicism. Some patients with hypomelanosis of Ito have hemimegalencephaly. Patients with hypomelanosis of Ito are at risk for seizures, including infantile spasms. Intellectual disability is common. Facial or limb asymmetry may be present. Eye, hair, and dental abnormalities can also occur.

Other causes of hemimegalencephaly are epidermal nevus syndrome, tuberous sclerosis complex, and Proteus syndrome.

10. A

Mutations in the filamin-A gene *(FLNA)* can cause X-linked dominant periventricular nodular heterotopia. Filamin-A is involved in initiation of migration. It is defective in some patients with periventricular nodular heterotopia. Some of the patients with this condition have an aortic aneurysm; therefore, an echocardiogram should be obtained at the time of diagnosis.

11. D

This patient has a mutation in *L1CAM* at chromosome Xq28. Mutations in *L1CAM*, which encodes for L1 cell adhesion molecule, cause hydrocephalus due to aqueductal stenosis; CRASH syndrome; MASA syndrome; and hydrocephalus with Hirschsprung disease. CRASH stands for corpus callosum hypoplasia, mental retardation, adducted thumbs, spastic paraplegia, and hydrocephalus.

MASA stands for mental retardation, aphasia, shuffling gait, and adducted thumbs. MASA syndrome is also known as spastic paraplegia-1.

There are multiple types of hereditary spastic paraplegia. In addition, argininemia, which is autosomal recessive, can cause spastic diplegia or quadriplegia. Argininemia is results from a deficiency of arginase in the urea cycle and is treated with a special diet. It is caused by mutations in the gene *ARG1*.

Congenital aqueductal stenosis is a common cause of neonatal hydrocephalus. Other causes include myelomeningocele, communicating hydrocephalus, and Dandy-Walker syndrome. These conditions also cause fetal hydrocephalus. In addition, holoprosencephaly is a major cause of fetal hydrocephalus.

Mutations in *ASPM* are a cause of primary microcephaly. *ASPM* encodes a protein that is involved in neural progenitor cell mitosis.

The gene *IKBKG*, which was formerly known as *NEMO*, is associated with incontinentia pigmenti, which is X-linked dominant.

12. D

Dandy-Walker syndrome is a triad of agenesis of the cerebellar vermis, cystic dilatation of the fourth ventricle, and an enlarged posterior fossa with an elevated tentorium. Other anomalies, such as agenesis of the corpus callosum, heterotopia, syringomyelia, and cardiac and urogenital anomalies, may also be present. Hydrocephalus can occur. Cognitive abilities are variable.

There are multiple forms of pontocerebellar hypoplasia (PCH). In PCH, the cerebellar hemispheres may be more affected than the vermis.

13. B

Myelomeningocele is caused by failure of the posterior neural tube to close. Folic acid helps to prevent this condition. In patients with myelomeningocele, the meninges and neural tissue protrude through a vertebral defect and may be visible on physical examination. A Chiari II malformation is common in patients with lumbar myelomeningocele. In patients with a Chiari II malformation, the medulla, cerebellum, and fourth ventricle are displaced into the upper cervical canal, and the tectum can appear beaked. Hydrocephalus can occur.

A Chiari I malformation is characterized by extension of the cerebellar tonsils at least 5 mm through the foramen magnum. Often, this is an incidental finding. Occipital headache can occur. Severe cases can cause cervical cord compression and lower cranial nerve deficits. Surgical decompression may be necessary for patients with significant symptoms.

Diastematomyelia refers to division of the spinal cord into two halves.

Klippel-Feil syndrome is characterized by abnormal fusion of cervical vertebrae. This can result in a short neck, low hairline, and decreased neck movement.

14. B

The patient has evidence of a central cord lesion, which manifests with sensory loss in a shawl-like pattern in the upper extremities. Symptoms result from involvement of crossing spinothalamic fibers. The posterior columns are spared; therefore, vibration, pinprick, and light touch sensation are intact. Given the history of Chiari I malformation, a syrinx is the most likely diagnosis.

Vitamin B12 deficiency causes a posterolateral column syndrome in which the dorsal columns and corticospinal tracts are affected. Pain and temperature are intact in this condition because the spinothalamic tracts are preserved.

15. A

The term *caudal regression* refers to abnormal development of the sacrum and coccyx. Abnormalities of the legs, gastrointestinal tract, or genitourinary tract may be present. Maternal diabetes is a risk factor.

16. D

A molar tooth is a midbrain abnormality seen in Joubert, COACH, CORS, and oral-facial-digital syndrome type VI (OFD-VI) syndromes. Lack of decussation of superior cerebellar tract fibers produces an abnormal configuration of the superior cerebellar peduncles, which gives the appearance of a molar tooth.

Patients with Joubert syndrome have developmental delay, hypotonia, ataxia, and hypoplasia of the vermis. Irregular breathing and abnormal eye movements can also be seen. There are multiple forms of Joubert syndrome, some of which are associated with other systemic abnormalities. For example, hepatic fibrosis can occur in Joubert syndrome due to mutations in *TMEM67*. Joubert syndrome is considered a ciliopathy, as are the Bardet-Biedl and Meckel syndromes.

COACH stands for cerebellar vermis hypo/aplasia, oligophrenia (intellectual disability), ataxia, ocular coloboma, and hepatic fibrosis.

CORS stands for cerebello-oculo-renal syndrome.

17. A

The most common type of plagiocephaly is positional plagiocephaly.

Premature closure of one or more sutures causes craniosynostosis. Craniosynostosis most often results from premature closure of the sagittal suture, which causes the skull to elongate in the anterior-posterior direction.

There are multiple causes of craniosynostosis. Systemic diseases such as hyperthyroidism and rickets can cause craniosynostosis. Lack of brain growth can result in craniosynostosis. In addition, mutations in fibroblast growth factor receptors cause multiple conditions with craniosynostosis, such as Apert and Crouzon syndromes.

18. B

This patient has neurofibromatosis type 1 (NF type 1). She has a bony deformity and the requisite size and number of café-au-lait patches, which are two of the criteria for diagnosis. (Since the patient is prepubertal, she must have at least six café-au-lait patches measuring at ≥5 mm to meet the criterion.) Other diagnostic criteria are optic glioma; iris hamartomas (Lisch nodules); axillary and inguinal freckling; neurofibromas and plexiform fibroma; and a positive family history. Patients with NF type 1 tend to have macrocephaly and learning problems. They are also at risk for brain tumors, peripheral nerve sheath tumors, and vasculopathy. Renal artery stenosis can occur. Blood pressure should be monitored.

NF type 1 is caused by mutations in the gene *NF1*. *NF1* is found on chromosome 17q and encodes for neurofibromin, which is a tumor suppressor that regulates Ras.

Pulmonary lymphangioleiomyomatosis can occur in tuberous sclerosis complex.

19. B

This patient has neurofibromatosis type 2 (NF type 2), which is caused by mutations in merlin on chromosome 22. (Merlin is also known as schwannomin.) Bilateral vestibular schwannomas are diagnostic of NF type 2. (These have also been referred to as acoustic neuromas, but they are in fact schwannomas of the vestibular nerve.) Patients with NF type 2 can also have posterior subcapsular lens opacities, astrocytomas, ependymomas, and meningiomas.

20. A

This patient has tuberous sclerosis complex (TSC). Brain neuroimaging is recommended. Cortical tubers and subependymal nodules are expected. Patients with TSC can also have subependymal giant cell astrocytomas (SEGAs). Enlarging SEGAs that could obstruct the foramen of Monro may require treatment with a mammalian target of rapamycin (mTOR) inhibitor or surgery.

Patients diagnosed with TSC should undergo MRI of the abdomen to evaluate for renal angiomyolipoma and renal cysts. Renal cell carcinoma can occur in adults with TSC but is rare. Pulmonary lymphangioleiomyomatosis (LAM) is also a concern in adults with TSC, particularly in women.

Mutations in the gene *TSC1* or *TSC2* cause TSC, which is autosomal dominant. *TSC1* encodes hamartin, and *TSC2* encodes tuberin.

21. D

Vigabatrin is preferred for the treatment of infantile spasms in patients with tuberous sclerosis complex. However, vigabatrin can cause visual field defects, so the US Food and Drug Administration has recommended frequent ophthalmology evaluations. Vigabatrin can also cause reversible hyperintensities on T2-weighted and diffusion-weighted brain MRI.

Patients with TSC should also be followed by ophthalmology because of the risk of retinal hamartomas and retinal depigmentation.

22. C

This patients has Sturge-Weber syndrome, which can be caused by somatic mosaic mutation in the *GNAQ* gene. Typically, patients with Sturge-Weber syndrome have a port-wine colored vascular nevus in the distribution of the ophthalmic branch of the trigeminal nerve. Patients with this syndrome are at risk for glaucoma. Most have seizures, and many develop a hemiparesis. Developmental delay is common. Sturge-Weber syndrome is associated with leptomeningeal venous angiomas, most often in the occipital or occipitoparietal region. These are associated with dystrophic calcification, often in a tram-track pattern.

23. A

This patient has ataxia-telangiectasia, which is caused by mutations in *ATM*. Ataxia-telangiectasia is autosomal recessive. Cerebellar symptoms, such as ataxia, dysarthria, or oculomotor apraxia, are present in early childhood. Dystonia or chorea may be present. Telangiectasias appear between 3 and 6 years of age. Patients with ataxia-telangiectasia often have a history of sinopulmonary infections. Neuropathy, premature aging, and diabetes may also be seen. Ataxia-telangiectasia is a disorder of DNA repair. Patients with ataxia-telangiectasia are sensitive to ionizing radiation and are at risk for lymphoma and leukemia. Laboratory studies show an elevated AFP and decreased IgA, IgG, and IgE.

Other DNA repair disorders include ataxia-telangiectasia–like disorder, Cockayne syndrome, xeroderma pigmentosa, spinocerebellar ataxia with axonal neuropathy, Nijmegen breakage syndrome, and trichothiodystrophy.

REFERENCES

1. Fry AE, Cushion TD, Pilz DT. The genetics of lissencephaly. *Am J Med Genet C Semin Med Genet* 2014;166C:198–210.
2. Bahi-Buisson N, Poirier K, Fourniol F, et al. The wide spectrum of tubulinopathies: What are the key features for the diagnosis? *Brain* 2014;137:1676–1700.

5.

CRITICAL CARE AND TRAUMA

QUESTIONS

1. A 15-year-old boy was struck in the head by a baseball. He briefly lost consciousness when it occurred but then recovered. In the emergency department, he begins to become confused and drowsy and then vomits repeatedly. Which of the following has most likely occurred?
   A. Aneurysmal rupture
   B. Laceration of the middle meningeal artery
   C. Post-traumatic seizure
   D. Post-traumatic migraine

2. Which of the following statements is *false*?
   A. Headgear does not prevent concussion in those playing sports but may help to prevent more serious brain injury.
   B. Loss of consciousness is required to diagnose concussion.
   C. An athlete with a suspected concussion should be removed from play to prevent additional injury.
   D. An apparently mild second head injury can be fatal if the patient has not recovered from the first head injury.

3. A boxer who has been knocked out repeatedly develops progressive cognitive decline. He has memory impairment and executive dysfunction. The symptoms began after retirement from the sport. Magnetic resonance imaging (MRI) shows diffuse cerebral atrophy, a cavum septum pellucidum, and thinning of the corpus callosum. What is the most likely diagnosis?
   A. Chronic neurocognitive impairment
   B. Chronic postconcussion syndrome
   C. Chronic traumatic encephalopathy
   D. Parkinson disease

4. A 24-year-old patient was involved in a motor vehicle accident 5 days ago and is not awakening. Pupils are reactive, and corneal and gag reflexes are present. Withdrawal responses are symmetric. Computed tomography (CT) scans have been negative, and intracranial pressure (ICP) is normal. What is the most likely MRI finding?
   A. A brainstem ischemic stroke
   B. Microbleeds in the corpus callosum and at the gray-white junction
   C. A subdural empyema
   D. A subdural hygroma

5. A 25-year-old woman presents with a severe traumatic brain injury due to a motor vehicle accident. Her Glasgow Coma Scale (GCS) score is 7, and her CT scan is abnormal. Which of the following is recommended?

   A. High-dose corticosteroids
   B. Erythropoietin
   C. Progesterone
   D. Intracranial pressure monitoring

6. In the context of increased ICP and the Monro-Kellie hypothesis, which of the following is usually the most important blood volume regulator?
   A. Arteriolar oxygen
   B. Arteriolar carbon dioxide
   C. Arteriolar lactic acid
   D. Venous oxygen

7. Which of the following treatments for elevated ICP is reserved primarily for *acute* treatment?
   A. Hyperventilation
   B. Mannitol
   C. Hypertonic saline
   D. Hypothermia

8. Which of the following conditions is characterized by extracellular edema due to injury to the blood-brain barrier?
   A. Cytotoxic edema
   B. Interstitial edema
   C. Vasogenic edema

9. Osmotic agents (mannitol and hypertonic saline) are most effective at treating which of the following types of edema?
   A. Cytotoxic edema
   B. Interstitial edema
   C. Vasogenic edema

10. Which of the following statements is *false*?
    A. Post-traumatic epilepsy is a common cause of acquired epilepsy.
    B. Administration of anti-epileptic medications immediately after a traumatic brain injury prevents patients from developing epilepsy later.
    C. The majority of patients who develop epilepsy from a traumatic brain injury do so within the first 2 years after the injury.
    D. Prophylactic anti-epileptic medication decreases the risk of early post-traumatic seizures.

11. Mutism, lack of emotion, and minimal movement may indicate an injury to which region?
    A. Dorsolateral frontal lobe
    B. Orbital-frontal region
    C. Superior mesial frontal lobe
    D. Inferior temporal lobe

12. A 67-year-old man with a history of prostate cancer presents to the emergency department with lower back pain and leg weakness. MRI shows spinal metastases. What is the *first* step?
    A. Administer high-dose dexamethasone.
    B. Arrange for spinal radiation therapy.
    C. Make arrangements for surgery.
    D. Order a CT myelogram to better define cord impingement.

13. Which of the following statements is *false*?
    A. Patients with a traumatic spinal cord injury above the C5 level that is complete should be intubated.
    B. A traumatic spinal cord injury in the upper thoracic spine that is complete typically causes early hypertension and tachycardia.
    C. A common cause of spinal cord infarction is surgery, such as aortic surgery.
    D. Cerebrospinal fluid (CSF) drainage is used to treat acute spinal cord infarction.

14. Which of the following features is *not* typical of metabolic encephalopathy?
    A. Nonreactive pupils
    B. Nonfocal neurologic examination
    C. Distractibility
    D. Waxing and waning alertness

15. The electroencephalogram (EEG) finding of 14- and 6-Hz positive spikes is classically associated with which condition?
    A. Benzodiazepine intoxication
    B. Cardiac arrest
    C. Renal failure
    D. Reye syndrome

16. A 60-year-old man in the intensive care unit (ICU) develops altered mental status and has a brief seizure. He is afebrile. His complete blood count and CSF studies are unremarkable. His complete metabolic profile shows a sodium level of 115 mEq/L. Which of the following is the best treatment?
    A. Intravenous fosphenytoin
    B. Intravenous levetiracetam
    C. Scheduled intravenous lorazepam
    D. Sodium correction

17. A patient who was admitted to the ICU with a frontal contusion becomes intermittently unresponsive. Laboratory studies are normal, and head CT findings are unchanged. Which of the following is most likely to yield the diagnosis?
    A. Continuous EEG monitoring
    B. Repeat MRI
    C. Magnetic resonance venography (MRV)
    D. Computed tomography angiography (CTA)

18. A neurosurgical patient develops confusion. Syndrome of inappropriate antidiuretic hormone secretion (SIADH) is suspected. Which of the following is *least* likely to be present?

    A. Sodium level >145 mEq/L
    B. Decreased urine output
    C. Concentrated urine
    D. Hypervolemia

19. A patient in the ICU develops hemiballism. Which of the following is the most likely etiology?
    A. Hypoglycemia
    B. Hypercalcemia
    C. Hypomagnesemia
    D. Nonketotic hyperglycemia

20. A patient presents with leg weakness and areflexia. Electromyography (EMG) shows a demyelinating polyneuropathy. The weakness progresses to the upper extremities after admission. In addition to treating the patient's underlying condition, which of the following is recommended?
    A. Perform a swallow study.
    B. Check forced vital capacity and negative inspiratory force.
    C. Repeat EMG on the following day to assess for worsening.
    D. Place a nasogastric tube.

21. A patient with a history of respiratory failure and sepsis cannot move when the paralytic agent is discontinued. Creatine kinase is elevated. Muscle biopsy shows selective loss of myosin filaments. What is the most likely diagnosis?
    A. Critical illness myopathy
    B. Critical illness polyneuropathy
    C. Hypothyroidism
    D. Periodic paralysis

22. A 30-year-old man presents with respiratory failure. He is found to have limb-girdle weakness. EMG shows myotonic discharges in the paraspinal muscles. What is the most likely cause?
    A. Acid maltase deficiency
    B. Myophosphorylase deficiency
    C. Mutation in *PHOX2B*
    D. Spinal muscular atrophy type 1 (Werdnig-Hoffman disease)

23. Which of the following is a medication that is sometimes used in the treatment of neuroleptic malignant syndrome but should not be given if calcium channel antagonists are being used?
    A. Amantadine
    B. Bromocriptine
    C. Dantrolene
    D. L-Dopa

24. Which of the following is a medication that should be avoided in patients with neuromuscular disease because of the risk of hyperkalemia?
    A. Atracurium
    B. Succinylcholine
    C. Rocuronium
    D. Vecuronium

25. **Typically, a poor pupillary response and absence of corneal reflexes on day 3 after a cardiac arrest indicates a poor prognosis. In which of the following situations should one wait past day 3 to decide the prognosis?**
    A. The patient is less than 50 years old.
    B. The patient was treated with hypothermia.
    C. The patient's ejection fraction is less than 10%.
    D. The patient has pericarditis.

26. **What is Cushing's triad?**
    A. Hypotension, bradycardia, apnea
    B. Hypertension, tachycardia, apnea
    C. Hypotension, tachycardia, tachypnea
    D. Hypertension (widened pulse pressure), bradycardia, and irregular respirations

27. **If a patient has been treated with neuromuscular blocking agents, how can one best determine whether they are affecting the brain death examination?**
    A. Check a serum level.
    B. Perform the train-of-four technique with maximal ulnar stimulation
    C. Do an EMG.
    D. Use a painful stimulus.

28. **Which of the following is *least* helpful as an ancillary test during brain death testing in adults?**
    A. Electroencephalography
    B. Transcranial Doppler ultrasonography
    C. Single-photon emission computed tomography (SPECT) nuclear scan
    D. Somatosensory evoked potentials (SSEPs)

29. **Which of the following can be present in brain death?**
    A. Wave I on brainstem auditory evoked potential testing
    B. A focal epileptiform discharge over the right occipital lobe
    C. A delayed, but present, P100 on visual evoked potential testing
    D. N20 on somatosensory evoked potential testing

CRITICAL CARE AND TRAUMA

ANSWERS

1. B

Given his lucid interval, the most likely etiology is an epidural hematoma, which is most often caused by laceration of the middle meningeal artery.

Subdural hematomas are typically caused by tearing of bridging veins.

The American Academy of Neurology position paper on concussion stated that indications for head computed tomography (CT) after a sports-related head injury include loss of consciousness, post-traumatic amnesia, Glasgow Coma Scale (GCS) score less than 15, focal deficits, evidence of skull fracture, or clinical worsening. Clues that a basilar skull fracture has occurred are hemotympanum, the Battle sign (ecchymosis over the mastoid process), bruising around the eyes, and cerebrospinal fluid leakage. Basilar skull fractures can cause pneumocephalus (see Fig. 5.1).[1]

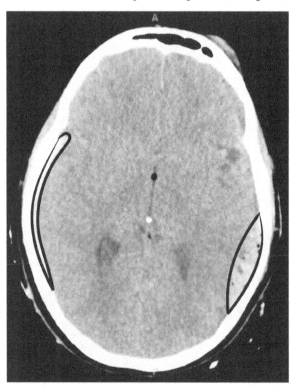

Figure 5.1 A subdural hematoma is present on the right side of the brain (*left side of image*) and an epidural hematoma on the left side of the brain (*right side of image*). (From Fisch A. *Neuroanatomy: Draw It to Know It,* 2nd ed, Fig. 2-2. New York: Oxford University Press, 2012.)

2. B

Loss of consciousness is *not* required to diagnose concussion. Headache is commonly reported. A patient with concussion commonly has anterograde or retrograde amnesia. Symptoms of concussion may not manifest immediately after the injury; they may appear later.

The sports with the greatest risk for head injury are football, rugby, lacrosse, ice hockey, and soccer. In some sports, such as soccer and basketball, the risk for concussion is higher in females than in males.

A player with a suspected concussion should be removed from play to prevent additional injury. The player should be cleared by a licensed health care provider before returning to play. The American Academy of Neurology (AAN) and the Centers for Disease Control and Prevention (CDC) have created resources for coaches and health care providers who evaluate athletes. When the player returns to play, graded physical activity may be recommended.

If a player has a concussion, he or she needs to be asymptomatic off medication before being cleared to return to play. A prior concussion is a risk factor for concussion. The term *second-impact syndrome* refers to massive brain edema after a second, apparently mild head injury that occurs when one is still recovering from a prior head injury.

Neuropsychological testing may help in decisions regarding return to play but is not required when a patient has had a concussion. If a player has had multiple concussions and reports cognitive impairment, neuropsychological testing may be helpful in deciding whether the player needs to retire from the sport.[1]

3. C

This patient has chronic traumatic encephalopathy (CTE). CTE is a neurodegenerative disease that is caused by repetitive traumatic brain injury. It may manifest with behavioral, motor, or cognitive signs or symptoms, and it is progressive. CTE tends to have a latency period, whereas chronic post-concussion syndrome does not. CTE is a tauopathy. There may be diffuse amyloid deposition or deposition of transactive response (TAR) DNA-binding protein 43 (TDP-43). Pathologic changes are seen in the superficial cortical layers, the perivascular regions, and the depths of sulci.

Chronic neurocognitive impairment typically follows multiple head injuries and is diagnosed with neuropsychological testing. It usually is not progressive.

Chronic postconcussion syndrome is diagnosed when a patient has postconcussive symptoms lasting longer than 1 year. It begins acutely after a single head injury. It usually is not progressive (see Table 5.1).[2]

Table 5.1 COMPARISON OF CHRONIC POSTCONCUSSION SYNDROME AND CHRONIC TRAUMATIC ENCEPHALOPATHY

	CHRONIC POSTCONCUSSION SYNDROME	CHRONIC TRAUMATIC ENCEPHALOPATHY
Injury	Single	Repetitive
Latent period	No latent period	Latent period is typically present
Progressive or not	Not progressive	Progressive

4. B

This patient has diffuse axonal injury from a motor vehicle accident. This can cause microbleeds in the brainstem and corpus callosum and at the gray-white junction, which may not be seen on CT. MRI with gradient echo/susceptibility-weighted imaging (SWI)/susceptibility-weighted angiography (SWAN) may be particularly helpful in detecting these lesions. At the microscopic level, axonal injury is manifested as axonal swellings (called retraction balls) in the white matter.

5. D

According to the 2007 Brain Trauma Foundation guidelines, indications for ICP monitoring in the intensive care unit (ICU) are a GCS score of 8 or less and an abnormal CT in a patient who can improve. If the CT is normal, ICP monitoring is indicated if the GCS score is ≤8 and at least two of the following criteria are present: age >40 years, posturing, and hypotension (systolic blood pressure <90 mm Hg.)[3]

6. B

The Monro-Kellie hypothesis states that the sum of the brain, cerebrospinal fluid (CSF), and intracranial blood volumes is constant. If there is a space-occupying lesion, the ICP increases. Typically, CSF volume decreases first in order to compensate. Also, venous blood may be pushed into the systemic circulation to compensate.

Cerebral perfusion pressure (CPP) is determined by the ICP and the mean arterial pressure (MAP): CPP = MAP – ICP.

The brain tries to maintain a certain amount of blood flow despite changes in perfusion pressure through cerebral autoregulation. Arterial carbon dioxide levels have an impact cerebral blood flow. Hypercapnia causes cerebral vasodilation and an increase in cerebral blood flow. Hypocapnia causes vasoconstriction and decreased cerebral blood flow.

The brain also tries to maintain a constant amount of oxygen delivery, so anemia, hemoglobin binding capacity problems, and severe hypoxia can raise cerebral blood flow; however, these abnormalities are much less commonly encountered. Acidosis can affect local flow.

In neurocritical care, the goal is to maintain adequate CPP, to avoid excessive ICP, and to avoid further brain injury.

7. A

Hyperventilation, elevation of the head of the bed to 30 degrees, mannitol, hypertonic saline, and hypothermia are all treatments for elevated ICP. Hyperventilation is reserved for acute treatment. Prolonged hypocapnia can cause excessive vasoconstriction and ischemia.

8. C

Patients with vasogenic edema have extracellular edema due to disruption of the blood-brain barrier (BBB). Vasogenic edema is seen in patients with tumors, hemorrhage, abscesses, malignant hypertension, or meningitis.

In patients with cytotoxic edema, the cells swell with fluid and the extracellular fluid space is reduced. The BBB is intact. Cerebral ischemia is the most common cause. In the setting of cerebral ischemia, the adenosine triphosphate (ATP)-dependent sodium-potassium membrane pump fails. Sodium accumulates in the cell, and water follows, resulting in swelling of the cell. There is an increased signal on diffusion-weighted imaging owing to restriction of free water diffusion.

Interstitial edema is seen with obstructive hydrocephalus. Cerebrospinal fluid (CSF) travels across the ependymal lining into the periventricular tissue (between cells and myelin).

9. C

Osmotic agents (mannitol and hypertonic saline) are most effective at treating vasogenic edema. They remove water from the brain when the blood-brain barrier (BBB) is intact. If the BBB is not intact, they can accumulate in the brain and cause rebound edema. Both mannitol and hypertonic saline can cause diuresis, metabolic acidosis, congestive heart failure, and pulmonary edema.

Hypertonic saline solutions stronger than 3% need to be given by central venous catheter. This can delay administration of the first dose. Hypertonic saline is a volume expander. Myelinolysis is a concern with hypertonic saline.

Mannitol decreases blood viscosity by its rheologic effect, as well as causing an osmotic diuresis. Initially, it increases the intravascular volume, but it can cause hypotension and hypovolemia due to diuresis. It also can cause nephrotoxicity.

10. B

Administration of anti-epileptic medications immediately after a traumatic brain injury does *not* prevent patients from developing epilepsy later. In an adult with severe traumatic brain injury, prophylaxis with an anti-epileptic drug can decrease the risk of *early* post-traumatic seizures.

11. C

Mutism, lack of emotion, and minimal movement may indicate a lesion in the superior mesial frontal lobe.

12. A

Dexamethasone should be administered as soon as possible in a patient with spinal metastases and neurologic symptoms. Then further arrangements for treatment can be made.

13. B

A common cause of spinal cord infarction is surgery, such as aortic surgery. Most commonly, the thoracic cord is affected by spinal cord infarction. The goal of treatment of spinal cord ischemia is to increase cord perfusion. Vasopressors and lumbar CSF drainage have been used for this purpose. In general, corticosteroids are not recommended for spinal cord infarction.

In traumatic spinal cord injury, respiratory failure occurs with complete spinal cord lesions at C5 and above. These patients need to be intubated. Complete lesions of the upper thoracic spine interrupt supraspinal control of sympathetic preganglionic neurons in the thoracic cord. Patients can have bradycardia and hypotension because the parasympathetic system is unopposed. Patients with major injury to the cord at the T6 level or above are at particular risk for neurogenic shock due to loss of control of the sympathetic nervous system. Neurogenic shock is characterized by hypotension and warm, dry skin. Late effects of thoracic spine infarction can include bouts of hypertension and tachycardia.

Typically, cord injury needs to be bilateral to affect bowel, bladder, and sexual functions. An annual renal ultrasound study is recommended for neurogenic bladder caused by spinal cord injury.

14. A

Typically, pupils are reactive in patients with metabolic encephalopathy. However, in severe metabolic encephalopathy, pupillary responses can be lost.

Usually, the examination is nonfocal; however, there may be focal findings in certain medical conditions, such as hypoglycemia and hyperglycemia.

15. D

The EEG finding of 14- and 6-Hz positive spikes is a normal variant. However, it is also classically associated with Reye syndrome.

16. D

This patient's altered mental status and seizure are caused by hyponatremia. Sodium correction is needed.

However, overly rapid correction can cause central pontine myelinolysis, which is also known as osmotic demyelination syndrome. Chronic hyponatremia requires even more slow correction than acute hyponatremia.

17. A

Nonconvulsive status epilepticus is relatively common in the neurointensive care unit. Fluctuating consciousness should raise suspicion for this diagnosis. Prolonged EEG monitoring may be necessary to diagnose and manage this condition. The initial treatment is with a benzodiazepine such as lorazepam.

18. A

SIADH causes hyponatremia. Urine output is decreased, and the urine is concentrated. There is water retention, and the patient is hypervolemic.

Cerebral salt wasting is associated with laboratory results similar to those of SIADH and can occur in similar conditions (e.g., subarachnoid hemorrhage, traumatic brain injury, neurosurgery). Volume status helps to differentiate the two conditions. Urine sodium is typically high in cerebral salt wasting. Patients with cerebral salt wasting need replacement of salt and water.

Diabetes insipidus (DI) is associated with hypernatremia, serum hyperosmolality, increased urine output, dilute urine, and hypovolemia. It may manifest as polyuria. There are many causes of DI, including brain tumor surgery, traumatic brain injury, and brain death. Central DI is treated with rehydration and desmopressin (DDAVP). Lithium causes nephrogenic DI.

19. D

Nonketotic hyperglycemia (e.g., in patients with diabetes) can cause hemiballism or hemichorea. Increased signal is seen in the basal ganglia on T1-weighted MRI sequences. Nonketotic hyperglycemia can also cause epilepsia partialis continua.

20. B

Given the progression of the weakness, the patient may be at risk for respiratory failure. The forced vital capacity and negative inspiratory force should be monitored closely.

21. A

This patient has critical illness myopathy, specifically thick-filament myopathy. There are three types of critical illness myopathy: thick-filament myopathy, diffuse (cachectic) myopathy, and necrotizing myopathy of intensive care. Creatinine kinase may or may not be elevated in critical illness myopathy.

The most common type of critical illness myopathy is thick-filament myopathy. Risk factors include corticosteroids, neuromuscular blockers, and sepsis. There is selective loss of myosin filaments on muscle biopsy.

Critical illness polyneuropathy is an axonal sensorimotor polyneuropathy. Patients have sensory loss and generalized weakness that is worse distally than proximally. Risk factors include sepsis, multiorgan failure, respiratory failure, systemic inflammatory response syndrome, and persistently elevated blood glucose levels.

Hypothyroidism can cause a necrotizing myopathy, but the biopsy in this case is consistent with critical illness myopathy.

22. A

This patient has glycogen storage disease type II (GSD II), or Pompe disease, which is caused by acid maltase deficiency, also known as acid α-glucosidase deficiency. Infantile-onset Pompe disease manifests with cardiac failure, macroglossia, hypotonia. Pompe disease can also manifest later in life with proximal muscle weakness and respiratory insufficiency. Creatinine kinase is elevated. EMG may show myotonic discharges in the paraspinal muscles. Enzyme replacement therapy is available.

Myophosphorylase deficiency causes glycogen storage disease type V (McArdle disease), which leads to exercise intolerance.

Mutations in *PHOX2B* cause congenital central hypoventilation. *PHOX2B* is a homeobox gene that is important in the formation of the autonomic nervous system.

Spinal muscular atrophy type 1 (Werdnig-Hoffman disease) manifests in infancy with hypotonia, progressive weakness, and feeding difficulties. Respiratory failure occurs in early childhood.

23. C

Dantrolene has been used to treat neuroleptic malignant syndrome and malignant hyperthermia. It inhibits intracellular calcium release. If dantrolene is given with calcium channel antagonists, the patient may experience cardiovascular collapse. Dantrolene can also cause hepatic toxicity.

L-Dopa, bromocriptine, and amantadine can increase serotonin centrally, so they should be avoided if serotonin syndrome has not been ruled out. Bromocriptine may worsen psychosis and may result in hypotension.

24. B

Succinylcholine can cause hyperkalemia and arrhythmia in patients with neuromuscular disease. Chronic immobility leads to massive potassium release from depolarization when succinylcholine is administered. The same issue occurs in patients with stroke who have been hemiplegic for more than a few days.

The other agents do *not* cause hyperkalemia, but their effect can be quite prolonged in patients with neuromuscular disease.

25. B

Alpha coma on EEG does *not* necessarily predict a poor outcome (see Box 5.1 and Fig. 5.2).

Box 5.1 PREDICTORS OF POOR OUTCOME IN COMATOSE PATIENTS AFTER CARDIOPULMONARY RESUSCITATION

- Absent pupillary light response or corneal reflexes
- Extensor posturing or no motor response to pain after 3 days
- Myoclonus status epilepticus within the first day
- Bilateral absent cortical responses on somatosensory evoked potential testing after 3 days
- Generalized suppression, burst suppression, or generalized periodic complexes on a flat background on EEG
- High serum neuron-specific enolase

It is more difficult to predict the prognosis of patients who have been treated with hypothermia after cardiac arrest.[4]

26. D

Cushing's triad is a late sign of intracranial hypertension. The triad is hypertension (widened pulse pressure), bradycardia, and irregular respirations. Many patients do not manifest all three components.

27. B

If a patient has been treated with neuromuscular blocking agents, the train-of-four technique with maximal ulnar stimulation should be performed.[5]

28. D

Computed tomographic angiography (CTA), magnetic resonance angiography (MRA), and SSEPs should not be used as ancillary tests to assist in the diagnosis of brain death. Cerebral angiography may be used. There are specific requirements for performing an EEG to assess for brain death.

Ancillary testing is not required if the patient can be declared brain dead based on clinical examination and apnea testing. In order to declare a patient brain dead, the cause of coma should be known and irreversible. Neuroimaging should support coma. Levels of central nervous system depressant drugs should be negligible. The patient should not be paralyzed. There should be no significant electrolyte or endocrine abnormalities. The patient should have a temperature greater than 36° C. Systolic blood pressure should be greater than or equal to 100 mm Hg. The patient should have no respirations. Spinal cord reflexes, such as the triple flexion response, may be present in a patient with brain death.[5]

29. A

Epileptiform discharges indicate cortical activity and rule out brain death.

The presence of wave I on brainstem auditory evoked potential testing does *not* rule out brain death. Any wave form afterward does.

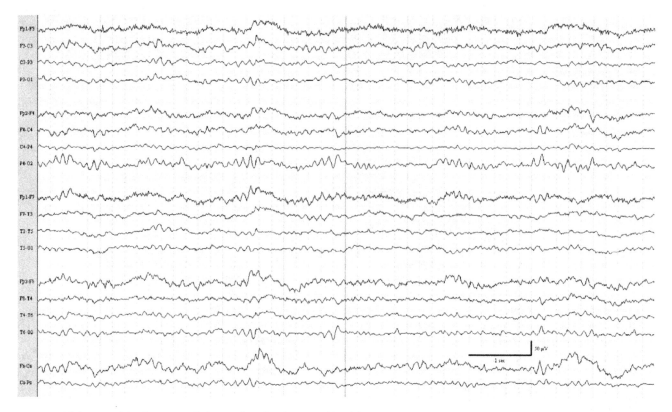

Figure 5.2 Alpha coma. The electroencephalogram (EEG) is dominated by alpha activity, which is nonreactive in a patient who is in a coma due to anoxia. (From Misulis KE. *Atlas of EEG, Seizure Semiology, and Management,* Fig. 4.73. New York, Oxford University Press, 2013.)

The presence of P100 on visual evoked potential testing rules out brain death.

N20 is a cortical waveform that is absent in brain death; however, somatosensory evoked potential testing is are not recommended for diagnosing brain death.

REFERENCES

1. Giza GC, Kutcher JS, Ashwal S, et al. Summary of evidence-based guideline update: Evaluation and management of concussion in sports. Report of the Guideline Development Subcommittee of the American Academy of Neurology. *Neurology* 2013;80:2250–2257.

2. Jordan BD. Chronic traumatic encephalopathy and other long-term sequelae. *Continuum (Minneap Minn)* 2014;20(6):1588–1604.

3. Brain Trauma Foundation, American Association of Neurological Surgeons, Congress of Neurological Surgeons. Guidelines for the management of severe traumatic brain injury. *J Neurotrauma* 2007;24(Suppl 1):S1–S106.

4. Wijdicks EFM, Hijdra A, Young GB, et al. Practice parameter: Prediction of outcome in comatose survivors after cardiopulmonary resuscitation (an evidence-based review). Report of the Quality Standards Subcommittee of the American Academy of Neurology. *Neurology* 2006;67:203–210.

5. Wijdicks EFM, Varelas PN, Gronseth GS, et al. Evidence-based guideline update: Determining brain death in adults. Report of the Quality Standards Subcommittee of the American Academy of Neurology. *Neurology* 2010;74:1911–1918.

6.

DEMENTIA

QUESTIONS

1. A 60-year-old man is brought to clinic by his daughter. He has been forgetful and loses objects. She suspects dementia. Which of the following best differentiates mild cognitive impairment from dementia?
   A. Preservation of executive function
   B. Preservation of language skills
   C. Preservation of visuospatial skills
   D. Preservation of activities of daily living

2. Which of the following is *not* an early finding in Alzheimer disease (AD)?
   A. Episodic memory loss
   B. Rapid forgetting
   C. Difficulty managing finances
   D. Impaired procedural memory

3. A college professor is concerned that he may have early AD. What is the most helpful evaluation?
   A. Clinical Dementia Rating scale
   B. Mini-Mental State Examination (MMSE)
   C. Montreal Cognitive Assessment
   D. Neuropsychological testing

4. A 60-year-old patient with a diagnosis of mild cognitive impairment (MCI) is concerned about progression to AD. Which of the following is *not* an indicator of more rapid progression from MCI to AD?
   A. Low Abeta42 and high tau in cerebrospinal fluid
   B. Carrier of ε4 allele of apolipoprotein E
   C. Positron emission tomography (PET) shows hypometabolism in the frontal lobes
   D. A positive amyloid scan

5. What is the greatest risk factor for AD?
   A. Family history of AD
   B. Head trauma
   C. Socioeconomic status
   D. Increasing age

6. A 50-year-old man presents with concerns about AD. His mother, maternal aunt, and maternal grandmother were diagnosed with AD. What is the most likely cause?
   A. Mutation in *APP*
   B. Mutation in *ApoE4*
   C. Mutation in *PSEN1*
   D. Mutation in *PSEN2*

7. In patients with AD, choline acetyltransferase is decreased in which structure?
   A. Basalis nucleus of Meynert
   B. Raphe nuclei
   C. Nucleus accumbens
   D. Locus ceruleus

8. Which of the following is *not* a characteristic pathologic finding in AD?
   A. Synaptic loss
   B. Alzheimer type II astrocytes
   C. Granulovacuolar degeneration
   D. Hirano bodies

9. Which of the following statements is *false*?
   A. The diagnoses of Alzheimer disease (AD) and vascular cognitive impairment (VCI) are mutually exclusive.
   B. Depression may contribute to cognitive symptoms in patients who have had a stroke.
   C. VCI is typically subcortical in nature.
   D. VCI can occur without memory deficits.

10. Which of the following is *not* recommended to prevent vascular cognitive impairment in at-risk individuals?
    A. Antioxidants
    B. Mediterranean diet
    C. Physical activity
    D. Treatment of hypertension

11. A 60-year-old, usually quiet college professor begins rolling her eyes when asked questions in class and yelling lewd comments at students. In the medical office, her examination is normal, but she is chewing on a pen. Which of the following is most likely her diagnosis?
    A. Alzheimer disease
    B. Creutzfeldt-Jakob disease
    C. Frontotemporal degeneration
    D. Progressive supranuclear palsy

12. Which of the following is *least* consistent with behavioral variant frontotemporal degeneration?
    A. Apathy
    B. Loss of sympathy
    C. Ritualistic behavior
    D. Visuospatial difficulties

13. Mutation in which of the following genes is the most common cause of familial frontotemporal dementia with amyotrophic lateral sclerosis (ALS)?
    A. *C9ORF72*
    B. *GRN*

C. *MAPT*
D. *SOD1*

14. **Which form of primary progressive aphasia is associated with AD?**
    A. Semantic variant
    B. Nonfluent/agrammatic variant
    C. Logopenic variant (logopenic phonological aphasia)

15. **Which of the following statements is *false*?**
    A. Attention difficulties and personality changes occur late in human immunodeficiency virus (HIV)-associated dementia.
    B. HIV-associated dementia may respond to antiretroviral therapy.
    C. Patients can develop HIV-associated neurocognitive disorders (HAND) even while receiving antiretroviral therapy.
    D. Neuropsychological testing is required to diagnose milder forms of HIV-associated neurocognitive disorders.

16. **A patient is brought in by his family because of dementia. The family members report that he has poor attention, forgetfulness, visual hallucinations, depression, falls, and strange behavior in his sleep. On examination, he has facial masking and bradykinesia. There is no tremor. Which disease is the most likely cause?**
    A. Alzheimer disease
    B. Parkinson disease
    C. Dementia with Lewy bodies
    D. Normal pressure hydrocephalus

17. **A 50-year-old patient presents with rapidly progressive cognitive problems and myoclonic jerks. Creutzfeldt-Jakob disease is suspected. Which of the following findings is *least* consistent with this diagnosis?**
    A. Elevated cerebrospinal fluid (CSF) tau
    B. Elevated CSF neuron-specific enolase
    C. Increased signal in the basal ganglia on magnetic resonance imaging (MRI)
    D. CSF pleocytosis

18. **Which of the following structures are most likely to be found in chronic traumatic encephalopathy?**
    A. Bunina bodies
    B. Lewy bodies

C. Neurofibrillary tangles
D. Aggregates of ubiquitin

19. **Which sleep disorder is characteristic of older adults with dementia?**
    A. Delayed sleep phase syndrome
    B. Irregular sleep-wake rhythm disorder
    C. Restless leg syndrome
    D. Short sleeper

20. **Which of the following is *not* recommended for patients with dementia?**
    A. Brief afternoon naps
    B. Music therapy
    C. Physical exercise
    D. Social engagement

21. **Which of the following is *not* recommended to reduce behavioral symptoms in patients with dementia?**
    A. Gently correct the patient each time the patient is mistaken.
    B. Avoid changes in routine.
    C. Avoid disturbing television programs and movies.
    D. Prevent fatigue.

22. **Prior to objective testing with an on-the-road driving test, which of the following is most helpful in deciding whether a patient with dementia can drive safely?**
    A. The Clinical Dementia Rating Scale
    B. The patient thinks it is safe.
    C. Neuropsychological testing
    D. Analysis of processing speed

23. **A patient taking rivastigmine is having significant vomiting. The family feels that the medication has been beneficial, however. Which of the following drugs is recommended?**
    A. Donepezil
    B. Galantamine
    C. Tacrine
    D. Transdermal rivastigmine

24. **What is the mechanism of action for memantine?**
    A. AMPA (α-amino-3-hydroxyl-5-methyl-4-isoxazole-propionate) receptor antagonist
    B. Cholinesterase inhibitor
    C. NMDA (*N*-methyl-D-aspartate) antagonist
    D. Reduces glutamate release at the synapse

DEMENTIA

ANSWERS

1. D

Some cognitive changes are normal with aging, such as misplacing objects and difficulty multitasking. Patients with mild cognitive impairment (MCI) have true cognitive decline. They can have problems with memory, language, visuospatial skills, or executive function, but they have preserved function in daily life. Impaired function in activities of daily living indicates dementia. Patients with MCI do have an increased risk for Alzheimer disease compared with others their age.

Cardiovascular risk factors, including smoking, are risk factors for dementia. Physical, cognitive, and social activities may help delay cognitive decline.

2. D

Episodic memory loss and rapid forgetting occur early in the course of AD. Difficulty with finances may be another early sign. Early impaired procedural memory is more characteristic of Parkinson disease.

3. D

In a highly educated individual, neuropsychological testing is the most helpful instrument for detecting early dementia.

4. C

Hypometabolism in the temporal and parietal lobes is consistent with a more rapid progression from mild cognitive impairment to AD (see Table 6.1).[1]

Table 6.1 INDICATORS OF MORE RAPID PROGRESSION FROM MILD COGNITIVE IMPAIRMENT TO ALZHEIMER DISEASE

TYPE OF INFORMATION	FINDING
Clinical	More severe clinical impairment
Cerebrospinal fluid	Low Abeta42, elevated tau
Genetic	Carrier of ε4 allele of apolipoprotein E
Magnetic resonance imaging	Atrophic hippocampi
SPECT/PET	Hypometabolism in temporal and parietal lobes, positive amyloid scan

PET = positron emission tomography; SPECT = single-photon emission computed tomography.

5. D

Increasing age is the primary risk factor for AD. After age, the greatest risk factor is a positive family history.

The major factor contributing to the development of sporadic AD is presence of the ε4 allele of apolipoprotein E.

6. C

Mutations in the genes encoding amyloid beta A4 precursor protein, presenilin 1, and presenilin 2 cause autosomal dominant AD.

Mutations in presenilin 1 are the most common cause of familial AD. They cause early onset of symptoms. *PSEN1*, which encodes presenilin 1, is located on chromosome 14.

Mutations in *APP* are the second most common cause of familial AD. The *APP* gene, which encodes amyloid precursor protein, is located on chromosome 21. Mutations in *APP* can also cause some familial forms of cerebral amyloid angiopathy (CAA).

PSEN2, which encodes presenilin 2, is located on chromosome 1. Patients with *PSEN2* mutations have the oldest age at onset among the familial forms of AD, but the age at onset is variable. One mutation in *PSEN2* is associated with seizures.

ApoE4 encodes apolipoprotein E and is located on chromosome 19. The apolipoprotein E ε4 allele usually causes late-onset AD. Having two copies of this allele increases the risk for younger age at onset.

7. A

In patients with AD, choline acetyltransferase is decreased in the basalis nucleus of Meynert.

8. B

Alzheimer type II astrocytes are not found in AD. They occur in hyperammonemia.

AD cannot be diagnosed definitively without pathology results. Neuropathologic features of AD include granulovacuolar degeneration, Hirano bodies, senile/neuritic plaques, neurofibrillary tangles, neuronal death, synaptic loss, and brain atrophy. Senile plaques consist of amyloid and neuritic processes. The major component of neurofibrillary tangles is tau protein, which is abnormally phosphorylated microtubule-associated protein. AD is a type of tauopathy.

9. A

AD and VCI can co-occur.

VCI is usually associated with subcortical symptoms. Cognitive slowing and abulia are more common than memory problems. Patients with VCI may just have executive function deficits. There is no specific cognitive profile that is diagnostic of VCI; patients with VCI can have any type of neuropsychological dysfunction. Micro-infarcts and white matter disease are thought to contribute more to VCI than macro-infarcts and large-vessel disease.

Depression is the most common psychiatric condition after stroke and needs to be ruled out in patients with cognitive impairment.

10. A

Treatment of cardiovascular risk factors is recommended to prevent vascular cognitive impairment. A Mediterranean diet and physical activity may help prevent cognitive decline. Antioxidants have not been proven to be helpful.

The American Heart Association/American Stroke Association guideline from 2011 regarding vascular contributions to cognitive impairment stated that donepezil can be used to improve cognition in vascular dementia and that galantamine may be helpful for patients with mixed AD and vascular dementia. At that time, studies did not indicate significant benefit from rivastigmine or memantine in patients with vascular dementia.[2]

11. C

This patient has behavioral variant frontotemporal degeneration (bvFTD), which is the most common cause of frontotemporal degeneration. Cholinesterase inhibitors and memantine are not recommended for this condition. Selective serotonin reuptake inhibitors (SSRIs) and serotonin norepinephrine reuptake inhibitors (SNRIs) have been used to treat behaviors in these patients.

12. D

Patients with behavioral variant frontotemporal degeneration (bvFTD) have disinhibition, which is often evident by socially inappropriate behaviors. Patients have a change in personality. They become apathetic and lose the ability to empathize and sympathize. Hyperorality, dietary changes, and obsessive-compulsive behaviors are seen. Neuropsychological testing indicates executive deficits. Memory and visuospatial functions are relatively spared. Frontal and/or anterior temporal atrophy, hypoperfusion, or hypometabolism supports the diagnosis. Genes that cause bvFTD include *MAPT, GRN,* and *C9ORF72.* Mutations in *MAPT* causes hyperphosphorylated tau deposition; mutations in *GRN* and *C9ORF72* cause deposition of the 43 kDa transactive response (TAR) DNA-binding protein (TDP-43). A smaller group of patients have inclusions containing the fused in sarcoma (FUS) protein.

Both the *MAPT* and *GRN* are located on chromosome 17q21. Mutations in *GRN* (also known as *PGRN*), which encodes granulin, can also cause nonfluent variant primary progressive aphasia and neuronal ceroid lipofuscinosis-11 (CLN11).

Psychosis can occur in patients with bvFTD caused by mutations in *C9ORF72* (chromosome 9, open reading frame 72).

Progressive supranuclear palsy (PSP) and corticobasal syndrome (CBS) can manifest with symptoms similar to those of bvFTD.

13. A

ALS can occur with any of the types of frontotemporal dementia (FTD), but it is most common in patients with behavioral variant FTD. Expansion of a GGGGCC hexanucleotide repeat in the noncoding region of the gene *C9ORF72* on chromosome 9 causes familial FTD and/or ALS.

The gene *SOD1* encodes superoxide dismutase-1. Mutations in the SOD1 protein can also cause ALS.

14. C

There are three types of primary progressive aphasia (PPA): logopenic, semantic, and nonfluent/agrammatic variants.

The logopenic variant is associated with AD. Patients with the logopenic variant of PPA have nonfluent speech and difficulty with repetition. Single-word comprehension is intact. There is atrophy at the left temporoparietal junction.

The semantic variant and the nonfluent/agrammatic variant are associated with frontotemporal dementia (FTD).

The semantic variant of PPA affects the anterior temporal lobes. Patients have a fluent aphasia with anomia. They have difficulty comprehending single words. Aggregates of TAR DNA-binding protein 43 (TDP-43) are most commonly found on neuropathology.

The nonfluent/agrammatic variant of PPA is associated with left perisylvian atrophy. Impaired grammar produces nonfluent speech. Tau-positive neuronal and glial inclusions are most commonly found on neuropathology, but TDP-43 has also been found. Mutations in the *GRN* gene can cause this variant.

Speech therapy is recommended for patients with PPA.

15. A

HIV-associated neurocognitive disorders (HAND) include HIV-associated dementia, HIV-associated mild neurocognitive disorder (MND), and HIV-associated asymptomatic neurocognitive impairment. HAND can occur at any stage of HIV infection and can occur despite treatment.

HIV-associated dementia is the most common neurologic condition in patients with acquired immunodeficiency syndrome (AIDS) and may be the presenting symptom. HIV-associated dementia is a subcortical dementia. Attention difficulties and personality changes occur early.

Neuropsychological testing is required to diagnose milder forms of HIV-associated neurocognitive disorders. Patients with mild neurocognitive disorder have mildly impaired function and deficits in at least two cognitive domains. The diagnosis of asymptomatic neurocognitive disorder also requires deficits in two cognitive domains. These patients have no difficulties with everyday activities.

If a patient has HAND, the physician may want to consider the central nervous system (CNS) penetration effectiveness (CPE) of the patient's medications. Efavirenz tends to cause CNS toxicity and therefore is not ideal for HIV-associated dementia.

16. C

This patient has dementia with Lewy bodies (DLB). Dementia is a prerequisite for the diagnosis of DLB. Other core features are fluctuations in cognition, especially attention and alertness; visual hallucinations; and parkinsonism. Patients with DLB can have bradykinesia, facial masking, and rigidity, similar to patients with Parkinson disease, but resting tremor is unusual. Suggestive features of DLB are rapid eye movement (REM) sleep behavior disorder, neuroleptic sensitivity, and low dopamine transporter uptake in the basal ganglia on single-photon emission computed tomography (SPECT) or PET. Cholinesterase inhibitors have been used to treat DLB. Symptomatic treatment may also be necessary. Traditional neuroleptics are avoided because of neuroleptic sensitivity. Dopamine agonists can worsen psychiatric symptoms in patients with DLB.[3]

Normal pressure hydrocephalus can cause dementia and a gait disorder, but facial masking does not occur.

17. D

CSF pleocytosis is rare in Creutzfeldt-Jakob disease (CJD) and should raise suspicion for another etiology.

American Academy of Neurology guidelines recommend checking for the presence of 14-3-3 protein in the CSF if a patient has rapidly progressing dementia of unknown etiology and there is strong suspicion of sporadic Creutzfeldt-Jakob disease.[4]

Patients with CJD may have elevated levels of tau, P-tau, and neuron-specific enolase in the CSF. Patients with sporadic CJD may have increased signal in the basal ganglia and/or cortical ribbon on fluid-attenuated inversion recovery (FLAIR) MRI and diffusion-weighted imaging sequences. Periodic sharp wave complexes occurring every 0.5 to 1 seconds are characteristic of sporadic CJD. Patients with variant CJD have increased signal in the pulvinar and do not have periodic sharp wave complexes.

18. C

Chronic traumatic encephalopathy (CTE) is a neurodegenerative disease that is caused by repetitive traumatic brain injury. It is a 3R and 4R tauopathy. Hyperphosphorylated tau accumulates in neurons and astrocytes. Neurofibrillary tangles (NFTs) and neuritic threads are seen. Abnormal TAR DNA-binding protein 43 (TDP-43) is often present in CTE. Abnormal axonal pathology is also seen in CTE.

Although it is a tauopathy, there are some neuropathologic features of CTE that separate it from AD and other tauopathies. In chronic traumatic encephalopathy, there are perivascular collections of hyperphosphorylated tau. Also, NFTs in CTE tend to start in the depths of the sulci. Rather than being found in layers IV and V, as in patients with AD, NFTs are found in the superficial layers (layers I and II). Also, the NFTs in CTE tend to be larger.

Dementia pugilistica is a type of CTE. It is a severe dementia caused by brain injury sustained during a boxing career.

The term *post-traumatic dementia* refers to dementia resulting from a single traumatic brain injury.

Bunina bodies are inclusions found in patients with ALS.

19. B

Older adults with dementia often have irregular sleep-wake rhythm disorder, which is characterized by loss of a normal circadian rhythm. The patient awakens and sleeps at variable times, naps intermittently during the day, and does not sleep for long periods.

A short sleeper is one who routinely sleeps less than 6 hours per night but functions normally and has no complaints of sleepiness. It is a normal variant.

20. A

Brief afternoon naps may disrupt sleep at night and are not recommended for patients with dementia.

21. A

Avoiding confrontation, unless safety is an issue, helps to reduce behavioral symptoms. Changes in routine should be avoided whenever possible.

If behavioral symptoms are not severe, they may respond to treatment of the dementia. Atypical antipsychotics can be used for psychosis, but antipsychotics increase the risk for cerebrovascular events in the elderly and for death in patients with dementia. There are caregiver training programs to teach caregivers how to prevent and handle behavioral symptoms.

22. A

According to American Academy of Neurology guidelines, the Clinical Dementia Rating Scale may be used to help determine whether a patient can drive safely. The fact that a patient feels his or her driving is safe does not predict safety. If a patient reports concern about driving, then there should be increased concern about the patient's ability to drive. If a caregiver thinks that the patient's driving is unsafe, the physician should be concerned that it is unsafe for the patient to drive. Motor vehicle accidents, reduced mileage driven, aggression, and impulsivity also raise concern that driving is unsafe. A Mini-Mental State Examination score of 24 or less is also concerning.[5]

23. D

The patient's medication can be changed to transdermal rivastigmine, which should reduce the vomiting.

Rivastigmine is a pseudo-irreversible cholinesterase inhibitor (acetylcholinesterase and butyrylcholinesterase). Donepezil, galantamine, and tacrine are also cholinesterase inhibitors.

Galantamine is a reversible, competitive acetylcholinesterase inhibitor and an allosteric nicotinic receptor modulator. Tacrine must be given four times per day and causes hepatotoxicity; therefore, the other medications are preferred.

Cholinesterase inhibitors can cause nausea, vomiting, diarrhea, anorexia, and weight loss. Syncope can also occur.

24. C

Memantine is a noncompetitive NMDA receptor antagonist.

REFERENCES

1. Peterson RC, Gill D. Update on mild cognitive impairment. Presented at the annual meeting of the American Academy of Neurology Institute, Philadelphia, 2014.
2. Gorelick PB, Scuteri A, Black SE, et al. Vascular contributions to cognitive impairment and dementia: A statement for healthcare professionals from the American Heart Association/American Stroke Association. *Stroke* 2011;42:2672–2713.
3. McKeith IG, Dickson DW, Lowe J, et al. Consortium on DLB: Diagnosis and management of dementia with Lewy bodies. Third report of the DLB Consortium. *Neurology* 2005;65:1863–1872.
4. Muayqil T, Gronseth G, Camicioli R. Evidence-based guideline: Diagnostic accuracy of CSF 14-3-3 protein in sporadic Creutzfeldt-Jakob disease. Report of the Guideline Development Subcommittee of the American Academy of Neurology. *Neurology* 2012;79:1499–1506.
5. Iverson DJ, Gronseth GS, Reger MA, et al. Practice parameter update: Evaluation and management of driving risk in dementia. Report of the Quality Standards Subcommittee of the American Academy of Neurology. *Neurology* 2010;74:16 1316–1324.

7.

DEMYELINATING DISEASES
AND NEUROIMMUNOLOGY

QUESTIONS

1. **A 25-year-old woman presents with eye pain and blurry vision. On examination, she has decreased visual acuity and an afferent pupillary defect. Brain magnetic resonance imaging (MRI) is normal apart from the eye. What is the treatment of choice?**
   A. Intravenous methylprednisolone followed by an oral prednisone taper
   B. Oral prednisone alone
   C. Therapeutic lumbar puncture
   D. Interferon-beta

2. **A patient presents with painless vision loss in one eye. He is found to have a centrocecal scotoma in that eye. His mother and brother experienced similar symptoms and eventually lost vision in both eyes. The patient's brain MRI is normal. Methylprednisolone does not improve his symptoms. What is his diagnosis?**
   A. Optic neuritis
   B. Leber hereditary optic neuropathy
   C. Myotonic dystrophy type 1
   D. Oculopharyngeal muscular dystrophy

3. **A patient involved in a motor vehicle accident has a brain MRI. Lesions consistent with multiple sclerosis are seen. The patient is asymptomatic from the lesions. What is the patient's diagnosis?**
   A. Clinically isolated syndrome
   B. Possible multiple sclerosis
   C. Probable multiple sclerosis
   D. Radiographically isolated syndrome

4. **Which of the following statements is *false*?**
   A. Multiple sclerosis can be diagnosed at the time of presentation of a clinically isolated syndrome (CIS) if the appropriate MRI findings are seen.
   B. A single MRI scan can demonstrate dissemination in time.
   C. Oligoclonal bands are pathognomonic of multiple sclerosis.
   D. In a patient with MS, brainstem symptoms at initial presentation suggest a worse prognosis.

5. **Which of the following statements about multiple sclerosis (MS) is true?**
   A. MS is more common in identical twins than in fraternal twins.
   B. MS has been linked to a polymorphism in the major histocompatibility class II locus on chromosome 6p.
   C. Geography affects the risk for MS.
   D. All of the above.

6. **Which of the following is most characteristic of MS?**
   A. Complete external ophthalmoplegia
   B. Complete third nerve palsy
   C. Sixth nerve palsy
   D. Vertical gaze palsy

7. **Which of the following is most likely to be seen in a patient with MS?**
   A. Diabetes insipidus
   B. Facial myokymia
   C. Livedo reticularis
   D. Retinopathy

8. **A patient presents with vision impairment, hearing loss, and headache. MRI demonstrates lesions in the middle of the corpus callosum. She also has lacunar infarcts. Branch retinal artery occlusions are seen with retinal fluorescein angiography. What is the most likely diagnosis?**
   A. Cerebral autosomal dominant arteriopathy with subcortical infarcts and leukoencephalopathy (CADASIL)
   B. Multiple sclerosis
   C. Neurosarcoidosis
   D. Susac syndrome

9. **A patient presents with headache, an abducens palsy, and pyramidal signs. She has a long history of mucosal ulcers and uveitis. What is the most likely diagnosis?**
   A. Behçet disease
   B. Multiple sclerosis
   C. Neurosarcoidosis
   D. Whipple disease

10. **Which of the following is most likely to be seen in a patient with MS?**
    A. Extrapyramidal signs
    B. Myorhythmia
    C. All the brain lesions enhance simultaneously
    D. Open ring sign

11. **Which of the following is *least* likely to occur in MS?**
    A. Depression
    B. Vitamin D deficiency
    C. Sexual dysfunction
    D. Seizures

12. **Which of the following is most abundant in an active MS plaque?**
    A. B cells
    B. Neutrophils

C. Eosinophils

D. T cells

13. Which of the following is the most specific characteristic of an active MS plaque?

A. Macrophages containing myelin debris

B. Astrocytic fibrillary gliosis

C. Almost no oligodendrocytes

D. Sharp margins on gross specimens

14. What are shadow plaques?

A. MS plaques with significant axon loss

B. Smaller MS plaques adjacent to a larger plaque

C. MS plaques with significant vasogenic edema

D. Remyelinating MS plaques

15. Which of the following is *least* likely to cause reappearance of prior deficits in a patient with MS?

A. Exercise

B. Fever

C. Pregnancy

D. Urinary tract infection

16. A young woman with relapsing remitting multiple sclerosis (RRMS) asks about having a child. Which of the following statements is *false*?

A. There is a decrease in the relapse rate during pregnancy.

B. There is an increased risk for miscarriage in RRMS.

C. In most patients with RRMS, there is no increase in delivery complications.

D. RRMS does *not* cause an increase in birth defects.

17. Which treatment for MS is safest during pregnancy?

A. Fingolimod

B. Glatiramer acetate

C. Dalfampridine

D. Natalizumab

18. Which medication for MS is pregnancy category X?

A. Dimethyl fumarate

B. Mitoxantrone

C. Rituximab

D. Teriflunomide

19. What is the reason for treating an MS exacerbation with methylprednisolone?

A. Prevention of future MS attacks

B. Delay in the next MS attack

C. More rapid improvement of symptoms

D. Reduction in the likelihood of permanent injury from an MS lesion

20. Which of the following statements is *false*?

A. Randomized controlled trials support the use of methylprednisolone to treat acute MS exacerbations in children.

B. Intravenous immunoglobulin (IVIG) can be used for acute MS exacerbations in adults if steroids are contraindicated.

C. Plasma exchange is a second-line treatment for adults with MS relapses.

D. Methylprednisolone can cause gastrointestinal bleeding.

21. Which of the following is the most likely to occur in a patient taking interferon?

A. Anemia

B. Flu-like symptoms

C. Leukopenia

D. Thrombocytopenia

22. Which of the following medications is contraindicated in patients with poor kidney function (i.e., a low glomerular filtration rate)?

A. Dalfampridine

B. Fingolimod

C. Natalizumab

D. Teriflunomide

23. Which of the following medications is a sphingosine-1-phosphate receptor modulator?

A. Dalfampridine

B. Fingolimod

C. Ocrelizumab

D. Teriflunomide

24. Which of the following medications is associated with cardiac arrhythmias, elevated liver enzymes, macular edema, skin cancer, and herpesvirus infections?

A. Cyclophosphamide

B. Fingolimod

C. Rituximab

D. Mitoxantrone

25. What is the mechanism of action of natalizumab?

A. It is a sphingosine-1-phosphate receptor agonist.

B. It interferes with the interaction between very late antigen-4 and vascular endothelial adhesion molecule-1.

C. It is an antibody to CD20.

D. It inhibits dihydro-orotate dehydrogenase.

26. Which of the following statements is *false*?

A. Mitoxantrone is a chemotherapeutic agent that decreases lymphocyte proliferation.

B. There is a limit for mitoxantrone dosing that should not be exceeded in a patient's lifetime.

C. There is a black box warning for mitoxantrone because of cardiotoxicity and treatment-associated leukemia.

D. If cardiotoxicity occurs with mitoxantrone, it occurs during the first months of treatment.

27. A patient who has been doing well on natalizumab presents with changes in behavior, gradually worsening left-sided weakness, and seizures. Which condition needs to be ruled out?

A. Progressive multifocal leukoencephalopathy (PML)

B. Immune reconstitution inflammatory syndrome

C. Hepatic encephalopathy

D. Reversible posterior leukoencephalopathy

28. Which of the following features is *least* consistent with the diagnosis of PML?

A. Areas of demyelination

B. Extensive perivascular cuffing and necrosis

C. Large astrocytes with bizarre nuclei

D. Oligodendrocytes with intranuclear inclusions

29. **Which of the following medications is a monoclonal antibody to CD52 and may carry a high risk for autoimmune complications?**
    A. Alemtuzumab
    B. Daclizumab
    C. Ocrelizumab
    D. Tocilizumab

30. **A 30-year-old woman is diagnosed with an asymmetric partial transverse myelitis. An inflammatory etiology is suspected. What is the best treatment?**
    A. Interferon-beta
    B. Intravenous immunoglobulin (IVIG)
    C. Methylprednisolone
    D. Plasma exchange

31. **True or False?**
    A patient with transverse myelitis and positive antinuclear antibodies (ANA) is presumed to have a rheumatologic cause for their transverse myelitis.

32. **A 20-year-old woman is diagnosed with transverse myelitis. Which of the following findings suggests that neuromyelitis optica spectrum disorder (NMOSD), *not* MS, is the etiology?**
    A. The presence of oligoclonal bands
    B. Longitudinally extensive transverse myelitis (i.e., the lesion involves at least three vertebral segments)
    C. Involvement of only the dorsolateral cord
    D. Involvement of less than one third of the cross-sectional area of the cord

33. **The presence of which of the following suggests that NMOSD, *not* MS, is the etiology of transverse myelitis?**
    A. Aquaporin-4 antibodies
    B. Myelin basic protein antibodies
    C. Proteolipid protein antibodies
    D. Elevated immunoglobulin G (IgG) index

34. **Which of the following is *not* associated with an increased risk for relapse of transverse myelitis according to the 2011 American Academy of Neurology evidence-based guideline regarding evaluation and treatment of transverse myelitis?**
    A. Neuromyelitis optica immunoglobulin G (NMO-IgG) antibodies
    B. Acute partial transverse myelitis
    C. Longer lesions (>3 vertebral segments)
    D. Male gender

35. **Which of the following statements is *false*?**
    A. In children, most cases of acute transverse myelitis are idiopathic, whereas in adults, a minority of cases are idiopathic.
    B. In children, acute transverse myelitis is more commonly associated with MS if fewer than three vertebral segments are involved.

C. Methylprednisolone is the treatment of choice for idiopathic acute transverse myelitis.

D. Infants have a better prognosis than other children with acute transverse myelitis.

36. **True or False?**
    NMOSD can manifest with intractable hiccups, vomiting, or narcolepsy.

37. **What is the target for neuromyelitis optica immunoglobulin G (NMO-IgG)?**
    A. A water channel protein
    B. A sodium channel
    C. A potassium channel
    D. A calcium channel

38. **Where is the target for NMO-IgG?**
    A. On astrocytes
    B. On oligodendrocytes
    C. On ependymal cells
    D. On the myelin sheath

39. **Which of the following potential treatments used for NMOSD is an anti-CD20 monoclonal antibody?**
    A. Aquaporumab
    B. Eculizumab
    C. Rituximab
    D. Tocilizumab

40. **Thiopurine methyltransferase levels are checked before NMOSD is treated with which agent?**
    A. Aquaporumab
    B. Azathioprine
    C. Mycophenolate mofetil
    D. Tocilizumab

41. **A 10-year-old girl presents with headache, sleepiness, and difficulty walking. She was normal until 2 weeks ago, when she had a virus with fever. MRI shows multiple lesions in the cerebral white matter, thalamus, and basal ganglia. Most of the lesions enhance. Analysis of the cerebrospinal fluid (CSF) shows 30 white blood cells (98% lymphocytes). Oligoclonal bands are negative. What is the most likely diagnosis?**
    A. Acute cerebellar ataxia
    B. Acute disseminated encephalomyelitis (ADEM)
    C. Multiple sclerosis
    D. Devic disease

42. **Which of the following is *least* typical of acute disseminated encephalomyelitis (ADEM)?**
    A. Severe axonal loss
    B. Perivenular demyelination
    C. The presence of lymphocytes around the veins
    D. The presence of macrophages around the veins

43. **Which of the following statements regarding demyelinating disorders in children is *false*?**
    A. For diagnosis of clinically isolated syndrome (CIS), the child should not have encephalopathy (that cannot be explained by fever).
    B. For diagnosis of CIS, the symptoms must be present for at least 1 week.

C. For diagnosis of CIS, the patient should not have had a prior central nervous system (CNS) demyelinating event.

D. Absence of encephalopathy with a first CNS demyelinating event indicates an elevated risk for MS.

44. Which of the following statements regarding demyelinating disorders in children is *false*?
    A. It is recommended that the term *recurrent ADEM* not be used.
    B. To fulfill criteria for multiphasic ADEM, the two events must occur at least 9 months apart.
    C. Younger children who are later diagnosed with MS are more likely to have a first event resembling ADEM than are adolescents with MS.
    D. If a child who has been diagnosed with ADEM is later diagnosed as MS, the onset of MS is said to have occurred when the ADEM event occurred.

45. Which of the following statements regarding demyelinating disorders in children is *false*?
    A. The presence of hypointense lesions on T1-weighted MRI is more suggestive of ADEM than of MS.
    B. Periventricular lesions are more consistent with MS than with ADEM.
    C. For diagnosis of MS, the two CNS demyelinating events have to occur at least 30 days apart.
    D. During childhood, MS usually follows a relapsing remitting course.

46. A 14-year-old girl presents with right arm weakness after an upper respiratory tract infection. MRI shows asymmetric lesions that have increased signal on T2-weighted and fluid-attenuated inversion recovery (FLAIR) sequences in the cortical gray-white junction of both hemispheres, in the deep white matter, and in the thalami and basal ganglia. There is relative sparing of the periventricular white matter. Cognition is normal. What is her diagnosis?
    A. Clinically isolated syndrome (CIS)
    B. Multiple sclerosis
    C. ADEM (monophasic)
    D. ADEM (multiphasic)

47. A 25-year-old woman with a recent upper respiratory tract infection presents with fever, confusion, and seizures. The C-reactive protein level is elevated. MRI shows diffuse, bilateral asymmetric lesions in the cerebral white matter. There is edema surrounding the lesions, and some of the lesions enhance. Some of the enhancing lesions are C-shaped. Susceptibility-weighted images show multiple punctate hemorrhages in the gray and white matter. She has a CSF pleocytosis. She subsequently becomes comatose and dies. What is the most likely diagnosis?
    A. Acute hemorrhagic leukoencephalitis
    B. Embolic stroke
    C. Malignant MS (Marburg disease)
    D. Marchiafava-Bignami disease

48. Which of the following causes an ADEM-like illness but is also associated with hepatosplenomegaly, lymphadenopathy, and increased levels of serum ferritin and triglycerides?
    A. Cerebrotendinous xanthomatosis
    B. Fabry disease
    C. Macrophage activation syndrome
    D. Metachromatic leukodystrophy

49. Which of the following cells are cytotoxic and kill cells infected with viruses?
    A. CD4+ T cells
    B. CD8+ T cells
    C. Gemistocytes
    D. Natural killer cells

50. True or False?
    Remyelination occurs more quickly in the peripheral nervous system than in the CNS.

51. Which of the following is found in CNS myelin?
    A. Proteolipid protein (PLP)
    B. Peripheral myelin protein 22 (PMP-22)
    C. Myelin protein zero (MPZ)

52. Patients with myasthenia gravis who test negative for acetylcholine receptor antibodies may have which of these antibodies?
    A. Anti-GQ1b antibodies
    B. Anti-GM1 antibodies
    C. Anti-MAG antibodies
    D. Anti-MuSK antibodies

53. Patients with myasthenia gravis with which of these antibodies often have a thymoma?
    A. Anti–striated muscle antibodies
    B. Anti-GQ1b antibodies
    C. Anti-MAG antibodies
    D. Anti-Hu antibodies

54. Which of the following statements is *false*?
    A. Plasmapheresis is recommended for patients with acute inflammatory demyelinating polyradiculoneuropathy (AIDP) who cannot walk or who require ventilatory support, and plasmapheresis can be considered in milder cases.
    B. Plasmapheresis is an option for treatment of chronic inflammatory demyelinating polyneuropathy (CIDP) in the short term.
    C. Plasmapheresis is indicated for treatment of polyneuropathy caused by immunoglobulin M (IgM) monoclonal gammopathy of undetermined significance (MGUS).
    D. Plasmapheresis can be considered in acute fulminant CNS demyelinating diseases.

55. Fill in the blank: Before giving intravenous immunoglobulin (IVIG), it is recommended that the _____ _____ level be checked.
    A. Albumin
    B. IgA
    C. IgE
    D. IgG

56. A patient presents with limbic encephalitis and neuromyotonia. Morvan syndrome is suspected. Which of the following conditions is most closely associated with Morvan syndrome?
   A. Breast cancer
   B. Malignant thymoma
   C. Small cell lung cancer
   D. Thyroid carcinoma

57. A 9-year-old boy presents with intractable focal clonic seizures of the left hand and arm. His left hand and arm are becoming progressively more weak. CSF analysis demonstrates no infection. MRI shows atrophy of the right hemisphere. Which of the following antibodies are most likely to be present?
   A. Antibodies to the calcium channel
   B. Antibodies to the γ-aminobutyric acid A (GABA A) receptor
   C. Antibodies to the glutamate receptor 3
   D. Antibodies to the sodium channel

58. Which of the following antibodies have been found in some patients with chronic relapsing inflammatory optic neuropathy and in some patients with ADEM who have prominent optic nerve involvement?
   A. Antibodies to GD1a
   B. Antibodies to MAG
   C. Antibodies to MOG
   D. Antibodies to sulfatide

59. Which of the following antibodies are most often associated with multifocal motor neuropathy?
   A. Monoclonal anti-MAG antibodies
   B. Monoclonal anti-GM1 antibodies
   C. Polyclonal anti-GM1 antibodies
   D. Polyclonal anti-GQ1b antibodies

DEMYELINATING DISEASES AND NEUROIMMUNOLOGY

ANSWERS

1. A

This patient has optic neuritis. The treatment of choice is methylprednisolone followed by prednisone according to the Optic Neuritis Treatment Trial.[1]

Brain MRI at the time of diagnosis with optic neuritis does help predict the risk for multiple sclerosis (MS). There is not enough information to warrant the diagnosis of MS or initiation of treatment with interferon-beta in this patient (see Box 7.1).

Box 7.1 FEATURES OF OPTIC NEURITIS

- It is painful.
- A relative afferent pupillary defect is present.
- Decreased contrast and color vision are often found.
- The optic disc may appear swollen.
- The patient may see light flashes with eye movements.
- It is usually unilateral but may be bilateral.
- Retinal hemorrhage and retinal exudates are unusual.

It is rare to have complete vision loss with optic neuritis due to MS. Severe vision loss and lack of response to steroids raise concern for neuromyelitis optica spectrum disorder (NMOSD). NMOSD also tends to cause simultaneous bilateral optic neuritis, to involve the chiasm, and to cause an altitudinal visual field defect.[2]

2. B

This patient and his family members have Leber hereditary optic neuropathy. This is a mitochondrial disorder that demonstrates maternal inheritance and is more common in males than in females. Patients initially develop unilateral symptoms and then progress to bilateral severe vision loss. This disease does not respond to methylprednisolone. It can be associated with cardiac conduction defects.

Oculopharyngeal muscular dystrophy causes ptosis but does not cause vision loss. It is associated with an expansion of a GCN trinucleotide repeat in the gene *PABPN1*.

The most common ophthalmologic findings in myotonic dystrophy type 1 are ptosis and cataracts.

The strong inheritance pattern and severe vision loss in the patient's family members make optic neuritis less likely.

3. D

This patient has radiographically isolated syndrome (RIS). Patients with RIS have MRI findings suggestive of MS that are found incidentally, without any clinical symptoms consistent with the disease.

Cervical cord lesions indicate increased risk for clinical conversion from RIS to MS.

4. C

The 2010 Revised McDonald criteria are used for the diagnosis of multiple sclerosis. The diagnosis of MS requires dissemination in time and space. A single MRI scan can demonstrate dissemination in time if there are both asymptomatic gadolinium-enhancing and nonenhancing lesions. A single MRI scan can also demonstrate dissemination in space if there are T2-weighted lesions in two of four characteristic locations for MS (i.e., periventricular, juxtacortical, infratentorial, and spinal cord). If a patient presents with brainstem or spinal cord symptoms, the symptomatic lesion should not be included (see Box 7.2).

Box 7.2 CHARACTERISTIC LOCATIONS OF MS LESIONS USED FOR DISSEMINATION OF SPACE CRITERIA

- Periventricular
- Juxtacortical
- Infratentorial
- Spinal cord

A positive CSF result is defined as the presence of oligoclonal bands in the CSF (but not in the serum) or an elevated CSF IgG index. In the 2010 Revised McDonald criteria, this is one of the criteria that can be used to aid in the diagnosis of MS in a patient with insidious neurologic progression suggestive of MS (i.e., primary progressive MS, or PPMS).

Although oligoclonal bands are common in patients with MS, they are also found in other conditions. For example, oligoclonal bands can be seen in CNS infections such as subacute sclerosing panencephalitis, herpes encephalitis, neurosyphilis, and Lyme disease. They can also be seen in neurosarcoidosis, cerebral lupus, and stroke.

The temporal profiles seen in MS are relapsing remitting MS (RRMS); secondary progressive (SPMS); and primary progressive MS (PPMS). (The term progressive relapsing MS is becoming obsolete.) RRMS is the most common type and has the least severe clinical course.

Motor, brainstem, or bowel/bladder symptoms with the initial attack suggest a worse prognosis. Also, failure to recover completely from the first attack suggests a worse prognosis (see Fig. 7.1).[3]

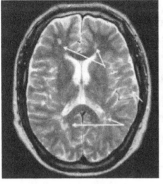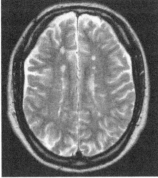

Figure 7.1 T2-weighted magnetic resonance imaging (MRI) scan showing white matter lesions *(arrows)* in a distribution typical of multiple sclerosis (MS). (From Scolding N, Wilkins A. *ONL Multiple Sclerosis*, Fig. 4.1. New York, Oxford University Press, 2012.)

5. D

Twin studies indicate a genetic component: MS is more common among identical twins than fraternal twins. Also, first-degree relatives of patients with MS have an increased risk for the disease.

MS susceptibility has been linked to polymorphisms in the DR gene, particularly *DRB1*1501*.

MS is less common near the equator. It is more common in northern latitudes. There is some evidence that vitamin D deficiency plays a role in this difference in prevalence.

6. C

Sixth nerve palsy and unilateral or bilateral internuclear ophthalmoplegia (INO) are typical in MS. One-and-a-half syndrome is less common but can occur in MS. Complete external ophthalmoplegia, a complete third nerve palsy, and vertical gaze palsies are *not* typical for MS.

Complete external ophthalmoplegia is found in mitochondrial DNA (mtDNA) deletion syndromes such as chronic progressive external ophthalmoplegia (CPEO), Kearns-Sayre syndrome, and Pearson syndrome. It is also seen in some *POLG*-related disorders.

7. B

Facial myokymia can be seen in patients with MS, but the other conditions are atypical for MS and suggest that there may be another diagnosis.

Sarcoidosis, histiocytosis, and neuromyelitis optica spectrum disorder (NMOSD) are mimickers of MS that can cause diabetes insipidus and other hypothalamic disturbances. Bone lesions occur in histiocytosis.

Lupus and antiphospholipid antibody syndrome are mimickers of MS that can cause livedo reticularis.

Retinopathy occurs in mitochondrial diseases and Susac syndrome, which can resemble MS.

8. D

This patient has Susac syndrome, which can mimic MS. Susac syndrome is a microangiopathy that affects the brain, retina, and cochlea, causing a triad of encephalopathy, sensorineural hearing loss, and vision loss. Focal neurologic signs, tinnitus, or vertigo may be present. Patients may have scotoma due to optic involvement. Branch retinal artery occlusions can be seen with retinal fluorescein angiography. On brain MRI, lacunar infarcts may be present. Susac syndrome causes lesions in the middle of the corpus callosum; the periphery of the corpus callosum tends to be spared. This helps to differentiate it from MS. Lesions can also be found in the basal ganglia, thalamus, brainstem, and cerebellum.

9. A

Patients with MS may have a history of uveitis, but this constellation of symptoms is most consistent with Behçet disease, which can mimic MS. Behçet disease is a type of vasculitis associated with recurrent oral and genital ulcers, uveitis, and skin lesions. It can affect multiple systems. In the CNS, Behçet disease can cause cerebral venous thrombosis or parenchymal involvement. It can cause recurrent meningoencephalitis, cranial nerve palsies, ataxia, and pyramidal signs. Brain MRI may show diffuse white matter involvement, infiltrating brainstem lesions, or atrophy of the brainstem.[4]

Chronic lymphocytic inflammation with pontine perivascular enhancement responsive to steroids (CLIPPERS) is another disease that affects the brainstem and resembles MS. It can cause diplopia and ataxia. The characteristic MRI finding is enhancing punctate lesions in the pons.[5]

10. D

Extrapyramidal signs are atypical for MS and raise concern for MS mimickers such as Whipple disease and Wilson disease. Whipple disease can cause oculomasticatory myorhythmia. Palatal tremor (palatal myoclonus) can occur in MS.

Simultaneous enhancement of all the brain lesions can be seen in vasculitis, lymphoma, and sarcoidosis. Sarcoidosis can also cause meningeal enhancement and lesions with persistent enhancement on MRI with gadolinium.

11. D

Seizures can occur in patients with MS but are not common. Seizures can occur in mimickers of MS, such as Whipple disease.

Depression, vitamin D deficiency, and sexual dysfunction are common in MS. Fatigue, spasticity, and bladder problems are also common issues. Pain may also need to be addressed.

12. D

T cells are the most abundant cells in an active MS plaque.

13. A

In an active MS plaque, there are perivascular and parenchymal lymphocytes and macrophages. There are also reactive astrocytes and macrophages containing myelin debris. Astrocytes become gemistocytes, which are plump cells with abundant fibrillary processes. Most inflammation is at the edge of the lesion. T cells are seen there.

Chronic plaques are characterized by astrocytic fibrillary gliosis and sharp margins on gross specimens. Almost no oligodendrocytes are present.

14. D

Shadow plaques are plaques where remyelination is occurring. They contain remyelinating axons, which have thin myelination.

15. C

There is a lower risk for an MS exacerbation during pregnancy, but there is a higher risk in the postpartum period.

16. B

RRMS does not increase the risk of miscarriage, delivery complications, or birth defects.

17. B

Glatiramer acetate (Copaxone) is pregnancy category B. It consists of a polymer that includes salt forms of four amino acids (L-glutamic acid, L-lysine, L-alanine, and L-tyrosine). It is administered by injection, and some patients have an immediate postinjection reaction. Lipoatrophy can occur with extended use.

Dalfampridine, fingolimod, interferon-beta, and natalizumab are pregnancy category C.

18. D

Teriflunomide is pregnancy category X. Teriflunomide reversibly inhibits dihydro-orotate dehydrogenase, which results in decreased proliferation of autoreactive T cells. Teriflunomide reduces progression of disability. It can cause diarrhea and hepatotoxicity. It potentially could reactivate tuberculosis. Initially, it can cause hair thinning. Clearance of teriflunomide takes months. There is an accelerated elimination procedure.

Mitoxantrone is pregnancy category D.

Rituximab and dimethyl fumarate are pregnancy category C. Dimethyl fumarate is taken orally twice daily and can cause flushing, vomiting, diarrhea, and abdominal pain.

19. C

Methylprednisolone produces more rapid clinical improvement, but it does not affect the long-term course of MS.

20. A

There are no randomized controlled trials of the use of methylprednisolone in children with MS exacerbations.

21. B

Injection site reactions, flu-like symptoms, elevated liver enzymes, and neutralizing antibodies can occur in patients taking interferon.

22. A

Dalfampridine (Ampyra) is the extended-release form of 4-aminopyridine, which is a potassium channel blocker. It is contraindicated in poor kidney function due to seizure risk. It improves ambulation.

23. B

Fingolimod (Gilenya) is a sphingosine-1-phosphate receptor modulator. It prevents egression of lymphocytes from lymphoid tissues.

24. B

Fingolimod has been associated with cardiac arrhythmias, elevated liver enzymes, macular edema, skin cancer, and herpesvirus infections. Electrocardiographic monitoring is recommended during the first administration of fingolimod, which can cause bradycardia or atrioventricular conduction delay.

25. B

Natalizumab is an antibody to α4 integrin. It interferes with the interaction between the integrin very late antigen-4 and vascular endothelial adhesion molecule-1. It prevents entry of lymphocytes into the central nervous system.

26. D

A maximum cumulative dose of mitoxantrone for a patient's lifetime has been determined. Mitoxantrone can cause acute myeloid leukemia and cardiotoxicity. In addition to checking cardiac function before initiating treatment and before each dose, the US Food and Drug Administration (FDA) has recommended annual cardiac function evaluations after completion of mitoxantrone therapy because there can be delayed cardiotoxicity. Cardiac toxicity is manifested as decreased left ventricular ejection fraction (LVEF) and/or congestive heart failure.[6]

27. A

This patient has symptoms that are concerning for PML. PML can cause subacute, progressive symptoms such as seizures, aphasia, hemiparesis, behavior changes, and retrochiasmal visual deficits. PML progresses over several weeks, rather than having an acute onset, as seen in MS. Unlike MS, PML usually does not affect the optic nerves or spinal cord.

If a patient develops PML while taking natalizumab, the drug must be permanently discontinued.

PML associated with natalizumab responds differently than other types of PML in regard to immune reconstitution. Immune function can be restored more quickly in patients with natalizumab-related PML. Immune reconstitution inflammatory syndrome can occur in patients with PML due to natalizumab when natalizumab is discontinued.

Patients who are human immunodeficiency virus (HIV) positive, have an immune disorder, or have a hematologic malignant condition should *not* be given natalizumab. Natalizumab should not be combined with immunosuppressants. A washout period is recommended before starting natalizumab if the patient has been taking an immunosuppressant.

Patients who are seronegative for anti-JC virus antibodies are at lower risk for PML (see Box 7.3).[7]

Box 7.3 RISK FACTORS FOR DEVELOPMENT OF PML IN PATIENTS TAKING NATALIZUMAB

- Antibodies to the JC virus
- Treatment with natalizumab for longer than 2 years
- Prior treatment with immunosuppressants

---

28. B

PML is caused by reactivation of the JC virus. The pathologic features of PML include intranuclear inclusions in oligodendrocytes; enlarged, bizarre astrocytes; and demyelination.

Extensive perivascular cuffing and necrosis indicates significant inflammation, as might be seen in encephalitis.

29. A

Alemtuzumab is a monoclonal antibody to CD52 that depletes mature lymphocytes and monocytes. Alemtuzumab carries a risk for autoimmune complications such as immune thrombocytopenic purpura, autoimmune thyroiditis, and glomerular nephropathy. It increases one's risk for malignancy. It can also cause an infusion reaction.

Daclizumab is an anti-IL2 receptor antibody.

Ocrelizumab is an anti-CD20 antibody.

Tocilizumab is an anti-IL6 receptor antibody (see Tables 7.1 and 7.2).

Table 7.1 MECHANISM OF ACTION OF MULTIPLE SCLEROSIS MEDICATIONS

MEDICATION	MECHANISM OF ACTION
Alemtuzumab (Lemtrada)	Monoclonal antibody to CD52; Decreases proliferation of autoreactive T cells
4-Aminopyridine/ Dalfampridine (Ampyra)	Potassium channel blocker
Dimethyl fumarate (Tecfidera)	Immunomodulation
Fingolimod (Gilenya)	Sphingosine-1-phosphate receptor agonist
Glatiramer acetate (Copaxone, Glatopa)	Immunomodulation
Interferon-beta 1a (Avonex, Rebif); peginterferon-beta 1a (Plegridy)	Immunomodulation
Interferon-beta 1b (Betaseron, Extavia)	Immunomodulation
Mitoxantrone (Novantrone)	Decreases lymphocyte proliferation
Natalizumab (Tysabri)	Antibody to $\alpha4$ integrin; prevents entry of lymphocytes into the central nervous system
Teriflunomide (Aubagio)	Inhibits dihydroorotate dehydrogenase; decreases proliferation of autoreactive T cells

---

Table 7.2 ROUTE OF ADMINISTRATION OF MULTIPLE SCLEROSIS MEDICATIONS

MEDICATION	ROUTE OF ADMINISTRATION
Alemtuzumab (Lemtrada)	Infusion
4-Aminopyridine/ Dalfampridine (Ampyra)	Oral
Dimethyl fumarate (Tecfidera)	Oral
Fingolimod (Gilenya)	Oral
Glatiramer acetate (Copaxone, Glatopa)	Injection
Interferon-beta 1a (Avonex, Rebif); peginterferon-beta 1a (Plegridy)	Injection
Interferon-beta 1b (Betaseron, Extavia)	Injection
Mitoxantrone (Novantrone)	Infusion
Natalizumab (Tysabri)	Infusion
Teriflunomide (Aubagio)	Oral

30. C

Methylprednisolone is the first-line treatment to improve symptoms. There is weak evidence that plasma exchange can be used in patients if treatment with methylprednisolone fails.[8]

31. False

ANA antibodies can be found in patients with neuromyelitis optica spectrum disorder (NMOSD) and in patients with MS.

32. B

Transverse myelitis (TM) that is longitudinally extensive (i.e., involving at least three vertebral segments) is more consistent with NMOSD than with MS. A complete spinal cord syndrome and centrally located lesions also raise suspicion for NMOSD. Paroxysmal tonic spasms can occur in myelitis patients with NMOSD.

The TM lesions in patients with MS tend to be more patchy, more peripheral, and shorter in length. MS cord lesions are usually less than two vertebral segments in length, involve less than half of the cross-sectional area, and most often involve the dorsolateral cord.

There is weak evidence that CSF oligoclonal bands differentiate patients with TM due to MS from those with TM due to other etiologies, including NMOSD.[2,8]

33. A

There is moderate evidence (level B) that neuromyelitis optica immunoglobulin G (NMO-IgG) antibodies are useful in differentiating patients with acute complete transverse myelitis due to NMOSD from other etiologies. Patients with NMOSD typically have antibodies to aquaporin-4.[8]

34. D

According to the 2011 AAN evidence-based guideline regarding the evaluation and treatment of transverse myelitis, NMO-IgG antibodies, acute partial transverse myelitis, and longer lesions have been associated with an increased risk for relapse. (There is moderate evidence for the antibodies, weak evidence for the others.) However, no demographic characteristics were predictive of relapse.[8] Since the publication of the AAN guideline, some studies have shown an increased risk for recurrence in females.

There is weak evidence that rituximab may be useful in preventing relapses in patients with transverse myelitis due to NMOSD.[8]

35. D

Most children with acute transverse myelitis (TM) have pain, sensory loss, autonomic disturbance, and urinary retention. Infants have a worse prognosis than other children with acute TM.

As in adults, acute TM is more commonly associated with MS if *fewer* than three vertebral segments are involved.

36. True

The core clinical characteristics of NMOSD are optic neuritis, acute myelitis, area postrema syndrome, acute brainstem syndrome, symptomatic narcolepsy or acute diencephalic syndrome with typical MRI lesions, and symptomatic cerebral syndrome with typical MRI lesions. The area postrema syndrome may manifest with intractable hiccups or vomiting.

A prolonged progressive course is not typical for NMOSD. Infection, sarcoidosis, and cancer can mimic NMOSD. Likewise, acute symptoms are not typical for NMOSD. Abrupt spinal cord symptoms raise concern for ischemia.[2]

37. A

Aquaporin-4 is a water channel protein. Patients without antibodies to aquaporin-4 can be diagnosed with NMOSD, but they must meet additional criteria.[2]

38. A

Aquaporin-4 is found on the foot processes of astrocytes.

39. C

Rituximab is an anti-CD20 monoclonal antibody. CD20 is a B lymphocyte antigen. Rituximab can increase one's risk for PML.

Eculizumab is an antibody to the terminal component of complement (complement protein C5). It is associated with a risk for meningococcal infection.

40. B

Azathioprine is a purine analog. It interferes with purine metabolism and DNA synthesis. Thiopurine methyltransferase is involved in the metabolism of azathioprine. Reduced levels cause accumulation of a toxic metabolite, which can lead to bone marrow suppression.

Aquaporumab blocks other antibodies from binding to aquaporin-4.

Mycophenolate mofetil prevents lymphocyte proliferation.

Tocilizumab is an anti-IL6 receptor antibody.

41. B

This patient has acute disseminated encephalomyelitis (ADEM). ADEM is an demyelinating condition caused by inflammation. It is typically monophasic. ADEM is characterized by multifocal neurologic signs, change in consciousness, and typical MRI findings. The brain MRI shows diffuse, bilateral, asymmetric lesions involving the gray and white matter. Lesions are primarily in the cerebral white matter but may also be seen in the thalamus or basal ganglia. Lesions can also be seen in the brainstem, cerebellum, or spinal cord. The lesions are not well demarcated, have increased signal on T2-weighted MRI, and may enhance. ADEM often occurs after a virus infection or vaccination.

Devic disease is now referred to as NMOSD.

42. A

ADEM causes perivenular demyelination. Lymphocytes and macrophages surround the veins as well.

43. B

For diagnosis of CIS, the symptoms need to be present for only 24 hours.[9]

44. B

To fulfill criteria for multiphasic ADEM, the two events must occur at least 3 months apart.[9]

45. A

Hypointense lesions on T1-weighted MRI are rare in ADEM; they are more likely to occur in MS. Periventricular lesions are also less common in ADEM than in MS.

Most children with MS have a relapsing remitting course. Children typically have more relapses than adults early in their disease course. A primary progressive course should raise concern for other diagnoses.[9]

46. A

This patient has clinically isolated syndrome (CIS). Although this MRI result is consistent with ADEM, the patient does not have encephalopathy; therefore, the diagnosis of ADEM cannot be made.

47. A

An incomplete rim of enhancement is consistent with demyelination. The patient also has punctate hemorrhages on susceptibility-weighted imaging. This occurs in acute hemorrhagic leukoencephalitis. Acute hemorrhagic leukoencephalitis, also known as acute necrotizing hemorrhagic encephalomyelitis, manifests with fever, headache, a stiff neck, and altered mental status. This progresses to focal seizures, weakness, and then coma. It can be fatal. Often there is a preceding upper respiratory tract infection. Pathology shows hemorrhagic demyelinating lesions with necrosis surrounding blood vessels. There is axonal injury and prominent edema.

An incomplete rim of enhancement, giving a C-shape, may also be seen in the MS variants tumefactive MS and malignant MS. Tumefactive MS is characterized by a demyelinating lesion resembling a tumor. Malignant MS, or Marburg disease, is a fulminant, monophasic condition. Demyelination, axon loss, and necrosis occur.

Baló concentric sclerosis is another MS variant. It is characterized by alternating rings of myelinated and demyelinated tissue.

Marchiafava-Bignami disease is demyelination of the corpus callosum associated with alcohol use.

48. C

Macrophage activation syndrome causes an ADEM-like illness that occurs in patients with rheumatic disease (e.g., systemic juvenile idiopathic arthritis). It is characterized by fever, hepatosplenomegaly, lymphadenopathy, increased levels of serum ferritin and triglycerides, and decreased levels of serum fibrin. It can cause purpura and mucosal bleeding. Multiorgan failure can occur. Hemophagocytosis (macrophages engulfing blood cells) is seen in the bone marrow.

49. B

CD8+ T cells are cytotoxic lymphocytes that kill cells infected with virus. CD8+ T cells have been found in patients with neuro-immune reconstitution inflammatory syndrome (neuro-IRIS) and Rasmussen encephalitis. Human immunodeficiency virus (HIV)-associated CD8+ T cell encephalitis has also been described. In polymyositis, CD8+ T cells infiltrate the muscle.

CD4+ T cells are helper cells. They are depleted in later stages of HIV infection.

Gemistocytes are a type of astrocyte.

Natural killer cells are a type of lymphocyte and may be involved in the mechanism of action of daclizumab.

50. True

After an injury, remyelination occurs more efficiently in the peripheral nervous system than the CNS.

Oligodendrocytes are the myelin-producing cells in the CNS; Schwann cells are the myelin-producing cells of the peripheral nervous system.

Oligodendrocytes produce many internodes of myelin on multiple axons, so injury to a few oligodendrocytes can produce a noticeable area of demyelination.

Schwann cells produce one internode of myelin and interact with one axon. Schwann cells are close in proximity to the internode of myelin, whereas the oligodendrocyte is connected by long processes (see Table 7.3).

Table 7.3 COMPARISON OF OLIGODENDROCYTES AND SCHWANN CELLS

OLIGODENDROCYTE	SCHWANN CELL
Central nervous system	Peripheral nervous system
Produce many internodes of myelin	Produce one internode of myelin, interact with one neuron
Connected to myelin by long processes	In close proximity to myelin
Remyelination is less efficient	Remyelination is more efficient

51. A

PLP is found in the CNS. It is defective in Pelizaeus-Merzbacher disease. Mutations in the gene that encodes PLP (located on the X chromosome) are also associated with hereditary spastic paraparesis.

Myelin basic protein is also found in CNS myelin.

PMP-22 is found in myelin in the peripheral nervous system. Duplication of *PMP22*, which encodes PMP-22, causes Charcot-Marie-Tooth disease type 1A. Deletion of one copy of *PMP22* causes hereditary neuropathy with liability to pressure palsies.

Myelin protein zero is the most prevalent protein in peripheral nervous system myelin. The gene *MPZ* encodes myelin protein zero. Mutations in this gene cause multiple genetic neuropathies. For example, mutations in *MPZ* can cause Charcot-Marie-Tooth disease types 1B, 2I, and 2J; Dejerine-Sottas disease; and congenital hypomyelinating neuropathy.

52. D

Most patients with myasthenia gravis (MG) have acetylcholine receptor antibodies (anti-AChR antibodies). Acetylcholine receptor antibodies may be measured in binding, blocking, or modulation assays. Many patients with acquired generalized MG or ocular MG have AChR-binding antibodies.

Patients with MG who test negative for acetylcholine receptor antibodies may have muscle-specific receptor tyrosine kinase antibodies (anti-MuSK antibodies). These antibodies are involved in clustering acetylcholine receptors at the neuromuscular junctions. Patients with these antibodies tend to be young females and have less ocular involvement than most patients with MG; their condition may worsen with edrophonium.

53. A

Myasthenia gravis (MG) patients with anti–striated muscle antibodies often have a thymoma. Modulating acetylcholine receptor antibodies are also found in MG patients with thymoma.

54. C

The American Academy of Neurology practice guideline regarding plasmapheresis states that plasmapheresis should

---

Box 7.4 AMERICAN ACADEMY OF NEUROLOGY PRACTICE GUIDELINES REGARDING PLASMAPHERESIS

- Plasmapheresis is recommended for patients with Guillain Barré syndrome (GBS), or AIDP, who cannot walk or who require ventilatory support, and plasmapheresis can be considered in milder cases.
- Plasmapheresis is an option for treatment of CIDP in the short term.
- Plasmapheresis can be considered in acute fulminant CNS demyelinating diseases.
- There is not enough evidence to make recommendations regarding treatment of myasthenic crisis or MG prior to thymectomy, pediatric autoimmune neuropsychiatric disorders associated with streptococcal infection (PANDAS), or Sydenham chorea with plasmapheresis.
- Plasmapheresis should not be used for chronic progressive or secondary progressive MS but can be offered for adjunctive treatment of an exacerbation in patients with relapsing forms of MS.

---

not be used for polyneuropathy due to IgM monoclonal gammopathy of undetermined significance (MGUS) but can be used for IgA or IgG MGUS (see Box 7.4).[10]

55. B

Before giving intravenous immunoglobulin (IVIG), it is recommended that the IgA level be checked to rule out IgA deficiency. Patients with IgA deficiency may develop anaphylactic shock if given IVIG, which typically contains IgA.

56. B

Morvan syndrome is characterized by limbic encephalitis, neuromyotonia, hyperhidrosis, and polyneuropathy. This is a paraneoplastic condition caused by malignant thymoma. Patients may have potassium channel antibodies.

57. C

This patient has epilepsia partialis continua due to Rasmussen encephalitis. It sometimes responds to IVIG. Refractory cases may require hemispherectomy. Some patients with Rasmussen encephalitis have antibodies to the glutamate receptor.

58. C

Myelin oligodendroglial glycoprotein (MOG) antibodies have been found in some patients with chronic relapsing inflammatory optic neuropathy (CRION) and in some patients with ADEM who have prominent optic nerve involvement.

Paraneoplastic optic neuropathy is associated with antibodies to collapsin response-mediating protein-associated (CRMP-5).

59. B

Monoclonal anti-GM1 antibodies are associated with multifocal motor neuropathy (MMN), which is a chronic acquired demyelinating polyneuropathy. Corticosteroids and plasma exchange are *not* helpful in its treatment.

Polyclonal anti-GM1 antibodies are associated with acute motor axonal neuropathies.

Monoclonal anti-MAG antibodies are associated with a demyelinating polyneuropathy.

Polyclonal antibodies to GQ1b are common in Miller-Fisher syndrome, which is characterized by the triad of areflexia, ophthalmoplegia, and ataxia. Polyclonal antibodies to GQ1b are also seen in Bickerstaff brainstem encephalitis.

REFERENCES

1. Beck RW, Cleary PA, Anderson MM, et al. A randomized, controlled trial of corticosteroids in the treatment of acute optic neuritis. *N Engl J Med* 1992;326:581–588.
2. Wingerchuk DM, Banwell B, Bennett JL, et al. International consensus diagnostic criteria for neuromyelitis optica spectrum disorders. *Neurology* 2015;85:177–189.

3. Polman CH, Reingold SC, Banwell B et al. Diagnostic criteria for multiple sclerosis: 2010 Revisions to the McDonald criteria. *Ann Neurol* 2011;69:292–302.
4. Kalra S, Silman A, Akman-Demir G, et al. Diagnosis and management of neuro-Behçet's disease: International consensus recommendations. *J Neurol* 2014;261:1662–1676.
5. Dudesek A, Rimmele F, Tesar S, et al. CLIPPERS: Chronic lymphocytic inflammation with pontine perivascular enhancement responsive to steroids—Review of an increasingly recognized entity within the spectrum of inflammatory central nervous system disorders. *Clin Exper Immunol* 2014;175: 385–396.
6. Marriott JJ, Miyasaki JM, Gronseth G, O'Connor PW. Evidence report: The efficacy and safety of mitoxantrone (Novantrone) in the treatment of multiple sclerosis. *Neurology* 2010;74: 1463–1470.
7. Kappos L, Bates D, Edan G, et al. Natalizumab treatment for multiple sclerosis: Updated recommendations for patient selection and monitoring. *Lancet Neurol* 2011;10:745–758.
8. Scott TF, Frohman EM, Seze JD, et al. Evidence-based guideline: Clinical evaluation and treatment of transverse myelitis. Report of the Therapeutics and Technology Assessment Subcommittee of the American Academy of Neurology. *Neurology* 2011;77: 2128–2134.
9. Krupp LB, Tardieu M, Amato MP, et al. International Pediatric Multiple Sclerosis Study Group criteria for pediatric multiple sclerosis and immune-mediated central nervous system demyelinating disorders: Revisions to the 2007 definitions. *Mult Scler* 2013;19:1261–1267.
10. Cortese I, Chaudhry V, So YT, et al. Evidence-based guideline update: Plasmapheresis in neurologic disorders. Report of the Therapeutics and Technology Assessment Subcommittee of the American Academy of Neurology. *Neurology* 2011;76:294–300.

8.

EPILEPSY

1. **A 24-year-old woman presents with an unprovoked seizure. Her family asks about workup. Which of the following statements is *false*?**
   A. An electroencephalogram (EEG) is recommended after the first unprovoked seizure.
   B. Neuroimaging is recommended after the first unprovoked seizure.
   C. Prolactin can help to differentiate generalized tonic-clonic from psychogenic nonepileptic seizures if measured within 10 to 20 minutes after an event.
   D. A complete metabolic profile (CMP), complete blood count (CBC), and lumbar puncture are recommended.

2. **A 4-year-old girl presents with her first nonfebrile seizure. Which of the following statements is *false*?**
   A. An EEG is recommended.
   B. Starting an anti-epileptic drug (AED) will impact her long-term prognosis.
   C. If the risks of medication are less than the risks associated with a second seizure, an AED can be prescribed after the first seizure.
   D. If imaging is performed, magnetic resonance imaging (MRI) is preferred to computed tomography (CT).

3. **A 19-year-old man presents with intractable generalized tonic-clonic (GTC) seizures. His seizures worsen with sleep deprivation. He reports morning twitching and jerks while taking carbamazepine. He said he had similar muscle twitching during his EEG when the light was flashing.**

a. **What are the expected EEG findings?**
   A. Generalized 4- to 6-Hertz (Hz) polyspike and wave discharges with a photoconvulsive response
   B. Generalized 3-Hz spike and wave discharges
   C. Generalized 2.0-Hz spike and wave discharges
   D. Left temporal focal epileptiform discharges

b. **What is the next step in treatment?**
   A. Add phenytoin.
   B. Change carbamazepine to oxcarbazepine.
   C. Change from carbamazepine to levetiracetam.
   D. Continue carbamazepine and add levetiracetam.

4. **A 6-year-old patient presents with nocturnal GTC seizures. A few seizures have been preceded by facial twitching, drooling, and speech arrest. What are the expected EEG findings?**
   A. Focal epileptiform discharges over the centrotemporal regions that increase during sleep.
   B. Focal epileptiform discharges over the right frontopolar region.
   C. Focal epileptiform discharges over the midline (at the Cz electrode).
   D. Generalized epileptiform discharges at 3 to 4 Hz.

5. **A 5-year-old patient presents with prolonged nocturnal seizures characterized by eye deviation to the right and unresponsiveness. Seizures are preceded by nausea and accompanied by headache and vomiting. Which of the following is the most likely diagnosis?**
   A. Benign rolandic epilepsy
   B. Childhood absence epilepsy
   C. Juvenile myoclonic epilepsy
   D. Panayiotopoulos syndrome

6. **An 11-year-old boy has recurrent seizures during the night characterized by hyperkinetic motor activity. Each seizure is brief and is not followed by a postictal period. His mother has a history of similar nocturnal seizures. A defect in which of the following structures is most likely?**
   A. Potassium channel
   B. Sodium channel
   C. Calcium channel
   D. Chloride channel
   E. Nicotinic acetylcholine receptor

7. **A family brings in their 1-week-old child for evaluation. The patient is having multiple brief focal clonic seizures per day. They started at 3 days of life. She has not had fever. The examination findings are normal. Her inter-ictal EEG is normal. The family reports that the patient's father, paternal uncle, and paternal grandmother had similar events, but their seizures resolved before 1 month of age and they had no further neurologic problems. A defect in which of the following structures is most likely?**
   A. Potassium channel
   B. Sodium channel
   C. Calcium channel
   D. Chloride channel
   E. Nicotinic acetylcholine receptor

8. **An 8-month-old girl has a GTC seizure associated with a temperature of 101°F. She has another GTC seizure 1 month later, in conjunction with an ear infection with fever. The EEG is normal. The patient's**

mother states that she herself had seizures with fever from 6 months to 7 years of age. Her sister did as well. They are both neurologically normal. What diagnosis should be considered?

A. Febrile seizures plus
B. Benign neonatal familial convulsions
C. Benign myoclonic epilepsy
D. Early infantile epileptic encephalopathy

9. A 2-year-old boy presents with daily seizures. He started having seizures at 8 months of age. He has had status epilepticus on three occasions. Two of those episodes occurred with fever. In one episode, the seizure activity was primarily left-sided; the other two times, it was primarily right-sided. He also has a history of myoclonic jerks and head drops. Inter-ictal EEG shows mild diffuse background slowing, a photoparoxysmal response, and generalized 3-Hz spike and wave discharges. What is the most likely diagnosis?

A. Dravet syndrome
B. Lennox-Gastaut syndrome
C. Early infantile epileptic encephalopathy
D. Early myoclonic encephalopathy

10. A 30-year-old man who has been seizing (left arm clonic activity) for the past 30 minutes arrives in the emergency department. He is given lorazepam and fosphenytoin, and the clonic activity stops. A CT scan of the head was normal, but the patient is difficult to arouse, and his eyes intermittently deviate to the left. What test should be considered?

A. Positron emission tomography (PET) scan
B. Single photon emission computed tomography (SPECT)
C. Electroencephalography (EEG)
D. Magnetoencephalography (MEG)
E. Computed tomography angiography (CTA)

11. A 26-year-old man has right temporal lobe epilepsy. His seizures have not responded to levetiracetam or lacosamide. What is the next step?

A. Referral to an epilepsy monitoring unit for an epilepsy surgery evaluation.
B. Treatment with oxcarbazepine, levetiracetam, and lacosamide.
C. Treatment with valproic acid, levetiracetam, and lacosamide.
D. Referral to neurosurgery for implantation of a vagus nerve stimulator.

12. A 32-year-old woman with a history of frequent migraines presents after having three focal-onset seizures. Her family history is remarkable for osteoporosis. Her EEG shows occasional right frontal epileptiform discharges. What do you recommend?

A. Monitor her clinically.
B. Start topiramate.
C. Start vigabatrin.
D. Start carbamazepine.

13. An 18-year-old female patient who is taking valproic acid for juvenile myoclonic epilepsy (JME) asks for a different medicine because she is gaining too much weight. The decision is made to transition her from valproic acid to lamotrigine. Three weeks later, she calls to report a rash that seems to be spreading. What is the next step?

A. Stop lamotrigine.
B. Send her to her primary care physician for a workup.
C. Check her levels of valproic acid and lamotrigine.
D. Discontinue valproic acid.

14. A 16-year-old boy with JME presents to the emergency department with increased seizures despite documented good serum levels of lamotrigine. The on-call physician suggests a schedule for starting valproic acid. Later in the week, the patient's mother calls to say that he is sleepy and his gait is unsteady. What should be done first?

A. Head CT
B. MRI with epilepsy protocol
C. Stat EEG
D. Toxicology screen
E. Verify that his lamotrigine dose was reduced when valproic acid was started.

15. A 24-year-old woman with epilepsy is considering having children. Which of the following statements is *false*?

A. Pregnancy is associated with a significantly increased risk for status epilepticus.
B. To reduce major congenital malformations, valproic acid and polytherapy should be avoided if possible.
C. Children born to mothers who are taking anti-epileptic medications have an increased risk of being small for gestational age.
D. Anti-epileptic medications such as valproic acid, phenytoin, carbamazepine, and topiramate are associated with an increased risk of facial clefts.

16. A 7-year-old boy presents with frequent staring episodes. The mother says he pauses during activities, stares off, and then returns to the activity. She can't get his attention during the episodes. He is normal afterward. This occurs multiple times per day. His mother states that he once had an episode while blowing a pinwheel. He is otherwise normal, and his neurologic examination is normal. What is the medication of choice?

A. Ethosuximide
B. Valproic acid
C. Lamotrigine
D. Carbamazepine
E. Levetiracetam

17. A 20-year-old woman with Lennox-Gastaut syndrome has daily myoclonic, atonic, and tonic seizures. Her seizures have not responded to levetiracetam, topiramate, zonisamide, clobazam, clonazepam, or rufinamide. Which medication should be considered?

A. Felbamate
B. Phenytoin

C. Carbamazepine

D. Gabapentin

18. Elementary auditory seizures, such as a humming or buzzing sound, arise from which area?
    A. Frontal lobe
    B. Mesial temporal lobe
    C. Lateral temporal lobe
    D. Parietal lobe

19. Unformed visual hallucinations, such as spots and flashing lights, arise from which area?
    A. Parietal lobe
    B. Mesial temporal lobe
    C. Lateral temporal lobe
    D. Temporal-occipital association cortex
    E. Occipital lobe

20. Formed visual scenes arise from which area?
    A. Parietal lobe
    B. Mesial temporal lobe
    C. Lateral temporal lobe
    D. Temporal-occipital association cortex
    E. Occipital lobe

21. Which of the following statements is *false*?
    A. Patients with juvenile absence epilepsy (JAE) tend to have fewer absence seizures than patients with childhood absence epilepsy (CAE).
    B. Absence seizures in JAE tend to be shorter than absence seizures in CAE.
    C. Patients with JAE are more likely to have myoclonic and GTC seizures than patients with CAE.
    D. Patients with JAE may need lifelong treatment.

22. What is the most common generalized epilepsy syndrome in adults?
    A. Juvenile absence epilepsy
    B. Juvenile myoclonic epilepsy
    C. Epilepsy with GTC seizures alone
    D. Childhood absence epilepsy

23. Which of the following is *not* a channelopathy?
    A. Absence epilepsy and episodic ataxia
    B. Benign familial neonatal seizures
    C. Generalized epilepsy with febrile seizures plus
    D. Familial lateral temporal lobe epilepsy

24. Autosomal dominant focal epilepsy with auditory features is associated with mutations in which gene?
    A. Nicotinic acetylcholine receptor
    B. GABA A receptor
    C. GABA B receptor
    D. Glycine receptor
    E. Leucine-rich glioma inactivated (LGI1) gene

25. Which of the following medications can exhibit zero-order kinetics?
    A. Levetiracetam
    B. Valproic acid
    C. Phenobarbital
    D. Phenytoin

26. Which of the following medications may be associated with polycystic ovary syndrome and fatal hemorrhagic pancreatitis?
    A. Levetiracetam
    B. Valproic acid
    C. Phenobarbital
    D. Phenytoin
    E. Oxcarbazepine

27. A 30-year-old woman presents in generalized status epilepticus. Which of the following medications should be administered intravenously first?
    A. Diazepam
    B. Fosphenytoin
    C. Levetiracetam
    D. Lorazepam

28. A 2-week-old child presents with tonic seizures. EEG shows burst suppression during wakefulness and sleep. MRI shows hemimegalencephaly. What is the most likely diagnosis?
    A. Doose syndrome (myoclonic-astatic epilepsy)
    B. Early myoclonic encephalopathy of infancy
    C. Ohtahara syndrome (early infantile epileptic encephalopathy)
    D. West syndrome

29. Most focal seizures in adults arise from which area?
    A. Frontal lobe
    B. Temporal lobe
    C. Parietal lobe
    D. Occipital lobe

30. Which of the following is *not* a common feature of seizures arising from the supplemental motor area?
    A. Prolonged duration
    B. Tendency to occur during sleep
    C. Often stereotypical
    D. Multiple occurrences in a single night

31. Which of the following medications is *least* likely to lower the seizure threshold?
    A. Bupropion
    B. Clonidine
    C. Tramadol
    D. Diphenhydramine
    E. Cetirizine

32. Which of the following anti-epileptic medications is *not* a T-type (low voltage-activated) calcium channel blocker?
    A. Ethosuximide
    B. Topiramate
    C. Valproic acid
    D. Zonisamide

33. Which of the following anti-epileptic medications is *not* usually associated with weight loss?
    A. Felbamate
    B. Levetiracetam
    C. Topiramate
    D. Zonisamide

34. Which of the following anti-epileptic medications is broad spectrum?
    A. Carbamazepine
    B. Ethosuximide
    C. Oxcarbazepine
    D. Valproic acid

35. Which of the following is the most effective medication for a patient with childhood absence epilepsy and GTC seizures?
    A. Ethosuximide
    B. Oxcarbazepine
    C. Tiagabine
    D. Valproic acid

36. Which of the following medications has high protein binding?
    A. Ethosuximide
    B. Gabapentin
    C. Levetiracetam
    D. Phenytoin
    E. Vigabatrin

37. A 75-year-old woman presents with confusion. Her laboratory studies show hyponatremia. Which of the following medications is most likely to cause this condition?
    A. Oxcarbazepine
    B. Lacosamide
    C. Clobazam
    D. Zonisamide

38. Which of the following anti-epileptic medications blocks the metabolism of γ-aminobutyric acid (GABA) by GABA transaminase?
    A. Clobazam
    B. Felbamate
    C. Tiagabine
    D. Vigabatrin

39. Which of the following anti-epileptic medications is *least* likely to affect the eye?
    A. Clobazam
    B. Ezogabine/retigabine
    C. Topiramate
    D. Vigabatrin

40. Which of the following medications can increase absence and myoclonic seizures?
    A. Carbamazepine
    B. Clonazepam
    C. Lamotrigine
    D. Valproic acid

41. Fill in the blank: Patients taking _____ require the slowest titration of lamotrigine.
    A. Carbamazepine
    B. Phenobarbital
    C. Phenytoin
    D. Valproic acid

42. Which of the following medications is *least* likely to cause weight gain?
    A. Pregabalin
    B. Gabapentin
    C. Valproic acid
    D. Lamotrigine

43. Which of the following medications places people of Asian descent with the *HLA-B*1502* antigen at higher risk for Stephens-Johnson syndrome than other patients taking the same medication?
    A. Carbamazepine
    B. Lacosamide
    C. Valproic acid
    D. Topiramate

44. Patients with short QT syndrome are advised not to take which of the following medications?
    A. Carbamazepine
    B. Zonisamide
    C. Rufinamide
    D. Ezogabine/retigabine
    E. Topiramate

45. Which of the following medications affects sodium channels differently than the others?
    A. Phenytoin
    B. Lamotrigine
    C. Oxcarbazepine
    D. Lacosamide

46. Which of the following medications acts on the alpha-2-delta subunit of high voltage-activated calcium channels?
    A. Ezogabine/retigabine
    B. Valproic acid
    C. Rufinamide
    D. Gabapentin

47. Which of the following medications modulates synaptic vesicle protein 2A (SV2A)?
    A. Levetiracetam
    B. Lacosamide
    C. Lamotrigine
    D. Valproic acid
    E. Perampanel

48. A 5-year-old patient presents with decreased speech and three seizures over the past 3 weeks. His parents report that he first started having problems with comprehension, then started speaking less. Which of the following EEG findings is most likely?
    A. Frequent left centrotemporal discharges with a horizontal dipole
    B. Electrical status epilepticus in sleep
    C. Left temporal focal epileptiform discharges
    D. Left parietal focal epileptiform discharges

49. True or False?
    Although it is usually not a first-line treatment, the ketogenic diet is an option for all patients with epilepsy.

50. **Which of the following features is more consistent with psychogenic nonepileptic seizures than with epilepsy?**
    A. Tongue-biting
    B. The event is stereotyped.
    C. Prolonged events occur only in public settings.
    D. Significant postictal confusion

EPILEPSY

ANSWERS

1. D

An EEG and neuroimaging are recommended after a first unprovoked seizure. Laboratory studies and lumbar puncture are not routinely indicated in the workup of the first unprovoked seizure.

It is recommended that the patient be informed that the risk for seizure recurrence is the highest during the first 2 years after a seizure. The patient should also be informed that prior brain injury or an EEG showing epileptiform activity increase the risk of recurrence. There is also evidence that other magnetic resonance imaging (MRI) abnormalities increase the risk of recurrence. In addition, if the first seizure was nocturnal, there is increased risk of recurrence.[1,2,3]

2. B

AEDs should not be prescribed to prevent epilepsy. Starting an AED will *not* impact the patient's long-term prognosis.

American Academy of Neurology (AAN) guidelines recommend that adults presenting with an unprovoked first seizure be advised that an AED may decrease the risk for seizure recurrence in the first 2 years after a seizure.

However, an AED can cause adverse events and will not change long-term prognosis.[3,4,5]

3a. A and 3b. C

This patient most likely has juvenile myoclonic epilepsy (JME). He is having myoclonic seizures in response to photic stimulation. The EEG will show generalized 4- to 6-Hz polyspike and wave discharges with a photoconvulsive response.

Generalized 3-Hz spike and wave discharges occur in childhood absence epilepsy. Generalized 2.0-Hz spike and wave discharges occur in Lennox-Gastaut syndrome.

Carbamazepine can exacerbate myoclonic seizures. Levetiracetam would be a better treatment option. Lamotrigine, topiramate, and valproic acid are also good options; however, lamotrigine can sometimes increase myoclonic seizures.

4. A

The description of this patient's seizures is consistent with benign rolandic epilepsy.

The EEG would be expected to show centrotemporal discharges, with a horizontal dipole, that increase in sleep (see Fig. 8.1).

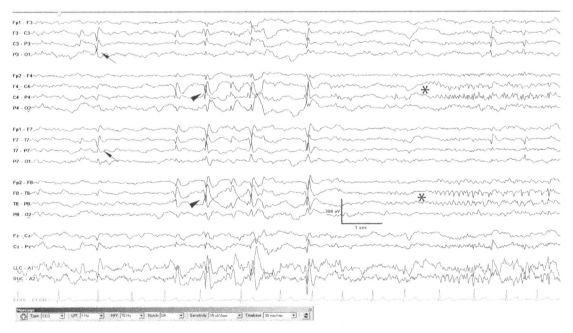

Figure 8.1 Typical focal epileptiform discharges seen in benign rolandic epilepsy *(arrows and arrowheads)*, followed by a seizure *(*)* arising from the right centrotemporal region. From Brazil CW, Chong J, Friedman G. *Epilepsy,* Fig. 2-1. New York, Oxford University Press, 2011.

5. D

This patient has Panayiotopoulos syndrome, which has also been referred to as "early-onset benign childhood occipital epilepsy (Panayiotopoulos type)." However, Dr. Panayiotopoulos prefers the term "Panayiotopoulos syndrome" because the symptoms and inter-ictal discharges are not necessarily occipital in origin. The peak age of onset is 4 or 5 years. Autonomic features, such as nausea and vomiting, are prominent in Panayiotopoulos syndrome. Seizures are often prolonged and are associated with tonic eye deviation.

Late-onset benign occipital epilepsy (Gastaut type) has a mean age at onset of 8 years. It is characterized by elementary visual hallucinations. A migraine-like headache may follow the seizure. Whereas seizures tend to be nocturnal and may be prolonged in Panayiotopoulos syndrome, seizures are brief and diurnal in late-onset benign occipital epilepsy. Temporary blindness may also occur in late-onset benign occipital epilepsy. Inter-ictal occipital discharges may increase significantly when the eyes are not fixated.[6]

6. E

This patient most likely has autosomal dominant frontal lobe epilepsy (ADNFLE), which is caused by defects in the genes that encode the nicotinic acetylcholine receptor on chromosomes 15q and 20q.

7. A

This patient most likely has benign neonatal familial convulsions, which are associated with defects in the potassium channel resulting from mutations in *KCNQ2* on chromosome 20q and *KCNQ3* on chromosome 8q.

Ezogabine (Potiga), one of the newer antiepileptic medications, acts on the potassium channel.

8. A

This family most likely has febrile seizures plus, previously known as generalized epilepsy with febrile seizures plus (GEFS+). It can occur with defects in *SCN1B* on chromosome 19q and *SCN1A* on chromosome 2q, resulting in sodium channel defects and defects in the GABA receptor.

Early infantile epileptic encephalopathy, otherwise known as Ohtahara syndrome, is a severe seizure disorder that manifests before 3 months of age. Patients have tonic seizures and a burst-suppression EEG.

Myoclonic jerks would be expected if the patient had benign myoclonic epilepsy.

9. A

The patient most likely has Dravet syndrome, also known as severe myoclonic epilepsy of infancy. The age at onset, multiple seizure types, photoparoxysmal response, and episodes of status epilepticus with fever support the diagnosis of Dravet syndrome, which is associated with *SCN1A* gene mutations on chromosome 2q. *SCN1A* gene mutations are also found in other types of epilepsy, such as febrile seizures plus.

Sodium channel blockers should be avoided in patients with Dravet syndrome. For example, carbamazepine, eslicarbazepine (Aptiom), lacosamide, lamotrigine, oxcarbazepine, phenytoin, and rufinamide should be avoided.

Preferred treatments for patients with Dravet syndrome are levetiracetam, topiramate, valproic acid, clonazepam, clobazam, and the ketogenic diet.

Lennox-Gastaut syndrome is also associated with multiple seizure types. Tonic, atonic, and atypical absence seizures are common, but any seizure type can occur in this syndrome. The EEG usually shows generalized slow spike and wave discharges at 1.5 to 2.5 Hz.

Early myoclonic encephalopathy and early infantile epileptic encephalopathy (Ohtahara syndrome) usually begin before 3 months of age and are associated with a burst-suppression pattern on the EEG.

10. C

Given the patient's prolonged seizure and intermittent eye deviation, an EEG is recommended to rule out ongoing seizure activity.

11. A

If first line anti-epileptic medications fail, the patient should be referred to an epilepsy surgery center. If the patient is a candidate for temporal lobe epilepsy surgery, it should be offered.[7]

12. B

This patient has had three seizures and has an abnormal EEG, so she is at risk for seizures in the future; therefore, treatment should be initiated. Topiramate can be used to prevent migraines and seizures and would be a good choice in this patient. Topamax is pregnancy category D, so risks should be discussed with the patient, and folate should be prescribed.[8]

Cytochrome P450 inducers, such as carbamazepine, are associated with increased risk for osteoporosis compared to noninducers. Vigabatrin carries a risk of permanent visual field defects and should not be used for initial treatment in this situation. However, vigabatrin is the preferred treatment for patients with infantile spasms due to tuberous sclerosis complex.

13. A

Due to the risk of life-threatening rash with lamotrigine, it should be discontinued when a rash occurs unless it is absolutely clear that the rash it is not drug related. This patient may see her primary care physician as well, but first lamotrigine should be stopped. It is helpful to have pictures of the rash if possible.

14. E

Valproic acid raises the level of lamotrigine. This is the reason that lamotrigine is increased more slowly if a patient is already taking valproic acid. It also means that lamotrigine should be decreased if valproic acid is added.

15. A

Pregnancy is *not* associated with a significantly increased risk for status epilepticus. Nor is it associated with a change in seizure frequency. However, levels of antiepileptic drugs (AEDs) may change during pregnancy. It is recommended that lamotrigine, carbamazepine, and phenytoin levels be monitored during pregnancy. Also, doses of these medications often requirement adjustment in the postpartum period.

It is recommended that women of child-bearing age taking AEDs take folate to prevent neural tube defects. To avoid the risk of major congenital malformations, it is recommended that polytherapy be avoided if possible. Consideration of avoidance of the use of valproic acid is also recommended because of the numerous birth defects with which it is associated. Also, maternal use of valproic acid during pregnancy is associated with a decrease in the child's intelligence quotient (IQ).[9,10]

16. A

Ethosuximide is the medication of choice for initial treatment of childhood absence epilepsy (CAE).

A double-blind, randomized, controlled trial was performed comparing ethosuximide, lamotrigine, and valproic acid in the treatment of CAE. Ethosuximide and valproic acid were more effective than lamotrigine. Valproic acid had more side effects than ethosuximide. Therefore, ethosuximide is the best choice if the patient does not have GTC seizures.[11]

17. A

As far as medications, felbamate is the most likely to help this patient. The ketogenic diet is also an option. If she's falling with her seizures, vagus nerve stimulation and/or corpus callosotomy should be considered.

18. C

Elementary auditory seizures, such as a humming or buzzing sound, arise from the lateral temporal lobe.

19. E

Unformed visual hallucinations arise from the occipital lobe.

20. D

Formed visual scenes arise from temporal-occipital association cortex.

21. B

Patients with JAE tend to have fewer seizures than patients with CAE, but the seizures are longer. Patients with JAE are also more likely to have myoclonic and GTC seizures than patients with CAE.

22. B

Juvenile myoclonic epilepsy is the most common generalized epilepsy syndrome in adults.

23. D

Familial autosomal dominant lateral temporal lobe epilepsy, which is also known as autosomal dominant focal epilepsy with auditory features, is not a channelopathy.

Absence epilepsy and episodic ataxia is caused by mutations in the gene *CACNA1A*, which encodes the principal subunit of the P/Q calcium channel.

Febrile seizures plus, previously known as generalized epilepsy with febrile seizures plus, can result from sodium channel mutations. Mutations in the GABA A receptor have also been associated with febrile seizures plus (see Table 8.1).

Table 8.1 CHANNELOPATHIES THAT CAUSE EPILEPSY

EPILEPSY SYNDROME	CHANNEL AFFECTED
Absence epilepsy and episodic ataxia	Calcium
Benign familial neonatal seizures	Potassium
Febrile seizures plus (generalized epilepsy with febrile seizures plus)	Sodium (or GABA A receptor)

GABA, γ-Aminobutyric acid.

24. E

Autosomal dominant focal epilepsy with auditory features is associated with mutations in the leucine-rich glioma inactivated (LGI1) gene.

25. D

Phenytoin exhibits first-order kinetics to a certain point, and then it exhibits zero-order kinetics. Initially, a certain percentage of the drug is eliminated in a specific time period (first-order kinetics). Then, when its metabolic pathways are saturated, metabolism of phenytoin changes to zero-order kinetics (i.e., a specific amount is metabolized in a specific time period). When this occurs, a small increase in dose will cause a large increase in the blood level.

Carbamazepine also has nonlinear metabolism. It induces its own metabolism.

26. B

Valproic acid is associated with polycystic ovary syndrome and fatal hemorrhagic pancreatitis.

27. D

Intravenous lorazepam is the first-line treatment for generalized status epilepticus in adults.

28. C

This patient has Ohtahara syndrome, which is also known as early infantile epileptic encephalopathy (EIEE). It manifests in the first 3 months of life with tonic seizures and a burst-suppression pattern on the EEG. Sometimes a structural lesion is present on brain MRI. Seizures are difficult to control.

Early myoclonic encephalopathy of infancy (EME) begins before 3 months of age, similar to EIEE. However, it typically manifests later than EIEE. Myoclonic seizures are prominent. The burst-suppression pattern is more prominent in sleep. Sometimes a metabolic etiology is found.

West syndrome refers to the triad of infantile spasms, developmental delay, and hypsarrhythmia. Infantile spasms typically manifest between 4 and 12 months of age.

Doose syndrome refers to myoclonic-astatic epilepsy. It presents in late infancy or early childhood. Tonic seizures do not usually occur in Doose syndrome. A patient with myoclonic, astatic, and tonic seizures is more likely to have Lennox-Gastaut syndrome than Doose syndrome.

29. B

Most focal seizures arise from the temporal lobe.

30. A

Seizures arising from the supplemental motor area tend to be brief, to begin and end quickly, and to occur outside of sleep. They may occur multiple times in a single night. Hypermotor activity with asymmetric tonic posturing is typical. A fencing posture may be seen. The patient may retain consciousness. Patients recover quickly, typically without postictal confusion. Ictal EEG findings are often less prominent than during other seizure types.

31. E

Cetirizine (Zyrtec) is *least* likely to lower the seizure threshold (see Box 8.1).

Box 8.1 MEDICATIONS THAT LOWER THE SEIZURE THRESHOLD

- Bupropion (Wellbutrin)
- Clonidine
- Clozapine
- Cyclosporin
- Diphenhydramine
- Imipenem
- Lithium
- Meperidine
- Theophylline
- Tacrolimus
- Tramadol

---

32. B

Topiramate is *not* a T-type calcium channel blocker.

Ethosuximide, valproic acid, and zonisamide are T-type calcium channel blockers. T-type calcium channels

are involved in the generation of absence seizures. Some patients with childhood absence epilepsy have mutations in *CACNA1H*, the gene encoding the calcium channel, voltage-dependent, T-type, alpha 1H subunit.

33. B

Levetiracetam usually does not affect weight.

Felbamate, topiramate, and zonisamide can all decrease appetite and cause weight loss.

34. D

Valproic acid is a broad-spectrum anti-epileptic drug. It can be used to treat focal and generalized seizures.

Ethosuximide is used for absence seizures.

Phenytoin, oxcarbazepine, and carbamazepine can exacerbate certain types of generalized seizures.

35. D

If a patient with childhood absence epilepsy has GTC seizures, valproic acid is preferred to ethosuximide. Both medications treat absence seizures; however, ethosuximide does not treat GTC seizures. Lamotrigine would be an alternative if valproic acid is contraindicated.

Tiagabine and vigabatrin can *cause* absence status.

36. D

Phenytoin has high protein binding (>75%). Ethosuximide, gabapentin, levetiracetam, and vigabatrin have low protein binding (<10%).

37. A

Of the options listed, oxcarbazepine is the most likely to cause hyponatremia. Carbamazepine and eslicarbazepine (Aptiom) also can cause hyponatremia.

38. D

Vigabatrin inhibits the breakdown of GABA by GABA transaminase.

Tiagabine blocks glial and presynaptic reputake of GABA.

39. A

Clobazam is *least* likely to affect the eye. It does carry a risk for Stevens-Johnson syndrome.

Ezogabine/retigabine can cause retinal pigment changes. It can also cause blue skin discoloration.

Topiramate can cause angle-closure glaucoma.

Vigabatrin can cause visual field defects; therefore, the US Food and Drug Administration (FDA) has recommended frequent ophthalmology evaluations. Vigabatrin can also cause hyperintensities on T2-weighted MRI. However, it is often used for patients with infantile spasms if adrenocorticotropic hormone (ACTH) is contraindicated or if the patient has tuberous sclerosis complex.

40. A

Carbamazepine can exacerbate absence and myoclonic seizures.

Lamotrigine can sometimes increase myoclonic seizures, but it is a treatment for absence seizures. It is used in some patients with JME even though there is a risk that myoclonic jerks may worsen.

Valproic acid treats both absence and myoclonic seizures.

Clonazepam can be used for myoclonic seizures, but it is not a first-line treatment for absence seizures.

41. D

Valproic acid inhibits the metabolism of lamotrigine. Therefore, lamotrigine is increased more slowly in these patients.

Carbamazepine, phenobarbital, and phenytoin are all inducers. Therefore, lamotrigine can be increased more quickly than it would be if given alone.

42. D

Lamotrigine does not usually cause weight gain or weight loss.

Gabapentin, pregabalin, and carbamazepine can cause weight gain. Gabapentin and pregabalin can also cause peripheral edema.

43. A

People of Asian descent with the *HLA-B*1502* antigen who take carbamazepine are at higher risk for Stephens-Johnson syndrome.

44. C

Patients with short QT syndrome are advised not to take rufinamide (Banzel).

Ezogabine (also known as retigabine) can prolong the QT interval.

45. D

Most anti-epileptic medications that affect the sodium channel act when it is in its fast-inactivated state. Lacosamide affects the slow-inactivated state of voltage-gated sodium channels.

46. D

Both gabapentin and pregabalin act on the alpha-2-delta subunit of high voltage-activated calcium channels.

Ezogabine (Potiga) acts on potassium channels.

47. A

Levetiracetam modulates SV2A, which is a synaptic vesicle protein. This effect is thought to be related to its mechanism of action.

Perampanel is a noncompetitive α-amino-3-hydroxyl-5-methyl-4-isoxazole-propionate (AMPA) receptor antagonist. It is approved for adjunctive therapy for partial-onset seizures and primary GTC seizures in patients 12 years of age and older. Homicidal and suicidal ideation are possible side effects.

48. B

This patient has Landau-Kleffner syndrome, which is associated with electrical status epilepticus in sleep. This is an epileptic encephalopathy with a peak age at presentation between 5 and 7 years. It is also known as acquired epileptic aphasia. Patients develop verbal auditory agnosia, and then expressive language deteriorates. Typically, the patient has seizures, but they are not frequent. High-dose diazepam is a common treatment, but many other medications have been used. Carbamazepine and phenytoin can exacerbate the EEG findings and should be avoided.

49. False

The ketogenic diet is a high-fat diet used to treat epilepsy. It is typically initiated in the hospital because of the risks of vomiting, hypoglycemia, and dehydration. Patients on this diet should not be given dextrose in their intravenous fluids. Possible side effects of the diet include kidney stones, constipation, hyperlipidemia, reduced bone mass, and decreased growth.

The ketogenic diet is not an option for all patients with epilepsy. The ketogenic diet can be lethal in certain metabolic conditions, such as pyruvate carboxylase deficiency. It is contraindicated in many other metabolic conditions, such as acute intermittent porphyria, cytochrome oxidase deficiency, carnitine deficiency, defects in oxidation of free fatty acids, and certain mitochondrial conditions.

The diet is particularly helpful for patients with glucose transporter type 1 deficiency and pyruvate dehydrogenase (E1) deficiency.

Topiramate and zonisamide should be used cautiously in patients on the ketogenic diet because these drugs can cause metabolic acidosis and kidney stones. Topiramate causes calcium phosphate (rather than calcium oxalate) stones.

Other dietary therapies include the low glycemic index diet and the modified Atkins diet.

In a 3:1 ratio ketogenic diet, the patient consumes three times as much fat as protein and carbohydrate combined (i.e., every 3 g of fat, there is 1 g of combined protein and carbohydrate).

50. C

Tongue-biting, stereotyped events, incontinence, occurrence during sleep, significant postictal confusion, and injuries during events support the diagnosis of epilepsy. Prolonged events that occur only in public settings raise concern for psychogenic nonepileptic seizures (PNES). However, the gold standard for diagnosing PNES is video-EEG monitoring.

REFERENCES

1. Krumholz A, Wiebe S, Gronseth G, et al. Practice parameter: Evaluating an apparent unprovoked first seizure in adults (an evidence-based review). Report of the Quality Standards Subcommittee of the American Academy of Neurology and the American Epilepsy Society. *Neurology* 2007;69:1996–2007.
2. Chen DK, So YT, Fisher RS. Use of serum prolactin in diagnosing epileptic seizures. Report of the Therapeutics and Technology Assessment Subcommittee of the American Academy of Neurology. *Neurology* 2005;65:668–675.
3. Krumholz A, Wiebe S, Gronseth G, et al. Evidence-based guideline: Management of an unprovoked first seizure in adults. Report of the Guideline Development Subcommittee of the American Academy of Neurology and the American Epilepsy Society. *Neurology* 2015;84:1705–1713.
4. Hirtz D, Ashwal S, Berg A, et al. Practice parameter: Evaluating a first nonfebrile seizure in children. Report of the Quality Standards Subcommittee of the American Academy of Neurology, the Child Neurology Society, and the American Epilepsy Society. *Neurology* 2000;55:616–623.
5. Hirtz D, Berg A, Bettis D, et al. Practice parameter: Treatment of the child with a first unprovoked seizure: Report of the Quality Standards Subcommittee of the American Academy of Neurology and the Practice Committee of the Child Neurology Society. *Neurology* 2003;60:166–175.
6. Panayiotopoulos CP. *A Clinical Guide to Epileptic Syndromes and Their Treatment*. New York, Springer Healthcare Ltd, 2010.
7. Engel JJr, Wiebe S, French J, et al. Practice parameter: Temporal lobe and localized neocortical resections for epilepsy. Report of the Quality Standards Subcommittee of the American Academy of Neurology, in association with the American Epilepsy Society and the American Association of Neurological Surgeons. *Neurology* 2003;60:538–547.
8. Harden CL, Pennell PB, Koppel BS, et al. Practice parameter update: Management issues for women with epilepsy. Focus on pregnancy (an evidence-based review): Vitamin K, folic acid, blood levels, and breastfeeding. Report of the Quality Standards Subcommittee and Therapeutics and Technology Assessment Subcommittee of the American Academy of Neurology and American Epilepsy Society. *Neurology* 2009;73:142–149.
9. Harden C, Hopp J, Ting T, et al. Practice parameter update: Management issues for women with epilepsy. Focus on pregnancy (an evidence-based review): Obstetrical complications and change in seizure frequency. Report of the Quality Standards Subcommittee and Therapeutics and Technology Assessment Subcommittee of the American Academy of Neurology and American Epilepsy Society. *Neurology* 2009;73:126–132.
10. Harden C, Meador K, Pennell P, et al. Practice parameter update: Management issues for women with epilepsy. Focus on pregnancy (an evidence-based review): Teratogenesis and perinatal outcomes. Report of the Quality Standards Subcommittee and Therapeutics and Technology Assessment Subcommittee of the American Academy of Neurology and American Epilepsy Society. *Neurology* 2009;73:133–141.
11. Glauser TA, Cnaan A, Shinnar S, et al. Ethosuximide, valproic acid, and lamotrigine in childhood absence epilepsy: Initial monotherapy outcomes at 12 months. *Epilepsia* 2013;54:141–155.

9.

METABOLIC DISORDERS

QUESTIONS

1. Which of the following conditions is *least* likely to cause hyperammonemia?
   A. Citrullinemia
   B. Isovaleric acidemia
   C. Maple syrup urine disease
   D. Medium-chain acyl-coenzyme A dehydrogenase (MCAD) deficiency

2. A neonate has seizures that do not respond to lorazepam, diazepam, fosphenytoin, phenobarbital, or levetiracetam. Which of the following medications should be administered next?
   A. Topiramate
   B. Zonisamide
   C. Pyridoxine
   D. Valproic acid

3. Fill in the blank: The conditions _____ and _____ have been found to be allelic disorders.
   A. Biotinidase deficiency and pyridoxine deficiency
   B. Folinic acid-responsive seizures and pyridoxine-dependent epilepsy
   C. Phenylketonuria and neopterin reductase deficiency
   D. Sepiapterin reductase deficiency and biopterin deficiency

4. A previously healthy 1-year-old boy presents with new-onset seizure. He has had vomiting, lethargy, and refusal to eat. He was diagnosed with a viral infection by his pediatrician on the day before admission. The examination is remarkable for hepatomegaly. Laboratory results show hypoketotic hypoglycemia, an elevated ammonia level, and hyperuricemia. What is the most likely diagnosis?
   A. Classic galactosemia
   B. Lowe syndrome
   C. Medium-chain acyl-coenzyme A dehydrogenase (MCAD) deficiency
   D. Glycogen storage disease type V (McArdle disease)

5. A 3-year-old macrocephalic boy presents with lethargy, dystonia, and hypotonia associated with a gastrointestinal illness. Magnetic resonance imaging (MRI) scan shows bilateral widening of the Sylvian fissures and increased T2 signal in the basal ganglia. What is the suspected diagnosis?
   A. Cerebral folate deficiency
   B. Glutaric aciduria type I

C. Miller-Dieker syndrome
D. Mowat-Wilson syndrome

6. A 5-year-old boy is adopted from another country. His mother would like him to be evaluated for developmental delay. On examination, he is microcephalic. He has pale blond hair, eczema, and a musty odor. MRI shows delayed myelination. What is the most likely diagnosis?
   A. Biotinidase deficiency
   B. Phenylketonuria
   C. Sulfite oxidase deficiency
   D. Thiamine deficiency

7. A 7-day-old infant presents with seizures, lethargy, opisthotonus, and sweet-smelling urine. Ketonuria is found on laboratory testing. MRI shows diffuse cerebral white matter edema. Which of the following treatments would be most successful?
   A. Administer carnitine.
   B. Administer riboflavin.
   C. Restrict branched-chain amino acids.
   D. Restrict glucose.

8. An infant presents with hypotonia, apnea, and intractable myoclonic seizures. He has a history of hiccups, perhaps even in utero. The electroencephalogram (EEG) shows burst suppression. What is the most likely diagnosis?
   A. Glucose transporter defect
   B. Infantile 3-phospholycerate dehydrogenase deficiency
   C. Molybdenum cofactor deficiency
   D. Nonketotic hyperglycinemia

9. An infant presents with new-onset seizures. He has a history of failure to thrive. He has axial hypotonia, and his reflexes are difficult to obtain. Although he is thin, he has a fat pad above his buttocks. His nipples are inverted. Which of the following analyses is most likely to yield the diagnosis?
   A. Cerebrospinal fluid (CSF) neurotransmitters
   B. Lipid panel
   C. Serum amino acids
   D. Transferrin isoform analysis

10. A 5-day-old newborn develops poor feeding, vomiting, and lethargy. Laboratory studies indicate acidosis, ketosis, hyperammonemia, and neutropenia. Which test is most likely to confirm his diagnosis?
    A. Chromosomal microarray
    B. Copper level

C. Lumbar puncture

D. Urine organic acids by gas chromatography–mass spectrometry

11. A 3-month-old patient presents with seizures. On examination, he is thin and hypotonic. His hair is light and sparse. Pili torti is seen when the hair is examined under light microscopy. Which of the following is the most likely cause?

A. A defect in copper-transporting adenosine triphosphatase (ATPase)

B. A defect in inositol polyphosphate 5-phosphatase OCRL-1

C. Mutation in the *PANK2* gene

D. Mutation in the *C19orf12* gene

12. A woman presents with altered mental status and hyperammonemia after being prescribed valproic acid. She has a history of recurrent vomiting attributed to a migraine variant. The patient and her mother are vegetarians. The patient's brother died in the newborn period of an unknown cause. What is the most likely diagnosis?

A. Hartnup disease

B. Ornithine transcarbamylase deficiency

C. Tangier disease

D. Wolman disease

13. Which of the following conditions is *least* likely to occur in mucopolysaccharidoses?

A. Carpal tunnel syndrome

B. Diabetes

C. Hydrocephalus

D. Cord compression

14. A 4-year-old child presents with loss of milestones. MRI demonstrates bilateral, symmetric, diffuse increased signal in the periventricular white matter. Nerve conduction studies show slowed conduction velocities. Nerve biopsy demonstrates lipid deposits. Which of the following is *not* typical of this condition?

A. Decreased arylsulfatase A activity

B. Decreased protein in the CSF

C. Delayed nerve conduction velocities

D. Increased urine sulfatide excretion

15. An 8-year-old boy is brought to the clinic because of worsening school performance. His mother reports that he was diagnosed with attention deficit hyperactivity disorder (ADHD) at age 6. However, he has had an increase in staring-off episodes despite stimulant medication. His handwriting has deteriorated, and he cannot follow oral instructions. MRI shows symmetric increased T2 signals in the parieto-occipital regions. Which laboratory test is most likely to be abnormal?

A. Cardiac echo

B. Lipid panel

C. Skeletal survey

D. Very-long-chain fatty acids

16. Which laboratory study or studies are useful in the diagnosis of peroxisome biogenesis disorders such as Zellweger disease?

A. Cathepsin D

B. Phytanic acid, pristanic acid, and pipecolic acid

C. Palmitoyl-protein thioesterase 1

D. Tripeptidyl-peptidase 1

17. A 15-month-old patient presents with seizures and loss of milestones. Examination shows macrocephaly, frontal bossing, hyperreflexia, and spasticity. Brain MRI shows increased T2 signal in the bifrontal white matter. A defect in which of the following genes is most likely?

A. *GFAP*

B. *PCDH19*

C. *PRICKLE1*

D. *STXBP1*

18. Which of the following is a neurodegenerative disease, caused by mutations in the proteolipid protein 1 (*PLP1*) gene, that results in nystagmus, stridor, hypomyelination, and initial hypotonia followed by spasticity?

A. Aicardi-Goutieres syndrome

B. Cerebrotendinous xanthomatosis

C. GM1 gangliosidosis

D. Pelizaeus-Merzbacher disease

19. Which of the following diseases is associated with mutations in the genes encoding subunits of the eukaryotic translation initiation factor 2B (eIF2B), foamy oligodendrocytes, decreased CSF asialotransferrin, and deterioration after stress?

A. Cerebrotendinous xanthomatosis

B. Childhood ataxia with central nervous system hypomyelination/vanishing white matter disease

C. Farber disease

D. 3-Hydroxy-3-methylglutaryl-coenzyme A (HMG-CoA) lyase deficiency

20. Which of the following conditions can mimic congenital infection and cause CSF lymphocytosis and calcifications in the basal ganglia?

A. Aicardi-Goutieres syndrome

B. Kearns-Sayre syndrome

C. Hereditary diffuse leukoencephalopathy with spheroids

D. Megalencephalic leukoencephalopathy with subcortical cysts

21. Which of the following leukodystrophies causes cataracts, dementia, ataxia, and elevated cholestanol?

A. Adult-onset polyglucosan body disease (APBD)

B. Cerebrotendinous xanthomatosis

C. HMG-CoA lyase deficiency

D. L2-hydroxyglutaric aciduria

22. An 8-month-old child presents with regression. The family reports that the patient became irritable at about 5 months of age. He stopped progressing developmentally and has been losing milestones recently. He has intermittent fever, but no infection been found. He is hypertonic and does not visually track. Lumbar puncture shows elevated protein. Which enzyme is deficient?

A. Ceramidase
B. Galactocerebrosidase
C. Neuraminidase
D. Sphingomyelinase

23. A 6-month-old boy presents with loss of milestones. He can no longer hold up his head or roll over. On examination, he has strabismus, stridor, hepatosplenomegaly, and hyperreflexia. During the examination, he repeatedly retroflexes his neck. Bone marrow analysis shows abnormal cells. What other finding is expected?
   A. Aromatic L-amino acid decarboxylase (AADC) deficiency
   B. Glucocerebrosidase deficiency
   C. Guanidinoacetate methyltransferase (GAMT) deficiency
   D. Creatine transporter (SLC6A8) deficiency

24. An infant presents with motor regression. She is macrocephalic and hypotonic. Canavan disease is suspected. Which test would aid in this diagnosis?
   A. Uric acid
   B. Urine N-acetyl aspartate (NAA)
   C. Urine oligosaccharides
   D. Urine glycosaminoglycans

25. A 1-year-old child presents with developmental delay. The family reports that she was normal at birth, but then they noticed a significant startle to noises. Due to concerns about her vision, she saw an ophthalmologist who "said something about fruit in her eye." On examination, she is hypotonic and hyperreflexic. What other findings might you expect?
   A. Hepatosplenomegaly
   B. Deficiency of hexosaminidase A
   C. Microcephaly
   D. Cardiomyopathy

26. A 15-year-old boy presents with lancinating extremity pain, which worsens in the summer. On review of systems, he lists abdominal pain. On examination, he has dark red dots near his umbilicus and on his thighs and buttocks. Which of the following conditions is *least* likely to occur in this disease?
   A. Deafness
   B. Hypertension
   C. Myocardial infarction
   D. Stroke

27. An 11-year-old girl presents with unsteadiness, seizures, and deteriorating school performance. On examination, she is unable to look upward, has dysarthria, and is ataxic. Bone marrow analysis reveals sea-blue histiocytes and foam cells. Filipin staining shows accumulation of cholesterol in lysosomes of cultured fibroblasts. Which other condition is associated with this disease?
   A. Cataplexy
   B. Conductive hearing loss
   C. Growth hormone deficiency
   D. Renal calculi

28. A 3-year-old boy presents with epilepsy and decreased vision. On electroencephalography (EEG), occipital spikes are seen at low-frequency stimulation. Visual evoked potentials are high in amplitude. The patient's sister had similar symptoms. She regressed, lost her vision, is ataxic, has action myoclonus, and has myoclonic epilepsy. She is scheduled for a biopsy. Which of the following findings is most likely?
   A. Electron-dense granules within the smooth muscle layer of small arterial vessels
   B. Curvilinear profiles within lysosomes
   C. Spheroids on nerve biopsy
   D. Ragged red fibers on muscle biopsy

29. A cherry-red spot, severe myoclonus, seizures, and night-blindness are found in which of the following diseases?
   A. Lafora disease
   B. Marinesco-Sjögren syndrome
   C. Sialidosis type I
   D. Unverricht-Lundborg disease

30. A child presents with weakness, myoclonus, and generalized seizures. The mother and maternal grandmother have optic atrophy and hearing loss. Which of the following is most likely to be present?
   A. Aggregates of polyglucosan in the apocrine and eccrine glands on skin biopsy
   B. Elevated lactate
   C. Potassium channel defect
   D. Scoliosis

31. Mutations in which of the following genes cause glucose transporter type 1 deficiency syndrome (also known as Glut1-DS or Glut-1 deficiency), early-onset absence epilepsy, alternating hemiplegia of childhood, paroxysmal choreoathetosis with episodic ataxia and spasticity (DYT9), and epilepsy with exercise-induced dyskinesia (DYT18)?
   A. *CACNA1A*
   B. *GABRAG2*
   C. *PLA2G6*
   D. *SLC2A1*

32. Which of the following is the best treatment for glucose transporter type 1 deficiency syndrome (Glut1-DS)?
   A. Carnitine
   B. Clonazepam
   C. Sulfonylurea
   D. The ketogenic diet

33. A 3-month-old infant presents with respiratory failure during a viral infection. She is hypotonic and developmentally delayed. MRI shows symmetric, increased signal in the basal ganglia. The CSF lactate level is elevated. What is the most likely diagnosis?
   A. Idiopathic basal ganglia calcification-1 (formerly called Fahr disease)
   B. Kernicterus
   C. Leigh syndrome
   D. Neurodegeneration with brain iron accumulation

34. Fill in the blank: Depakote is contraindicated in patients with _____.
    A. *CHRNA2* mutations
    B. *POLG* mutations
    C. *SCN1A* mutations
    D. Type II hyperprolinemia

35. A 5-year-old boy presents with a history of cerebral palsy. He has a history of hypotonia and delayed milestones. Currently, he has hyperreflexia and dystonia. He has scars from biting his hands and banging his head. Which of the following abnormalities is suspected?
    A. Deficiency of cystathionine β-synthase
    B. Deficiency of GTP cyclohydrolase 1
    C. Deficiency of hypoxanthine-guanine phosphoribosyltransferase
    D. Mutation in *ATP1A3*

36. A newborn in the nursery has microcephaly. He also has ptosis, epicanthal folds, cleft palate, polydactyly, and ambiguous genitalia. His serum cholesterol level is low. What diagnostic test would support his diagnosis?
    A. Serum amino acids
    B. Serum concentration of 7-dehydrocholesterol

C. Very-long-chain fatty acids
D. Urine organic acids

37. In which disease(s) does lactate fail to increase as expected during forearm exercise testing?
    A. Phosphofructokinase deficiency
    B. Myophosphorylase deficiency
    C. Phosphoglycerate mutase deficiency
    D. All of the above

38. Enzyme replacement therapy is available for which of the following diseases?
    A. Gaucher disease
    B. Fabry disease
    C. Pompe disease (glycogen storage disease type II)
    D. All of the above

39. Which of the following findings help to differentiate ataxia with vitamin E deficiency (AVED) from Friedreich ataxia (FA)?
    A. Nystagmus is present in FA but not in AVED.
    B. Posterior column dysfunction is present in FA but not in AVED.
    C. Cardiac conduction defects occur in FA but not in AVED.
    D. Titubation is more common in FA.

METABOLIC DISORDERS

ANSWERS

1. C

Maple syrup urine disease, which is a branched-chain aminoacidopathy, is least likely to cause hyperammonemia.

Citrullinemia is caused by a urea cycle defect, which results in hyperammonemia.

Isovaleric acidemia is an organic acidemia that cause hyperammonemia.

MCAD deficiency is the most common fatty acid oxidation disorder. It can cause hyperammonemia.

2. C

Pyridoxine deficiency can cause refractory seizures in the neonatal period. A trial of oral or intravenous pyridoxine aids in the diagnosis of pyridoxine-dependent epilepsy. Intravenous pyridoxine can cause apnea, so it should be used with caution.

There is an increased risk for fatal hepatoxicity when valproic acid is used in patients younger than 2 years of age.

3. B

Folinic acid-responsive seizures and pyridoxine-dependent epilepsy are allelic conditions. Both are caused by mutations in the *ALDH7A1* gene,

which encodes α-aminoadipic semialdehyde dehydrogenase (AASDH), also known as antiquitin. It is involved in lysine catabolism (the pipecolic acid pathway). Abnormalities in antiquitin/AASDH cause inactivation of pyridoxal phosphate, which results in seizures. α-Aminoadipic semialdehyde is increased in the plasma, urine, and CSF of these patients. In addition, pipecolic acid is elevated in the plasma and CSF.

Newborns with epilepsy who partially respond to pyridoxine and do not have a mutation in *ALDH7A1* may have a mutation in *PNPO*, which causes pyridoxal phosphate-responsive epilepsy. These patients respond to pyridoxal-5-phosphate.

4. C

Hypoglycemia after a short fast suggests a defect in carbohydrate metabolism. Hypoglycemia after a prolonged fast suggests a disorder of fatty acid oxidation.

The enzyme MCAD participates in mitochondrial fatty acid β-oxidation, which is required for production of ketones in the liver. Hepatic ketogenesis is important during prolonged fasting and in conditions in which there are increased energy demands.

Classically, MCAD deficiency manifests in an infant or young child with vomiting and lethargy during an illness resulting in fasting. The child may have a seizure. Coma may occur. The patients often have hepatomegaly. Laboratory studies show hypoketotic hypoglycemia, hyperammonemia, and hyperuricemia.

Classic galactosemia manifests in the newborn period after exposure to breast milk or lactose-containing formula.

Lowe syndrome, or oculocerebrorenal syndrome, causes cataracts, hypotonia, and areflexia at birth. Patients have developmental delays and renal complications such as aminoaciduria and renal tubular acidosis. Lowe syndrome occurs primarily in males; it has a X-linked inheritance pattern.

Glycogen storage disease type V, or McArdle disease, causes a myopathy that manifests as exercise intolerance.

5. B

This patient has glutaric aciduria type I, which is an organic acidemia. It can manifest acutely at the time of illness or surgery, or it can occur as a chronic condition. Imaging may show bilateral widening of the Sylvian fissures, abnormal signal in the basal ganglia, bitemporal arachnoid cysts, or subdural hemorrhages. This is one of the mimickers of child abuse. Other neurologic diseases that are mimickers of child abuse include Menkes kinky hair disease and tuberous sclerosis complex.

Glutaric aciduria type I also causes macrocephaly. Other metabolic diseases that cause macrocephaly include Canavan disease, Alexander disease, and Tay-Sachs disease.

Glutaric acidemia type II, as opposed to type I, is caused by a defect in the electron transfer flavoprotein or the electron transfer flavoprotein dehydrogenase in the mitochondrial respiratory chain. It causes a defect in fatty acid and amino acid oxidation. It can result in metabolic crisis. Some of these patients have a "sweaty feet" odor. (Isovaleric acidemia also causes this type of odor.)

Cerebral folate deficiency manifests at approximately 4 months of age. It causes deceleration of head growth, epilepsy, irritability, ataxia, and dyskinesia. CSF levels of 5-methyltetrahydrofolate (5MTHF) are low. It may be caused by mutations in *FOLR1*, which encodes folate receptor-α, or by autoantibodies against the folate receptor. It is treated with folinic acid (*not* folic acid, which can exacerbate the condition). Low CSF levels of 5MTHF can also be found in other neurologic conditions, such as atypical Aicardi-Goutières syndrome, Rett syndrome, and mitochondrial encephalomyopathies.

Miller-Dieker syndrome is characterized by microcephaly, lissencephaly, distinctive facial features, and cardiac anomalies.

Mowat-Wilson syndrome causes microcephaly, distinctive facial features, Hirschsprung disease, and cardiac anomalies.

6. B

This child has phenylketonuria (PKU), which is an aminoacidopathy caused by phenylalanine hydroxylase (PAH) deficiency. Children with PKU are microcephalic and have developmental delay, pale skin, pale hair, eczema, and a mousy/musty smell. In adulthood, patients can have hyperreflexia, tremor, paraplegia, or psychiatric conditions such as depression or anxiety.

There are other causes of hyperphenylalaninemia than PKU. Some of these are responsive to tetrahydrobiopterin, which is a cofactor for the hydroxylation reactions of phenylalanine, tyrosine, and tryptophan.

Biotinidase deficiency, sulfite oxidase deficiency, and PKU can all cause an eczematous rash.

Biotinidase deficiency causes alopecia; sulfite oxidase deficiency causes fine hair; and PKU causes fair hair and pale skin. Both biotinidase deficiency and sulfite oxidase deficiency can cause an epileptic encephalopathy.

Biotinidase deficiency is a type of multiple carboxylase deficiency. It causes seizures, hypotonia, developmental delay, and ataxia. Optic atrophy and hearing loss can occur. Alopecia, rash, and candidiasis are characteristic features. The rash is often perioral. Intermittent metabolic acidosis is seen, as well as lactic acidemia and propionic acidemia. Biotinidase deficiency is treated with biotin.

Sulfite oxidase deficiency may occur in isolation or as part of molybdenum cofactor deficiency. It causes microcephaly, failure to thrive, epilepsy, and lens dislocation. Lens dislocation is also seen in Marfan syndrome and homocystinuria (see Table 9.1).

7. C

This is maple syrup urine disease (MSUD). In the classic form of MSUD, the cerumen may have a sweet odor on the first day of life. If MSUD is left untreated, encephalopathy, abnormal movements (opisthotonus, bicycling), and seizures are seen, followed by coma and respiratory failure. MSUD is caused by a defect in branched-chain α-ketoacid dehydrogenase (BCKD). BCKD is required to break down leucine, isoleucine, and valine. Treatment is restriction of these three amino acids. One form of MSUD is responsive to thiamine.

8. D

This child had nonketotic hyperglycinemia (NKH), also known as glycine encephalopathy. It is caused by impaired glycine degradation. NKH and molybdenum cofactor deficiency both cause seizures and a burst suppression pattern on EEG, but the history of hiccups is typical of NKH.

Molybdenum cofactor is required for the function of sulfite oxidase, xanthine dehydrogenase, and aldehyde oxidase. Molybdenum cofactor deficiency causes an epileptic encephalopathy. Subtle dysmorphic features may be present. Sulfite, S-sulfocysteine, xanthine, and hypoxanthine are elevated in the urine. High levels of xanthine contribute to kidney stones. Serum uric acid is low. MRI shows brain edema followed by cystic lesions in the white matter.

The first step in serine synthesis requires 3-phospholycerate dehydrogenase. Deficiency of this enzyme causes intrauterine growth retardation, congenital microcephaly, and seizures in infancy reminiscent of a congenital infection.

9. D

This child has a congenital disorder of N-linked glycosylation, specifically PMM2-CDG (formerly known as congenital disorder of glycosylation type Ia, or CDG-Ia), which is the most common form of this disease.

PMM2-CDG causes failure to thrive, developmental delay, and axial hypotonia. There may be cerebellar hypoplasia. Patients may have inverted nipples and fat pads in unusual locations (e.g., suprapubic, above the buttocks). Multiple systems may be affected. Transaminases are often elevated, and patients can have a coagulopathy or endocrine dysfunction. A pericardial effusion may be present. Transferrin isoform analysis is diagnostic.

Table 9.1 FEATURES OF BIOTINIDASE DEFICIENCY, PHENYLKETONURIA, AND SULFITE OXIDASE DDEFICIENCY

	BIOTINIDASE DEFICIENCY	PHENYLKETONURIA	SULFITE OXIDASE DEFICIENCY
Skin	Eczema, perioral rash	Eczema, pale skin	Eczema
Hair	Alopecia	Light, blond hair	Fine hair
Neurologic features	Epileptic encephalopathy, hypotonia, developmental delay, ataxia, hearing loss	Microcephaly, developmental delay	Epileptic encephalopathy, microcephaly
Characteristic features	Candidiasis, episodic metabolic acidosis, lactic and propionic acidemia	Mousy/musty odor	Lens dislocation

10. D

This patient has an organic acidemia. Some examples of organic acidemias are glutaric acidemia type I, propionic acidemia, methylmalonic acidemia, multiple carboxylase deficiency, and isovaleric acidemia. Organic acidemias manifest with poor feeding, vomiting, lethargy, ketosis, acidosis, hyperammonemia, and neutropenia. The vomiting may be severe enough to be misdiagnosed as pyloric stenosis (i.e., in propionic acidemia, isovaleric acidemia, and methylmalonic acidemia). Hypoglycemia may be present. Patients with isovaleric acidemia may have a "sweaty feet" odor. Maple syrup urine disease may also be included in the organic acidemias, but it does not usually cause hyperammonemia or acidosis.

11. A

This child has Menkes disease, which is caused by mutations in the *ATP7A* gene, which encodes a transmembrane copper-transporting ATPase. Menkes disease is X-linked recessive. Newborns may have cephalohematomas, hypoglycemia, hypothermia, or inguinal hernias, but patients typically present with seizures, developmental delay or regression, and failure to thrive at a few months of age. Cheeks appear to sag; skin may be loose; hair is sparse, friable, and resembles steel wool. Pili torti (twisted hair shafts) is a distinctive feature of Menkes disease. Patients are hypotonic. Wormian bones are seen in the cranial sutures. Brain MRI shows abnormal myelination and tortuous vessels. The patient may have subdural hematomas. Menkes disease can be mistaken for child abuse because of associated rib fractures and subdural hematomas.

Both Menkes disease and Wilson disease are caused by defects in copper-transporting ATPase. Wilson disease is caused by a mutation in the *ATP7B* gene on chromosome 13. In Menkes disease, there is a copper deficiency. Copper transport from the intestine into the blood is impaired. It is treated with copper replacement. In Wilson disease, there is excess copper. Copper excretion from the liver into the bile is impaired. It is treated with chelation. In both Menkes disease and Wilson disease, serum copper and ceruloplasmin are low. Liver copper is low in Menkes disease but high in Wilson disease (see Table 9.2).

Table 9.2 COMPARISON OF MENKES DISEASE AND WILSON DISEASE

MENKES DISEASE	WILSON DISEASE
Copper deficiency	Copper excess
Defective absorption	Defective excretion
Treat with copper replacement	Treat with chelation

Mutations in the *OCRL* gene cause a defect in inositol polyphosphate 5-phosphatase OCRL-1. This results in oculocerebrorenal syndrome, also known as Lowe syndrome. As indicated by the name, patients have eye, brain, and kidney involvement. Patients have congenital cataracts and may have infantile glaucoma. At birth, patients are hypotonic with absent deep tendon reflexes. Development is delayed, and intellectual disability is common. Kidney involvement results in renal Fanconi syndrome. Lowe syndrome demonstrates X-linked inheritance.

Mutations in *PANK2* cause pantothenate kinase-associated neurodegeneration, which is a type of neurodegeneration with brain iron accumulation (NBIA).

Mutations in the *C19orf12* gene also cause a form of NBIA.

12. B

This is ornithine transcarbamylase (OTC) deficiency, which is the most common urea cycle disorder. It is X-linked. In males, it can manifest in the newborn period with hyperammonemic coma. The presentation in females is typically less severe and is variable. Females may avoid protein and be asymptomatic. Recurrent vomiting is another presentation. Females may develop altered mental status and hyperammonemia at the time of illness. Valproic acid is also a trigger.

Hartnup disease is caused by mutations in the *SLC6A19* gene, which encodes a neutral amino acid transporter expressed in the proximal renal tubules and in the intestine. Patients with Hartnup disease have pellagra-like skin changes and neurologic or psychiatric symptoms. Intermittent recurrent ataxia is one of the major neurologic manifestations.

Tangier disease is associated with reduced levels of high-density lipoprotein (HDL) in the blood. Cholesterol esters accumulate in tissues. Patients have premature atherosclerosis, orange tonsils, neuropathy, lymphadenopathy, and hepatosplenomegaly. They may also have corneal opacities.

Wolman disease, which is caused by lysosomal acid lipase deficiency, results in deposition of fat in multiple organs. Calcified adrenal glands are characteristic of the disorder.

13. B

Mucopolysaccharidoses (MPS) are a type of lysosomal storage disease. In MPS, glycosaminoglycans are stored in tissue and found in urine.

Patients with MPS are at risk for odontoid hypoplasia and cord compression, hydrocephalus, carpal tunnel syndrome, and obstructive sleep apnea. (Patients with trisomy 21 also have atlanto-axial instability and an increased risk for obstructive sleep apnea.) Seizures may occur with MPS type IIIA (Sanfilippo syndrome A).

There are many types of MPS. Skeletal defects are typical; dysostosis multiplex is characteristic. Many types are associated with cognitive impairment, cloudy corneas, hearing loss, coarse facial features, short stature, heart disease, and hepatosplenomegaly. Hunter syndrome, which is X-linked, is not associated with corneal clouding. Retinal degeneration may occur in some types. Enlarged perivascular spaces are often seen on brain MRI in patients with MPS.

Besides mucopolysaccharidoses, the lysosomal storage diseases include glycogen storage disease type II, lipidoses, mucolipidoses, oligosaccharidoses/glycoproteinoses, and sphingolipidoses (see Box 9.1).

Box 9.1 TYPES OF LYSOSOMAL STORAGE DISEASES

- Glycogen storage disease type II (Pompe disease)
- Lipidoses (neuronal ceroid lipofuscinoses, Niemann-Pick disease types C and D, Wolman disease)
- Mucolipidoses
- Mucopolysaccharidoses
- Oligosaccharidoses/glycoproteinoses
- Sphingolipidoses

---

14. B

CSF protein is increased in this condition. This patient has metachromatic leukodystrophy (MLD), which is a lysosomal storage disease. It is a disorder of sphingolipid metabolism.

The late infantile form is the most common form of MLD. It manifests between 1 and 2 years of age. Symptoms may appear to begin after an infection or anesthesia. Patients have motor regression. Reflexes are decreased, but there is an extensor plantar response. Initially, patients with MLD may be hypotonic, but they develop spastic quadriplegia and optic atrophy resulting in blindness. The patient may have seizures. Intestinal bleeding and gallbladder papillomatosis can occur with MLD. MRI shows bilateral, symmetric signal changes in the periventricular white mater with sparing of the U fibers. Patients have a demyelinating neuropathy resulting in slowed nerve conduction velocities and prolonged F-waves. Laboratory studies show an increase in urine sulfatide excretion. Nerve and brain biopsies show metachromatic lipid deposits. Arylsulfatase A is decreased.

If the patient has the MLD phenotype but arylsulfatase A activity is normal, then the patient may have saposin B deficiency. Saposin B acts as a cerebroside sulfatase activator.

There are milder adult forms of MLD that manifest with psychiatric or motor symptoms.

Multiple sulfatase deficiency manifests similar to MLD, but the patient also has features of mucopolysaccharidosis (MPS) as well as ichthyosis. Sulfatide and mucopolysaccharides are increased in the urine of patients with multiple sulfatase deficiency.

Like MLD, Krabbe disease can also cause elevated CSF protein and delayed nerve conduction velocities. Nerve specimens from patients with Krabbe disease and MLD contain deposits of sphingolipids.

15. D

This is X-linked adrenoleukodystrophy (ALD), which is the most common peroxisomal disorder. Very-long-chain fatty acids are elevated in ALD. The gene responsible for ALD is *ABCD1* (ATP-binding cassette, subfamily D, member 1).

This patient has the childhood cerebral form of X-linked ALD. It manifests in school-age children with symptoms resembling those of ADHD. Patients eventually develop dementia, visual and hearing impairments, quadriplegia, and adrenal insufficiency. MRI shows symmetric involvement of the posterior periventricular white matter. Garland-like contrast enhancement may be present at the periphery of the signal abnormality. Lorenzo's oil and bone marrow transplantation have been tried for treatment.

Adrenomyeloneuropathy (AMN) is another form of X-linked ALD. It manifests in the third decade of life with progressive spastic paraparesis and adrenal insufficiency.

X-linked ALD may also manifest as Addison disease without neurologic symptoms (initially).

Neonatal ALD is a different entity. Neonatal ALD is one of the peroxisome biogenesis disorders, Zellweger syndrome spectrum. These disorders are autosomal recessive and are caused by mutations in *PEX* genes.

16. B

Very-long-chain fatty acids, phytanic acid, pristanic acid, and pipecolic acid aid in diagnosis of the Zellweger syndrome spectrum of peroxisome biogenesis disorders, which includes Zellweger disease, neonatal adrenoleukodystrophy (ALD), and infantile Refsum disease. These diseases are caused by mutations in *PEX* genes. *PEX* genes encode peroxins, which are required for normal peroxisome assembly.

Zellweger syndrome is the most severe form; neonatal ALD is the intermediate form; and infantile Refsum disease is the least severe form.

Zellweger syndrome manifests in the newborn period with hypotonia, seizures, and poor feeding. Patients with Zellweger syndrome may have polymicrogyria, heterotopia, subependymal cysts, or a hypoplastic corpus callosum. Patients have a large fontanelle, a high forehead, flattened facies, a flat occiput, epicanthal folds, and a broad nasal bridge. There may be redundant skin folds on the neck. Some cases have been misdiagnosed as Down syndrome. Multiple systems are involved. Patients with Zellweger syndrome have hepatic dysfunction, renal cysts, and chondrodysplasia punctata (bony stippling) of the patellae.

Like patients with Zellweger syndrome, patients with neonatal ALD have hypotonia and may have seizures, but they are less likely to have cortical malformations and craniofacial abnormalities. In addition, stippled epiphyses are more characteristic of Zellweger syndrome.

Infantile Refsum disease is even less severe and may not manifest until later in life.

Patients with diseases in the Zellweger syndrome spectrum are at risk for coagulopathy and can develop intracranial hemorrhage.

Zellweger syndrome spectrum is one of two groups of peroxisome biogenesis disorders. Rhizomelic chondrodysplasia punctata type 1 is in the other group.

Palmitoyl-protein thioesterase 1 (PPT-1) is deficient in CLN1, one of the types of neuronal ceroid lipofuscinoses (NCL). CLN2 (classic late infantile NCL) is caused by mutations in *TPP1*, which encodes tripeptidyl-peptidase 1. Mutations in *CSTD*, which encodes cathepsin D, cause CLN10.

17. A

This is Alexander disease, which is a leukodystrophy. The infantile form is the most common form. Patients have developmental regression, macrocephaly, and spasticity. Some patients have seizures. Brain MRI shows increased T2 signal in the cerebral white matter with frontal predominance. Signal abnormality may also be seen in the basal ganglia and in the brainstem. Some patients have aqueductal stenosis and develop hydrocephalus. Alexander disease is caused by defects in the *GFAP* gene, which encodes the glial fibrillary acidic protein and is autosomal dominant. Mutations in the *GFAP* gene result in an abnormal glial fibrillary acidic protein that forms Rosenthal fibers within astrocytes. (Rosenthal fibers are also seen in pilocytic astrocytoma.)

Alexander disease can cause brainstem lesions that resemble a tumor. It can also mimic multiple sclerosis.

PCDH19 mutations cause an early infantile epileptic encephalopathy in females. (It is found on the X chromosome.)

STXBP1 mutations cause another early infantile epileptic encephalopathy.

PRICKLE1 mutations cause a progressive myoclonic epilepsy (EPM1B) with ataxia; however, intellect is spared.

18. D

Mutations in the proteolipid protein 1 (*PLP1*) gene cause Pelizaeus-Merzbacher disease. Proteolipid protein (PLP) is a component of myelin in the central nervous system.

Pelizaeus-Merzbacher disease is an X-linked recessive hypomyelinating disorder. Classic Pelizaeus-Merzbacher disease manifests with nystagmus in the first few months of life, stridor, and hypotonia. Patients then develop titubation, ataxia, and spasticity. Athetosis may be present.

MRI shows persistent hypomyelination without significant cortical atrophy. Alternating areas of myelination (around penetrating vessels) and demyelination may produce a "tigroid" appearance. (This can be seen in other conditions as well.) Pelizaeus-Merzbacher disease has a distinct pattern on magnetic resonance spectroscopy.

There is a severe connatal form of PMD that manifests at birth or within the first few weeks of life.

Mutations in gene *PLP1* also cause spastic paraplegia 2 (SPG2).

β-Galactosidase deficiency causes GM1 gangliosidosis. The most severe form is the infantile form, which manifests by 1 year of age with developmental regression and hypotonia. The patient may have an exaggerated startle. Patients develop a macular cherry-red spot, facial coarsening, hypertrophic gums, macroglossia, hepatosplenomegaly, scoliosis, and dysostosis. Some patients have mild corneal clouding. Some have cardiomyopathy. Ultimately, patients lose vision and develop seizures, decerebrate rigidity, and beaked vertebral bodies. Although this patient has features of mucopolysaccharidosis (MPS), there is no mucopolysacchariduria.

19. B

This is childhood ataxia with central nervous system hypomyelination/vanishing white matter (CACH/VM), also known as leukoencephalopathy with vanishing white matter. There are variable forms, and it can manifest at multiple ages. It may manifest with ataxia or spasticity. Some patients have optic atrophy. A distinct feature is significant deterioration occurring after minor head trauma or infection. Patients may have seizures, hypotonia, and vomiting and may become comatose in these settings. Brain MRI shows progressive white matter destruction with replacement by CSF. CSF asialotransferrin is decreased. CACH/VM is caused by mutations in the genes encoding subunits of the eIF2B.

20. A

The condition is Aicardi-Goutieres syndrome.

Some patients with Aicardi-Goutieres syndrome are normal initially. They present with encephalopathy, irritability, and sterile pyrexia. Loss of milestones occurs. Patients develop spasticity and microcephaly. They may have seizures or dystonia. Some patients develop chilblain lesions on the digits. MRI shows calcifications in the basal ganglia, cerebral atrophy, and increased T2 signal in the white matter. CSF shows increased interferon-alpha or lymphocytosis.

Some patients with Aicardi-Goutieres syndrome have a presentation similar to that of a patient with a congenital infection. They have fever, hepatosplenomegaly, elevated liver function enzymes, and thrombocytopenia at birth.

Aicardi-Goutieres syndrome results from mutations in genes encoding nucleases. For example, mutations in the *TREX1* gene are one cause of Aicardi-Goutieres syndrome. Mutations in this gene also cause retinal vasculopathy with cerebral leukodystrophy, chilblain lupus, and susceptibility to systemic lupus erythematosus (SLE).

Kearns-Sayre syndrome is a mitochondrial disease characterized by ptosis, progressive external ophthalmoplegia, and pigmentary retinopathy. Patients may have dementia, ataxia, cardiac conduction defects, sensorineural hearing loss, or endocrine abnormalities (e.g., diabetes). Blood and CSF lactate levels may be elevated. CSF protein is often elevated. MRI shows increased signal in the subcortical white mater and may show cerebral, brainstem, or cerebellar atrophy. Patients may have calcifications in the basal ganglia. Magnetic resonance spectroscopy shows elevated lactate.

In patients with megalencephalic leukoencephalopathy with subcortical cysts, the white matter is abnormal diffusely and cysts are consistently found in the anterior temporal region but may be found elsewhere as well.

Hereditary diffuse leukoencephalopathy with spheroids is a genetic leukoencephalopathy that can mimic multiple sclerosis.

21. B

Cerebrotendinous xanthomatosis is a disorder of lipid storage. Specifically, bile acid synthesis is defective because of a mutation in the gene that encodes sterol 27-hydroxylase. It may manifest with neonatal cholestasis, chronic diarrhea, or cataracts. During adolescence and young adulthood, tendon xanthomas appear. They are often found on the Achilles tendon. Patients have premature atherosclerosis and neurologic deterioration. They develop spasticity and ataxia. Some may have neuropsychiatric symptoms (including dementia), peripheral neuropathy, or seizures. MRI shows cerebellar white matter hyperintensity. The dentate may demonstrate T2 hyperintensity or hypointensity. Treatment is chenodeoxycholic acid.

Adult-onset polyglucosan body disease causes upper and lower motor neuron symptoms and can be clinically mistaken for amyotrophic lateral sclerosis (ALS). Brain MRI shows white matter abnormalities that can be mistaken for multiple sclerosis (MS). HMG-CoA lyase deficiency and L2-hydroxyglutaric aciduria are other genetic leukoencephalopathies that can cause multifocal white matter lesions mimicking MS.

22. B

This patient has Krabbe disease, which is also known as globoid cell leukodystrophy. It is a lysosomal storage disease, specifically a sphingolipidosis. It results from a deficiency of galactocerebrosidase (also known as galactosylceramidase or galactosylceramide β-galactosidase), which is caused by mutations in *GALC*. Most patients with Krabbe syndrome present by 6 months of age with irritability, sensitivity to external stimuli, and fever without infection. Patients have spasticity and vision loss. Krabbe disease affects the white mater of the central and peripheral nervous systems, causing leukodystrophy and a peripheral neuropathy. Multinucleated globoid cells are found in the white matter of the brain. Like metachromatic leukodystrophy (MLD), Krabbe disease can cause elevated CSF protein and delayed nerve conduction velocities.

Ceramidase deficiency causes Farber disease, which is also known as Farber lipogranulomatosis. This is a sphingolipidosis and one cause of a macular cherry-red spot.

Sphingomyelinase deficiency causes Niemann-Pick disease types A and B, which are also sphingolipidoses.

The sphingolipidoses also include Fabry disease, Gaucher disease, GM1 gangliosidoses, multiple sulfatase deficiency, Sandhoff disease, and Tay-Sachs disease (see Box 9.2).

Neuraminidase deficiency causes sialidosis type I, which is discussed later.

Box 9.2 SPHINGOLIPIDOSES

- Fabry disease
- Farber disease
- Gaucher disease
- GM1 gangliosidosis
- GM2 gangliosidoses (Sandhoff disease and Tay-Sachs disease)
- Krabbe disease
- Metachromatic leukodystrophy
- Multiple sulfatase deficiency
- Niemann-Pick disease types A and B

---

23. B

This patient has Gaucher disease type 2, which is one of the sphingolipidoses. It is caused by a mutation in *GBA*, which results in glucocerebrosidase (glucosylceramidase) deficiency. Patients have bulbar signs such as stridor and dysphagia; pyramidal signs such as opisthotonus and spasticity; and oculomotor abnormalities such as strabismus. Squinting and oculomotor apraxia may also be seen. Trismus can occur. Patients may have seizures. Hepatosplenomegaly is present. Gaucher cells may be seen in the bone marrow.

AADC deficiency, which is an inborn error in neurotransmitter metabolism, can also cause opisthotonus and hyperreflexia. It leads to oculogyric crises and can cause autonomic dysfunction. Hepatosplenomegaly would not be expected.

GAMT deficiency, SLC6A8 deficiency, and L-arginine:glycine amidinotransferase (AGAT or GATM) deficiency are cerebral creatine deficiency syndromes. They are characterized by seizures and intellectual disability. Patients with GAMT deficiency may also have autistic behaviors and dystonia. Some demonstrate self-mutilation.

24. B

Canavan disease is a leukodystrophy caused by aspartoacylase deficiency. Infants with Canavan disease present with developmental delay. They have macrocephaly, head lag, and hypotonia. Later, spasticity develops. Urine NAA is elevated. MRI shows bilateral diffuse white matter involvement including the U fibers (increased signal on T2, decreased signal on T1). Magnetic resonance spectroscopy shows an elevated NAA peak.

25. B

This patient has Tay-Sachs disease, which is a lysosomal storage disease. More specifically, it is a type of GM2 gangliosidosis. It is caused by deficiency in hexosaminidase A. Patients present with increased startle. Initially, they are weak and hypotonic. Later, they become hypertonic, macrocephalic, and blind. Patients also have seizures and a macular cherry-red spot.

Sandhoff disease, which is also a type of GM2 gangliosidosis, is caused by deficiency of hexosaminidase A and B. It has neurologic features similar to those of Tay-Sachs disease, including a cherry-red spot. However, hepatosplenomegaly occurs in Sandhoff disease; whereas patients with Tay-Sachs have normal-sized organs. Patients with Sandhoff disease may also have bony abnormalities.

26. A

This is Fabry disease, which is a X-linked lysosomal disease caused by deficiency of α-galactosidase A. This results in accumulation of glycosphingolipids, specifically globotriaosylceramide in cells. (Fabry disease is the only X-linked sphingolipidosis.) Patients with Fabry disease are at risk for early stroke, usually in the vertebrobasilar circulation. Fabry disease is also associated with dolichoectasia of cerebral vessels, white matter abnormalities, cardiac conduction defects, and cardiomyopathy. In addition, it causes a small-fiber peripheral neuropathy and autonomic dysfunction. Patients have hypohidrosis, painful acroparesthesias, and intestinal dysmotility. Other systemic manifestations include renal failure and corneal opacities. Angiokeratoma are one of the earliest findings. Enzyme replacement therapy is available.

27. A

This patient has Niemann-Pick type C disease, which is a lysosomal lipid storage disease caused by impaired cholesterol esterification. Clinical features include cataplexy, dysarthria, dementia, vertical gaze-palsy, ataxia, seizures, and hepatosplenomegaly. Movement disorders including dystonia, chorea, athetosis, and parkinsonism also occur in Niemann-Pick type C disease. Foam cells, which stain with filipin, and sea-blue histiocytes may be found in bone marrow.

28. B

This patient has classic late infantile neuronal ceroid lipofuscinosis (CLN2), which causes progressive myoclonic epilepsy. Curvilinear profiles are found within lysosomes.

Neuronal ceroid lipofuscinoses (NCL) are a type of lysosomal storage disease. There are multiple types, which manifest at different ages. Patients with NCL have seizures and regress in motor skills and cognition. Often they have vision impairment as well.

CLN1 (infantile NCL) is caused by mutations in *PPT1*, which encodes palmitoyl-protein thioesterase 1. Granular osmiophilic deposits (GROD) are found within lysosomes. These are seen in some other forms of NCL as well.

CLN2 is caused by mutations in *TPP1*, which encodes tripeptidyl-peptidase 1.

CLN3 (classic juvenile NCL) manifests in school-age children. Fingerprint profiles are found within lysosomes.

Ragged red fibers are found on muscle biopsy in mitochondrial diseases.

Electron-dense granules within the smooth muscle layer of small arterial vessels are found in cerebral autosomal dominant arteriopathy with subcortical infarcts and leukoencephalopathy (CADASIL).

Spheroids are found on nerve biopsy in patients with infantile neuroaxonal dystrophy.

29. C

Sialidosis type I, Lafora body disease, neuronal ceroid lipofuscinoses (NCL), and Unverricht-Lundborg disease all cause progressive myoclonic epilepsy (PME). In addition to PME, patients with sialidosis type I have a cherry-red spot and progressive vision loss. Sialidosis type I is caused by deficiency of neuraminidase. It is a type of lysosomal storage disease. Specifically, it is one of the oligosaccharidoses/glycoproteinoses.

A number of other diseases can cause a cherry-red spot, including Niemann-Pick type A disease, Sandhoff disease, and Tay-Sachs disease.

Marinesco-Sjögren syndrome is characterized by cataracts, cerebellar ataxia, and myopathy.

30. B

This patient has myoclonic epilepsy associated with ragged red fibers (MERFF), which is a progressive myoclonic epilepsy. Most commonly, it is caused by mutations in the mitochondrial DNA gene *MT-TK*, which encodes tRNA^{Lys}. Wolff-Parkinson-White (WPW) syndrome and cardiomyopathy can occur in MERRF. Patients may also have dementia, myopathy, polyneuropathy, ataxia, hearing loss, optic atrophy, short stature, and lipomas. Lactate is elevated.

Aggregates of polyglucosan (long, insoluble strands of glycogen) in the apocrine and eccrine glands are found on skin biopsy of patients with Lafora disease with the use of periodic acid-Schiff staining. Lafora disease is another progressive myoclonic epilepsy. It is caused by mutations in either the *EPM2A* gene, which encodes laforin, or the *NHLRC1* gene (previously known as *EPM2B*), which encodes malin. Lafora disease manifests in adolescence. Visual seizures are often the first sign. In addition to focal seizures arising from the occipital region, patients have GTC and myoclonic seizures. Dementia occurs early.

31. D

Classic glucose transporter type 1 deficiency syndrome (Glut1-DS) manifests as refractory epilepsy in infants. CSF glucose is low compared with serum glucose. If Glut1-DS is left untreated, it causes microcephaly, developmental delays, and movement disorders. The gene responsible for Glut1-DS is *SLC2A1*, which stands for solute carrier family 2 (facilitated glucose transporter), member 1. *SLC2A1* encodes a glucose transporter in the blood-brain barrier.

The gene *CACNA1A* encodes the calcium channel, voltage-dependent, P/Q type, alpha 1A subunit. Mutations in *CACNA1A* cause episodic ataxia type 2, familial hemiplegic migraine type 1, and spinocerebellar ataxia type 6.

Mutations in *GABRAG2*, which encodes the γ-aminobutyric acid (GABA) receptor type A gamma 2 subunit, are one cause of childhood absence epilepsy.

Mutations in the *PLA2G6* gene, which encodes A2 phospholipase, cause infantile neuroaxonal dystrophy. Mutations in this gene also cause neurodegeneration with brain iron accumulation type 2B and Parkinson disease type 14.

32. D

The ketogenic diet is used to treat Glut1-DS.

Sulfonylurea has been used in the treatment of developmental delay, epilepsy, and neonatal diabetes, which is caused by a potassium channel mutation.

33. C

This patient has Leigh syndrome, which is also known as subacute necrotizing encephalomyelopathy. There are several causes of Leigh syndrome. The most common cause is mutations in the gene *SURF1*, a mutation in nuclear DNA that result in disruption of the cytochrome *c* oxidase complex. Leigh syndrome can also be caused by mutations in mitochondrial DNA, most commonly *MT-ATP6*, which encodes the ATP synthase protein complex (complex V). Defects in pyruvate dehydrogenase complex and other enzymes involved in energy production also cause Leigh syndrome.

Leigh syndrome is a neurodegenerative condition that usually manifests before 1 year of age, often at the time of a viral infection. Patients have seizures, hypotonia, developmental delay, failure to thrive, and vomiting. Patients have psychomotor regression and develop movement disorders, ophthalmoplegia, peripheral neuropathy, respiratory disturbances, and swallowing dysfunction. Some patients have epilepsy. MRI shows symmetric necrosis in the thalamus, basal ganglia, and brainstem. Lactate is elevated.

Idiopathic basal ganglia calcification-1 (IBGC1), formerly known as Fahr disease, typically manifests in adulthood but can occur in the second decade of life. It causes parkinsonism and choreoathetosis. Some patients have hypoparathyroidism. It is caused by a mutation in the *SLC20A2* gene.

Kernicterus, or bilirubin encephalopathy, causes choreoathetoid cerebral palsy, vertical gaze disturbance, and hearing loss.

Neurodegeneration with brain iron accumulation (NBIA) includes multiple disorders characterized by the accumulation of iron in the basal ganglia. This results in symptoms such as parkinsonism, dystonia, and choreoathetosis. Most types of NBIA are autosomal recessive.

However, β-propeller protein-associated neurodegeneration (BPAN), which is caused by mutations in *WDR45*, is X-linked dominant. Also, neuroferritinopathy, caused by mutations in *FTL*, is autosomal dominant.

Pantothenate kinase-associated neurodegeneration, or PKAN, is the most common form of NBIA. It is caused by mutations in the gene *PANK2*. It produces an "eye of the tiger" sign on MRI. There is decreased T2 signal in the globus pallidus and substantia nigra with an area of hyperintensity in the center.

34. B

Valproic acid is contraindicated in patients with hepatic disease, urea cycle defects, and mitochondrial disease. Valproic acid can cause liver failure and death in patients with mutations in the mitochondrial DNA polymerase-γ (POLG) gene. POLG conditions include Alpers-Huttenlocher syndrome, childhood myocerebrohepatopathy spectrum disorders, myoclonic epilepsy myopathy sensory ataxia, POLG-related ataxia neuropathy spectrum disorders, and progressive external ophthalmoplegia.

Valproic acid is safe to use in patients with Dravet syndrome who have a *SCN1A* mutation and in patients with type II hyperprolinemia. It is also safe to use in patients with autosomal dominant nocturnal frontal lobe epilepsy caused by a mutation in *CHRNA2*; however, these patients are often treated with oxcarbazepine or carbamazepine.

35. C

This is Lesch-Nyhan disease, which is a disorder of purine metabolism. It is an X-linked recessive condition caused by a mutation in the *HPRT1* gene. Initially, patients with Lesch-Nyhan disease have hypotonia and developmental delay. Later they develop spasticity, extrapyramidal movements (such as choreoathetosis or dystonia), and self-mutilating behaviors. Patients often have cognitive impairment. Uric acid is elevated in blood and urine, and hypoxanthine-guanine-phosphoribosyltransferase (HGPRT) levels are low. Excess uric acid can cause arthritis and kidney and bladder stones. Orange crystals may be seen in the diaper of babies with Lesch-Nyhan disease.

Cystathionine β-synthase deficiency is a cause of homocystinuria.

Deficiency of GTP cyclohydrolase 1 causes dopa-responsive dystonia.

Mutations in *ATP1A3* cause rapid-onset dystonia-parkinsonism (DYT12).

36. B

The clinical and laboratory findings in this patient are suggestive of Smith-Lemli-Opitz syndrome, which is a condition associated with multiple congenital anomalies such as cleft palate, cardiac defects, ambiguous genitalia, postaxial polydactyly, and syndactyly of the second and third toes. Patients have growth retardation, microcephaly, and intellectual disability. Patients can have a range of central nervous system abnormalities such as malformations of the cerebellum, corpus callosum malformation, Dandy-Walker malformation, or holoprosencephaly. Smith-Lemli-Opitz syndrome is caused by abnormal cholesterol metabolism resulting from a deficiency of 7-dehydrocholesterol (7-DHC) reductase. This leads to elevated levels of 7-DHC in the serum. Cholesterol is often low, but it can be in the normal range.

This syndrome does share some features with risomy 13 and trisomy 18. Like patients with trisomy 13, patients with Smith-Lemli-Opitz syndrome can have holoprosencephaly, cleft palate, cardiac defects, and polydactyly; however, they also have ambiguous genitalia and may have a low serum cholesterol level. Patients with Smith-Lemli-Opitz syndrome may also have photosensitivity.

Other metabolic conditions that cause photosensitivity include phenylketonuria, Hartnup disease, and porphyria. Patients with Cockayne syndrome, ataxia-telangiectasia, xeroderma pigmentosum, and Bloom syndrome also have photosensitivity. Pellagra is a nutritional disorder that causes photosensitivity.

37. D

Patients with phosphofructokinase deficiency or myophosphorylase deficiency do not have a rise in lactate during forearm testing. Patients with phosphoglycerate mutase deficiency have reduced lactate elevation.

(Ischemia is no longer included in forearm exercise testing.)

38. D

Enzyme replacement therapy is available for Fabry disease (α-galactosidase A deficiency), Gaucher disease (glucocerebrosidase deficiency), Pompe disease (acid maltase deficiency), and certain mucopolysaccharidoses.

39. C

AVED has also been called Friedreich-like Ataxia. Given that AVED is treatable, it is important to differentiate it from Friedreich ataxia (FA). Cardiac conduction defects, cavus foot deformity, muscle weakness, and diabetes mellitus are more likely in FA than in AVED. Patients with AVED are more likely to have titubation.

10.

MOVEMENT DISORDERS

QUESTIONS

1. The subthalamic nucleus activates which inhibitory structure?
   A. Globus pallidus internal segment
   B. Nucleus accumbens
   C. Striatum
   D. Thalamus

2. Fill in the blank: In the basal ganglia direct pathway, the striatum sends GABAergic projections to the _____.
   A. Globus pallidus externa
   B. Globus pallidus internal segment and substantia nigra pars reticularis
   C. Subthalamic nucleus
   D. Thalamus

3. Fill in the blank: The basal ganglia indirect pathway involves _____ and then the _____.
   A. The globus pallidus externa and then the subthalamic nucleus
   B. The globus pallidus interna and then the subthalamic nucleus
   C. The substantia nigra pars compacta and then the substantia nigra pars reticularis
   D. The raphe nucleus and then the substantia nigra pars compacta

4. Which of the following disorders is most likely to be suppressible?
   A. Chorea
   B. Stereotypies
   C. Tics
   D. Tremor

5. Which of the following disorders is most likely to occur during action rather than during rest?
   A. Athetosis
   B. Chorea
   C. Tics
   D. Stereotypies

6. Which is the most accurate term for the occurrence of an unintentional movement along with a voluntary movement?
   A. Athetosis
   B. Overflow
   C. Myoclonus
   D. Ballism

7. Which of the following descriptions is more characteristic of rigidity than spasticity?
   A. There is velocity-independent resistance to passive movement.
   B. It has a "clasp-knife" quality.
   C. It affects upper extremity flexors more than extensors.
   D. Resistance is delayed if the direction of passive movement is reversed rapidly.

8. Which of the following descriptions is *not* characteristic of tics?
   A. They can be suppressed but tend to increase after a period of suppression.
   B. They can occur during sleep.
   C. They worsen in the cold.
   D. They are suggestible.

9. A 10-year-old boy with a history of attention deficit hyperactivity disorder (ADHD) is brought to the clinic for unusual movements and noises. Two years ago, he began making sniffing noises and clearing his throat. Allergy medications did not work. He then started blinking his eyes. His eye examination was normal. During the visit, he intermittently shrugs his shoulders for no apparent reason. He says he can stop it briefly, but then it is worse when it restarts. Which other condition is the patient most likely to have?
   A. Delusions
   B. Hallucinations
   C. Obsessive-compulsive disorder
   D. Panic attacks

10. Which of the following is *not* required for the diagnosis of Tourette syndrome?
    A. Onset before age 18 years
    B. Coprolalia
    C. Duration of at least 1 year
    D. At least one vocal tic

11. An 11-year-old boy with Tourette syndrome is having significant difficulties in school due to ADHD. His tics are embarrassing him. He also has problems with impulse control. Which of the following medications is most likely to treat all of his symptoms?
    A. Atomoxetine
    B. Clonidine
    C. Fluphenazine
    D. Risperidone

12. A 59-year-old man presents with right-hand tremor. On examination, the patient has bradykinesia,

cogwheel rigidity, a resting tremor, and reduced arm swing when walking. When he reaches a doorway or needs to turn, he freezes. Which of the following findings is expected?

A. Decreased pigmented neurons in the substantia nigra
B. Loss of neurons in the substantia nigra pars compacta that are immunoreactive with tyrosine hydroxylase
C. Intraneuronal inclusions that immunostain with antibodies to alpha-synuclein
D. All of the above

13. Which of the following features suggests that a patient may have a diagnosis other than Parkinson disease (PD)?

A. Asymmetric tremor
B. Early gait instability
C. Tremor improves with action
D. Tremor worsens with mental tasks

14. What is the function of carbidopa?

A. It inhibits aromatic amino acid decarboxylase.
B. It results in increased dopamine synthesis.
C. It causes dopamine release.
D. It prevents dopamine metabolism.

15. Which of the following effects is more likely with levodopa than with dopamine agonists?

A. Dyskinesias
B. Peripheral edema
C. Hallucinations
D. Hypotension

16. The wife of a man with PD complains that her husband has developed a gambling addiction. Which of the following medications is likely responsible?

A. Selegiline
B. Entacapone
C. Ropinirole
D. Amantadine

17. Which medication is useful for reducing dyskinesias but can cause confusion, hallucinations, myoclonus, peripheral edema, and livedo reticularis?

A. Amantadine
B. Benztropine
C. Rotigotine
D. Selegiline

18. Trihexyphenidyl has been used for treatment of PD. What is its mechanism of action?

A. It is an adenosine receptor antagonist.
B. It is a catechol-*O*-methyltransferase (COMT) inhibitor.
C. It is a monoamine oxidase B inhibitor.
D. It is a muscarinic antagonist.

19. What is the mechanism of action of rasagiline?

A. It is an adenosine receptor antagonist.
B. It is a catechol-*O*-methyltransferase (COMT) inhibitor.
C. It is a dopamine agonist.
D. It is a monoamine oxidase B inhibitor.

20. A patient with PD presents with diarrhea and discolored urine. Which medication is most likely responsible?

A. Amantadine
B. Apomorphine
C. Entacapone
D. Ropinirole

21. Which of the following medications has been approved for treatment of dementia in PD?

A. Memantine
B. Pramipexole
C. Risperidone
D. Rivastigmine

22. Deep brain stimulation (DBS) of which of the following structures is used to treat PD that is refractory to medication?

A. Bilateral caudate
B. Bilateral globus pallidus externa
C. Bilateral putamen
D. Bilateral subthalamic nucleus

23. Which of the following proteins is abnormal in Parkinson disease 1 (PARK1) and Parkinson disease 4 (PARK4)?

A. Alpha-synuclein
B. Leucine-rich repeat serine/threonine-protein kinase 2
C. Parkin
D. Serine/threonine-protein kinase

24. Which of the following is *least* likely to be associated with PD?

A. Anosmia
B. Depression
C. Oculogyric crisis
D. Rapid eye movement (REM) sleep behavior disorder

25. Which of the following is a meperidine derivative that can cause symptoms similar to those of PD?

A. 1-methyl-4-phenyl-1,2,3,6-tetrahydropyridine (MPTP)
B. Normeperidine
C. Dynorphin
D. Diphenoxylate

26. A welder presents with personality change and tremor. On examination, he has dystonia and an abnormal gait. He walks on his toes with his spine erect and his elbows flexed. Magnetic resonance imaging (MRI) shows increased signal in the pallidum on T1-weighted images. What is the most likely etiology?

A. Parkinson disease
B. Manganese toxicity
C. Mercury exposure
D. Neurodegeneration with brain iron accumulation

27. A 59-year-old man presents with falls. He also has had erectile dysfunction. On examination, he has orthostatic hypotension. He also has antecollis and a shuffling gait. He reports that he was given levodopa by

another neurologist but it didn't work. Which MRI finding is the most likely?

- A. "Mickey Mouse" appearance of the midbrain
- B. Midbrain atrophy
- C. Midcallosal atrophy
- D. Hypointense putamen on T2-weighted scans

28. Which of the following is the most specific pathologic marker of multiple system atrophy?
- A. Glial cytoplasmic inclusions (GCIs)
- B. Globose neurofibrillary tangles
- C. Loss of cells in the basal nucleus of Meynert
- D. Neocortical ballooned neurons

29. A 60-year-old man presents with difficulties swallowing and falls. On examination, he has a wide-eyed stare, decreased down-gaze, rigidity, and retropulsion. Which of the following genes has been associated with this condition?
- A. *ATM*
- B. *HTT*
- C. *PARK7*
- D. *MAPT*

30. Which of the following conditions is *least* likely to cause significant autonomic dysfunction?
- A. Dementia with Lewy bodies
- B. Parkinson disease
- C. Progressive supranuclear palsy
- D. Spinocerebellar ataxia type 2

31. A 60-year-old man is brought to the clinic by his wife because of cognitive problems and because he is not using his left arm. She says he does not seem to know that it is his. He has mild rigidity, decreased sensation, and brisk reflexes in the arm. He also has an upgoing toe on the left. Which of the following is the abnormal protein?
- A. Tau
- B. Alpha-synuclein
- C. Amyloid
- D. TDP-43

32. Which infectious cause of parkinsonism is associated with supranuclear ophthalmoplegia and oculomasticatory myorhythmia?
- A. Human immunodeficiency virus
- B. Saint Louis encephalitis
- C. West Nile virus
- D. Whipple disease

33. A 70-year-old man presents with cognitive decline. The family reports urinary incontinence. On examination, his gait is slow. His feet have the appearance of being fixed to the ground. He does not have tremor. MRI of the brain shows enlarged ventricles. Which of the following is most likely to yield the diagnosis?
- A. Check for mutations in the gene *HTT*
- B. Large-volume lumbar puncture
- C. A trial of carbidopa-levodopa
- D. A trial of pramipexole

34. A 38-year-old man is brought to the office by his wife. She complains that he has been depressed, clumsy, and fidgety. On examination, his saccades are slowed, and he has brisk reflexes including ankle clonus. MRI shows caudate atrophy.

a. Which of the following disease does *not* have the same triplet-repeat gene sequence found in this patient?
- A. Dentatorubral-pallidoluysian atrophy (DRPLA)
- B. Kennedy disease (bulbospinal muscular atrophy)
- C. Spinocerebellar ataxia type 3 (SCA3)
- D. Spinocerebellar ataxia type 10 (SCA10)

b. Which cells are particularly vulnerable to this disease?
- A. Astrocytes
- B. Interneurons of the striatum
- C. Medium spiny neurons
- D. Pyramidal cells

35. Tetrabenazine has been used to treat chorea in Huntington disease. What is its mechanism of action?
- A. It blocks dopamine receptors.
- B. It inhibits acetylcholinesterase.
- C. It inhibits monoamine oxidase.
- D. It inhibits a vesicle monoamine transporter.

36. A 14-year-old girl presents with facial tics, clumsiness, difficulty sitting still, and recent obsessive-compulsive behaviors. She has a darting tongue and spooning of her fingers. She is taking no medications. She was prescribed penicillin for a streptococcal throat infection 2 months ago but took only a few pills. What type of condition is causing her movements?
- A. Autoimmune
- B. Genetic
- C. Metabolic
- D. Trauma

37. Which of the following medications is *least* likely to cause chorea?
- A. Lithium
- B. Oral contraceptives
- C. Reserpine
- D. Methylphenidate

38. A 20-year-old man presents with bilateral hand tremor. He notices it more with movement than at rest. His mother has head and hand tremor. She reports that her tremor improves after a glass of wine. Which treatment should be prescribed?
- A. Botulinum toxin A injection
- B. Clonazepam
- C. Propranolol
- D. Levetiracetam

39. Which movement disorder is associated with a wing-beating tremor, risus sardonicus, sunflower cataracts, and increased signal on T2-weighted MRI in the basal ganglia?
- A. Dentatorubral-pallidoluysian atrophy
- B. Fahr syndrome

C. Rapid-onset dystonia-parkinsonism

D. Wilson disease

40. **Which of the following proteins is abnormal in the most common form of genetic dystonia?**
    A. Epsilon-sarcoglycan
    B. Myofibrillogenesis regulator 1
    C. TATA-binding protein-associated factor-1 (TAF1)
    D. TorsinA

41. **A 7-year-old girl presents with a diagnosis of cerebral palsy. Her main complaint is difficulty walking. She has abnormal leg posturing when she walks in the evening. A medication trial leads to significant improvement. Which medication was used?**
    A. Baclofen
    B. Edrophonium
    C. Carbamazepine
    D. Levodopa-carbidopa

42. **What is the mechanism of action of onabotulinumtoxinA (Botox)?**
    A. It inactivates synaptosomal-associated protein 25 (SNAP-25).
    B. It inactivates vesicle-associated membrane protein (VAMP).
    C. It inactivates syntaxin-1.
    D. It is a glycine agonist.

43. **Patients with severe primary dystonia that does not respond to treatment with medications may respond to deep brain stimulation (DBS) of which of the following areas?**
    A. Globus pallidus interna
    B. Subthalamic nucleus
    C. Thalamus
    D. Globus pallidus externa

44. **Which of the following conditions is responsive to alcohol?**
    A. Early-onset generalized torsion dystonia (DYT1)
    B. Myoclonus-dystonia (DYT11)
    C. Orthostatic myoclonus
    D. Rapid-onset dystonia-parkinsonism (RDP)

45. **Which of the following medications is *least* likely to cause myoclonus?**
    A. Bismuth (Pepto-Bismol)
    B. Gabapentin
    C. Meperidine
    D. Sodium oxybate

46. **A mother brings her 15-month-old son to the clinic because of unusual eye movements. She says that his eyes are "jumping all over the place." On examination, sudden arm jerks are also noted. What is the most appropriate next step?**
    A. Reassure the mother that these are temporary symptoms caused by a virus.
    B. Perform computed tomography (CT) of the chest, abdomen, and pelvis.

C. Refer the patient to ophthalmology.

D. Perform bone marrow biopsy.

47. **A 20-year-old man presents with difficulty moving his neck, which is in an unusual posture. He denies trauma. His medical history is remarkable for gastroesophageal reflux disease, for which he recently started taking metoclopramide. What is the best treatment?**
    A. Amantadine
    B. Botulinum toxin
    C. Diphenhydramine
    D. Risperidone

48. **A 5-year-old boy presents with an abnormal gait and falling grades. On examination, he has dystonia, spasticity, and hyperreflexia. MRI shows decreased signal in the globus pallidus except in the anteromedial portion, which has increased signal. Which of the following findings is expected in this condition?**
    A. Iron deposition in the basal ganglia
    B. Golden ring in Descemet's layer of the cornea
    C. A cherry-red spot
    D. Deafness

49. **Which autosomal dominant familial ataxia demonstrates an anticipation pattern of inheritance and is associated with seizures and blindness?**
    A. Spinocerebellar ataxia type 3 (SCA3)
    B. Spinocerebellar ataxia type 5 (SCA5)
    C. Spinocerebellar ataxia type 6 (SCA6)
    D. Spinocerebellar ataxia type 7 (SCA7)

50. **Which type of spinocerebellar ataxia is associated with anticipation but is *not* caused by a repeat expansion mutation?**
    A. Spinocerebellar ataxia type 1 (SCA1)
    B. Spinocerebellar ataxia type 3 (SCA3)
    C. Spinocerebellar ataxia type 5 (SCA5)
    D. Spinocerebellar ataxia type 7 (SCA7)

51. **Which of the following conditions can cause recurrent attacks of ataxia?**
    A. Argininosuccinate synthase deficiency
    B. Glucose transporter type 1 deficiency
    C. Hartnup disease
    D. All of the above

52. **Which of the following conditions is associated with myokymia?**
    A. Episodic ataxia type 1
    B. Episodic ataxia type 2
    C. Paroxysmal kinesigenic dyskinesia
    D. Paroxysmal non-kinesigenic dyskinesia

53. **Mutations in the calcium channel can cause which of the following conditions?**
    A. Episodic ataxia type 1
    B. Episodic ataxia type 2
    C. Paroxysmal kinesigenic dyskinesia
    D. Paroxysmal non-kinesigenic dyskinesia

54. A 50-year-old man presents with unsteadiness. On examination, he has ataxia and intention tremor. The patient's MRI shows T2 hyperintensities in the middle cerebellar peduncles. The patient's daughter had difficulties in school, and his grandson has intellectual disability and autism. What is the cause of this patient's ataxia?
   A. Dentatorubral-pallidoluysian atrophy
   B. Fragile X tremor-ataxia syndrome (FXTAS)
   C. Friedreich ataxia
   D. Spinocerebellar ataxia type 2

55. A mother brings her infant to the clinic for brief episodes of weakness involving either side of the body. These are triggered by fatigue, baths, or heat. They last for 1 hour unless the patient naps, in which case they resolve during sleep. What is the most likely diagnosis?
   A. Alternating hemiplegia of childhood
   B. Basilar migraine
   C. Periodic paralysis
   D. Todd's paralysis

56. A 14-year-old boy plays a long soccer game and then indulges in a large pasta meal. The following morning, he has difficulty moving. What is the most likely diagnosis?
   A. Glycogen storage disease type V
   B. Mitochondrial neurogastrointestinal encephalopathy (MNGIE)
   C. Periodic paralysis
   D. Stiff person syndrome

57. A 28-year-old pregnant woman reports discomfort in her legs, especially in the evenings. She has difficulty describing the feeling but she says it improves when she shakes her legs or paces. The physical examination is remarkable for mild pedal edema. What is the most likely diagnosis?
   A. Peripheral neuropathy
   B. Restless leg syndrome
   C. Discomfort due to pedal edema
   D. Preeclampsia

58. A 40-year-old woman presents with uncontrolled throwing-like movements in her right arm. What is the most likely site of her lesion?

   A. Caudate
   B. Putamen
   C. Subthalamic nucleus
   D. Globus pallidus external segment

59. A 5-year-old boy has frequent dystonic posturing of the arm. It typically occurs when he gets up from his chair at school. He remains alert, and the events last less than 1 minute. A mutation in which of the following genes is most likely responsible?
   A. *MR-1*
   B. *NKX2.1*
   C. *PRRT2*
   D. *SLC2A1*

60. A child is brought to clinic because of frequent startling. The family reports the child was stiff at birth and becomes stiff after being startled. On examination, the child has an exaggerated head retraction reflex. The patient's father also has a history of increased startle. A defect in which of the following receptors is most likely?
   A. Glycine receptor
   B. Glutamate receptor
   C. GABA-B receptor
   D. Adenosine receptor

61. A 40-year-old woman presents with worsening muscle cramps, leg stiffness, and falls. Loud noises trigger severe leg cramps, which sometimes cause her to fall. On examination, she has muscle rigidity and lumbar hyperlordosis. Which of the following antibodies are associated with this condition?
   A. Antibodies to glutamic acid decarboxylase 65 (GAD 65)
   B. Antibodies to collapsin response mediator protein 5 (CRMP-5)
   C. Antibodies to the metabotropic glutamate receptor 5 (mGluR5)
   D. Purkinje cell antibody-1 (PCA-1)

62. Which of the following medications is *least* likely to cause tardive dyskinesia?
   A. Pimozide
   B. Risperidone
   C. Tetrabenazine
   D. Ziprasidone

MOVEMENT DISORDERS

ANSWERS

1. A

The hyperdirect pathway is the cortico-subthalamo-pallidal pathway. The hyperdirect pathway is from the cerebral cortex (frontal lobe) to the subthalamic nucleus. The subthalamic nucleus activates the globus pallidus internal segment. It also sends fibers to the globus pallidus externa.

2. B

The basal ganglia direct pathway is the cortico-striato-pallidal pathway. In the direct pathway, the striatum sends inhibitory (GABAergic) projections to the globus pallidus internal segment and substantia nigra pars reticularis (GPi/SNr), which send inhibitory (GABAergic) projections to the thalamus. The result is excitation of the thalamus and, ultimately, the cortex.

3. A

The basal ganglia indirect pathway involves the globus pallidus externa and then the subthalamic nucleus. The indirect pathway is also known as the cortico-striato-GPe-subthalamo-GPi pathway. Excitation of the indirect pathway results in inhibition of the thalamus.

Injury to the indirect pathway causes decreased inhibition of the pallidum, which ultimately results in hyperkinetic movements (see Fig. 10.1).

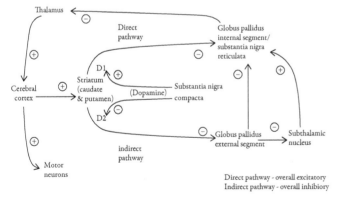

Figure 10.1 Direct and indirect pathways: circuitry. (From Fisch A. *Neuroanatomy: Draw It to Know It,* 2nd ed, Drawing 18-4. New York, Oxford University Press, 2012.)

4. B

Stereotypies are repetitive, purposeless behaviors such as hand flapping or body rocking. They are the most suppressible disorder listed.

5. B

Chorea and dystonia occur more during movement than during rest. The other disorders listed tend to occur more during rest than movement.

6. B

The term *overflow* is used when an unintentional movement accompanies a voluntary movement.

7. A

Resistance to passive movement that is independent of velocity is characteristic of rigidity.

Lesions of the basal ganglia can cause rigidity, whereas spasticity is caused by lesions of the corticospinal tract. Rigidity affects both agonist and antagonist muscles. Spasticity tends to affect flexors more than extensors in the upper extremity and extensors more than flexors in the lower extremity. Spasticity has a clasp-knife quality. There is increased resistance during early acceleration and then less resistance with continued passive movement. Spasticity is more apparent with fast movement. It is also associated with increased deep tendon reflexes. Rigidity may have a lead pipe or cogwheel quality. Superimposed tremor can cause the cogwheel quality.

Dystonia has qualities similar to rigidity. As in rigidity, resistance is not influenced by speed of passive movement, and rapid reversal of passive movement causes immediate resistance. However, patients with dystonia often have an abnormal posture when awake and improvement during sleep. In addition, performing voluntary movements with the opposite extremity causes a noticeable increase in resistance and abnormal posture of the dystonic extremity.

8. C

Tics are rapid, stereotyped, nonrhythmic movements. There is an urge to perform the tic, which is relieved when the tic is performed. Tics can temporarily be suppressed but then may increase after the period of suppression. Tics are suggestible. If the tic is mentioned or demonstrated, the patient may then have the tic. Tics worsen when patients are hot, under stress, fatigued, bored, or excited. Tics can persist during sleep.

9. C

This patient has Tourette syndrome. ADHD and obsessive compulsive disorder (OCD) are common comorbidities.

Patients with Tourette syndrome also have an increased incidence of generalized anxiety disorder and depression. They may also demonstrate aggression and oppositional behavior and have academic difficulties. Tourette syndrome can be seen in patients with autism spectrum disorder.

10. B

Coprolalia is not required for the diagnosis of Tourette syndrome.

Patients need to have multiple motor tics and at least one vocal tic to meet criteria. The symptoms must begin before age 18 years, must last at least 1 year, and must not be attributable to a medication, substance, or another medical condition. Tics tend to wax and wane.

11. B

Clonidine can be used to treat ADHD, tics, and impulse control problems. Guanfacine is also an option. Both are α_2-agonists.

Atomoxetine is helpful for ADHD and would not worsen this patient's tics, but clonidine is a better option in this case. Atomoxetine is useful for treatment of ADHD in patients whose tics have worsened on stimulants. It is a selective norepinephrine reuptake inhibitor.

Fluphenazine and risperidone would treat this patient's tics but not his ADHD.

Behavioral therapy, specifically Comprehensive Behavioral Intervention for Tics (CBIT), is also being used to treat tics.

12. D

This patient has PD, which causes loss of neurons in the substantia nigra containing melanin. These neurons are immunoreactive with tyrosine hydroxylase, which catalyzes the rate-limiting step in dopamine synthesis. Also, patients with PD have Lewy bodies, which are intraneuronal inclusions that primarily consist of alpha-synuclein.

13. B

There are many parkinsonian syndromes. Early gait instability raises concern for a parkinsonian syndrome other than idiopathic PD, such as multiple system atrophy (MSA) or progressive supranuclear palsy (PSP).

The tremor of PD is a resting tremor; it briefly improves with action. For example, if the arms are outstretched, there is brief improvement, but after a few seconds, the tremor may again be seen. The tremor worsens with mental tasks (see Boxes 10.1 and 10.2).

Box 10.1 PARKINSONIAN SYNDROMES

- Idiopathic Parkinson disease
- Corticobasal degeneration
- Multiple system atrophy
- Progressive supranuclear palsy
- Vascular parkinsonism
- Toxin-induced parkinsonism

Box 10.2 CHARACTERISTICS OF TREMOR IN PARKINSON DISEASE

- Asymmetric
- Frequency is 4 to 6 Hz
- More prominent at rest
- Improves with action
- More prominent during mental tasks, during walking, and with contralateral movement

14. A

Carbidopa is an inhibitor of aromatic L-amino acid decarboxylation (AADC), which converts levodopa to dopamine. Carbidopa prevents metabolism of levodopa to dopamine peripherally.

15. A

Levodopa is very efficacious at treating bradykinesia and rigidity in PD. However, dyskinesias are more common with levodopa than with dopamine agonists. Sustained-release levodopa does not prevent dyskinesias. Levodopa can also cause hallucinations, nausea, vomiting, orthostatic hypotension, and peripheral edema.

16. C

Ropinirole, a dopamine agonist, is most likely responsible. Dopamine agonists can cause disorders of impulse control (e.g., gambling, hypersexuality), sudden sleep attacks, peripheral edema, hallucinations, and hypotension. Dopamine agonists include pramipexole, ropinirole, and rotigotine. Rotigotine is administered as a patch.

Apomorphine is also a dopamine agonist. It can cause sedation and orthostatic hypotension.

17. A

Amantadine, which has been used as an antiviral agent, may be helpful in reducing dyskinesias in patients with PD with motor fluctuations. Its mechanism is unknown. It can cause confusion, hallucinations, myoclonus, peripheral edema, and livedo reticularis.

18. D

Trihexyphenidyl is an anticholinergic medication. Specifically, it is a muscarinic antagonist. Anticholinergic medications can cause multiple side effects in the elderly, so trihexyphenidyl is more commonly used in younger patients. It is more helpful for tremor than for the other symptoms of PD.

Benztropine is also anticholinergic.

Anticholinergic medications can cause confusion, hallucinations, blurred vision, dry mouth, constipation, and urinary retention.

19. D

Dopamine is metabolized by monoamine oxidase (MAO) and COMT. Rasagiline and selegiline are MAO-B inhibitors. They can reduce the off time. Selegiline, but not rasagiline, has an amphetamine metabolite that can cause hallucinations and sleep disturbance.

20. C

This patient most likely is taking entacapone. Entacapone and tolcapone are COMT inhibitors that prevent dopamine metabolism and therefore prolong its action. Both can cause diarrhea and discolored urine. Tolcapone has a risk of fatal fulminant liver failure.

If a COMT inhibitor is added to levodopa, the dose of levodopa may need to be reduced. COMT inhibitors potentiate levodopa (including its side effects).

21. D

Rivastigmine was approved for treatment of dementia in PD. Dopamine agonists may worsen psychiatric symptoms. Risperidone can worsen motor symptoms.

22. D

DBS of the bilateral subthalamic nucleus and DBS of the bilateral globus pallidus interna have been used to treat PD.

Unilateral DBS of the ventral intermediate thalamic nucleus (VIM) has been used to treat tremor in PD and essential tremor.

23. A

Mutations in the gene *SCNA*, which encodes for alpha-synuclein, are responsible for PARK1 and PARK4. Alpha-synuclein is found in Lewy bodies.

PARK1, PARK8, and PARK17 are autosomal dominant diseases. PARK8 is caused by mutations in the gene *LRRK2*, which encodes for leucine-rich repeat serine/threonine-protein kinase 2.

PARK2 is autosomal recessive. It is caused by mutations in the *PARK2* gene, which encodes for parkin. Parkin is a ubiquitin ligase. Mutations in *PARK2* cause early-onset PD.

Serine/threonine-protein kinase is the abnormal protein in PARK6, which is caused by mutations in *PINK1*. Mutations in *PINK1* also cause early-onset, autosomal recessive PD.

24. C

Oculogyric crisis is an exclusion criterion for PD. It can be seen in postencephalitic parkinsonism. It also is a type of dystonic reaction that occurs with neuroleptic use. It can also be seen in aromatic L-amino acid decarboxylase (AADC) deficiency and in Wilson disease.

Other exclusion criteria for PD are poor response to levodopa, cerebellar signs, a stepwise progression of symptoms, early cognitive problems, early autonomic symptoms, pyramidal signs, and supranuclear palsy.

25. A

MPTP can cause symptoms similar to those of PD.

Normeperidine is a derivative of meperidine. It is proconvulsant and can cause seizures.

26. B

This patient has manganese toxicity, which is a risk for welders. Manganese toxicity causes parkinsonism. It is associated with a "cock-walk" gait.

27. D

This is multiple system atrophy (MSA) parkinsonism associated with autonomic dysfunction. Autonomic dysfunction precedes motor dysfunction. MRI shows hypointense putamen on T2-weighted scans. Iron deposition can occur in the putamen, which may atrophy.

In the cerebellar form of MSA, a "hot cross bun" sign may be seen. The pontocerebellar fibers in the pons atrophy and have increased signal. Atrophy of the cerebellum and pons is also seen.

MSA is associated with iris atrophy, stridor, myoclonus, and early antecollis and gait instability. Rapid-eye-movement (REM) sleep behavior disorder may precede motor symptoms of MSA.

Midcallosal atrophy occurs in corticobasal degeneration.

Midbrain atrophy and a Mickey Mouse appearance of the midbrain are seen in progressive supranuclear palsy.

28. A

Glial cytoplasmic inclusions (GCIs), which are characteristic of multiple system atrophy (MSA), have alpha-synuclein immunoreactivity. Alpha-synuclein is also found in Lewy bodies. MSA, PD, and dementia with Lewy bodies are synucleinopathies. Rapid-eye-movement (REM) sleep behavior disorder is associated with synucleinopathies.

Globose neurofibrillary tangles are seen in progressive supranuclear palsy.

Loss of cells in the basal nucleus of Meynert is seen in Alzheimer disease.

Neocortical ballooned neurons are found in corticobasal degeneration.

29. D

This patient has progressive supranuclear palsy (PSP), which can be caused by mutations in *MAPT*. *MAPT* encodes tau. Features of PSP include a wide-eyed stare, postural instability, and retropulsion. Square wave jerks and slowing of vertical saccades may precede supranuclear vertical gaze palsy. Frontotemporal dementia can occur in some patients with PSP. Midbrain atrophy is seen on MRI in patients with PSP. This causes a hummingbird sign on sagittal images and the Mickey Mouse sign on axial images of the midbrain.

Mutations in the gene *ATM* cause ataxia-telangiectasia.

PARK7 encodes DJ-1.

HTT is discussed later.

30. C

Progressive supranuclear palsy is the least likely of the listed conditions to cause significant autonomic dysfunction.

Multiple system atrophy (MSA), dementia with Lewy bodies, and spinocerebellar ataxia type 2 (SCA2) can cause autonomic dysfunction and parkinsonism.

31. A

This patient has corticobasal degeneration (CBD), which is a neurodegenerative disease, specifically a tauopathy. Patients with CBD have limb rigidity, akinesia, dystonia, or myoclonus; alien limb phenomenon; and cortical sensory loss. Limb apraxia or mirror movements may be present. MRI shows midcallosal atrophy and asymmetric atrophy of the parietal cortex. Pathology shows achromatic neurons, ballooned neurons, and astrocytic plaques containing accumulated tau.

Besides progressive supranuclear palsy (PSP) and CBD, other tauopathies are Alzheimer disease, chronic traumatic encephalopathy, and frontotemporal dementia.

32. D

Whipple disease is caused by the bacterium *Tropheryma whipplei*. Whipple disease tends to affect middle-aged men. In addition to systemic manifestations such as diarrhea, fever, and polyarthritis, Whipple disease can cause neurologic conditions such as dementia, supranuclear ocular palsy, parkinsonism, and oculomasticatory myorhythmia. Intestinal biopsy aids in the diagnosis; periodic acid-Schiff (PAS)-positive bacteria are seen within macrophages.

33. B

This patient has normal pressure hydrocephalus (NPH). NPH is a potentially treatable cause of parkinsonism. It is characterized by the triad of dementia, gait disturbance, and urinary incontinence. All three conditions may not be present. Gait impairment is typically present and is often the first sign. The gait is described as a magnetic gait. A large-volume lumbar puncture aids in the diagnosis. Patients with NPH may have improved gait after the lumbar puncture.

34a. D and 34b. C

This patient has Huntington disease, which is caused by an increase in the number of CAG repeats in the *HTT* gene. This results in an abnormally long polyglutamine (polyQ) sequence. *HTT*, which is on chromosome 4, encodes the protein huntingtin. Expanded CAG repeats are also found in dentatorubral-pallidoluysian atrophy (DRPLA); Kennedy disease (bulbospinal muscular atrophy); and spinocerebellar ataxia types 1, 2, 3, 6, 7, 12, and 17.

Spinocerebellar ataxia type 10 (SCA10) is a pentanucleotide repeat disease (ATTCT).

Huntington disease is autosomal dominant. Anticipation occurs. Inheritance from the father is associated with worse prognosis, including earlier onset. Huntington disease causes a subcortical dementia, but changes in mood are seen first.

Medium spiny neurons, which are GABAergic, are particularly vulnerable to Huntington disease.

If Huntington disease manifests in childhood (Westphal variant), behavior issues and learning problems may be the earliest signs. Patients also have bradykinesia, rigidity with or without dystonia, myoclonus, and seizures. Chorea manifests later.

35. D

Tetrabenazine inhibits vesicle monoamine transporter type 2. This prevents transport of dopamine, serotonin, and norepinephrine into the presynaptic terminal and reduces dopamine transmission. Tetrabenazine can cause depression, suicidality, parkinsonism, and akathisia.

Tetrabenazine is metabolized by the cytochrome P450 enzyme CYP2D6. Patients taking an inhibitor of CYP2D6, such as fluoxetine, should be placed on a smaller dose of tetrabenazine.

The glutamatergic-modifying drugs amantadine and riluzole can also be used to treat chorea in Huntington disease. Riluzole can affect liver function tests.[1]

36. A

This is Sydenham chorea, which is a poststreptococcal autoimmune condition. A darting tongue and spooning of the fingers are classic signs. Milkmaid's grip is another classic sign. The MRI is normal. Sydenham chorea is a consequence of group A β-hemolytic streptococci (GABHS) infection. Elevated antistreptolysin O (ASO) and anti-DNAse B titers indicate prior infection. Sydenham chorea is a form of rheumatic disease. The patient should be assessed for arthritis and a cardiac murmur and should be treated with penicillin. The chorea can be treated with valproic acid or dopamine receptor antagonists. Benzodiazepines and steroids have also been used in patients with Sydenham chorea. Symptoms may recur during pregnancy.

Chorea can also occur in other autoimmune conditions, such as systemic lupus erythematosus, antiphospholipid antibody syndrome, and Sjögren syndrome. Chorea can also be a paraneoplastic phenomenon.

37. C

Multiple medications can cause chorea. Dopaminergic medications, stimulants, and lithium are examples. Antiepileptic medications such as gabapentin, carbamazepine, phenytoin, and valproic acid can cause chorea. Oral contraceptives can also cause chorea, as can pregnancy (chorea gravidarum).

Reserpine has been used to treat chorea, but has more side effects than some of the other treatment options.

38. C

This patient has essential tremor, which is the most common movement disorder. It is autosomal dominant. Essential tremor is bilateral, tends to occur with movement, and improves after alcohol. It can be treated with propranolol or primidone, which have the best evidence. There is less evidence for atenolol, sotalol, gabapentin, and topiramate. There is risk for abuse with clonazepam. Botulinum toxin A injection is reserved for refractory cases. Deep brain stimulation of the ventral intermediate thalamic nucleus has also been used to treat medically refractory limb tremor caused by essential tremor.[2]

39. D

Wilson disease causes sunflower cataracts, risus sardonicus, and a wing-beating tremor. Wilson disease, which is also known as hepatolenticular degeneration, results from a defect in copper-transporting adenotriphosphatase (ATPase). Specifically, it is caused by a mutation in the *ATP7B* gene on chromosome 13. Copper excretion from the liver into the bile is impaired, resulting in high levels of copper in the liver. Serum copper and ceruloplasmin are low. Urinary copper is high.

Wilson disease can manifest as liver disease or with neurologic or psychiatric symptoms. Wilson disease can cause rigidity or movement disorders such as tremor and chorea. A unique finding in Wilson disease is the Kayser-Fleischer ring, which is caused by deposition of copper in Descemet's membrane of the cornea. Sunflower cataracts are less common.

Wilson disease is associated with increased signal on T2-weighted MRI in the basal ganglia. In some patients, the face of the giant panda sign can be seen in the midbrain.

Wilson disease is treated with chelation.

Basal ganglia calcification characterizes Fahr syndrome, which can cause parkinsonism and choreoathetosis.

40. D

Early-onset generalized torsion dystonia (DYT1) is the most common form of primary genetic dystonia. It is caused by a GAG deletion in the *TOR1A* gene on chromosome 9. This deletion causes an abnormality in the adenosine triphosphate (ATP)-binding protein torsinA. DYT1 is autosomal dominant. It begins in a limb, usually in the second decade of life; symptoms then become more generalized.

TATA-binding protein-associated factor-1 (TAF1) is abnormal in dystonia-parkinsonism (DYT3), which is X-linked.

Myofibrillogenesis regulator 1 is abnormal in paroxysmal nonkinesigenic dyskinesia (DYT8).

Epsilon-sarcoglycan is abnormal in myoclonus-dystonia (DYT11).

41. D

This patient has dopa-responsive dystonia, or DYT5. The autosomal dominant form, which is the most common form, is caused by a deficiency of guanosine triphosphate (GTP) cyclohydrolase 1 (GTPCH1). The autosomal recessive form is caused by tyrosine hydroxylase deficiency. Dopa-responsive dystonia may also be caused by sepiapterin reductase deficiency.

GTPCH1 catalyzes the first step in the synthesis of tetrahydrobiopterin (BH$_4$). Sepiapterin reductase is involved later in production of BH$_4$. BH$_4$ is a cofactor for tyrosine hydroxylase, which converts tyrosine to L-dopa. This is the rate-limiting step in catecholamine synthesis.

Other types of dystonia may be treated with anticholinergic medications such as trihexyphenidyl. Baclofen, dopamine depleters, and benzodiazepines have also been used. Botulinum toxin can be helpful for focal or segmental dystonia.

42. A

Onabotulinumtoxin A, or Botox, inactivates SNAP-25.

Some botulinum toxins, such as botulinum toxin B, inactivate vesicle-associated membrane protein (VAMP).

Syntaxin-1 is the target for botulinum toxin C.

43. A

Patients with severe primary dystonia that does not respond to treatment with medications may respond to DBS of the globus pallidus interna.

44. B

DYT11 is alcohol responsive. Myoclonus usually affects the arms and neck. Dystonia is mild. Myoclonic jerks may occur only during hand-writing. DYT11 is caused by mutations in the epsilon-sarcoglycan gene (*SGCE*) on chromosome 7q. DYT11 is autosomal dominant. There is complete paternal inheritance but reduced maternal penetrance due to imprinting. DYT15 also results in myoclonus-dystonia.

Rapid-onset dystonia-parkinsonism (RDP) can be triggered by drinking alcohol. It can also be triggered by infection or other stressors. It is caused by mutations in *ATP1A3*. Mutations in this gene also cause some cases of alternating hemiplegia of childhood.

45. D

Sodium oxybate is least likely to cause myoclonus. It has been used to treat myoclonus but is not a first-line treatment.

46. B

This case is concerning for opsoclonus-myoclonus, which is associated with neuroblastoma. CT of the chest, abdomen, and pelvis should be performed to look for the tumor. Some patients with neuroblastoma have periorbital ecchymoses (raccoon eyes) resulting from metastasis to the orbit. Heterochromia of the iris can occur with a cervicothoracic neuroblastoma. Urine catecholamines and nuclear medicine scans may aid in the diagnosis.

47. C

This patient has an acute dystonic reaction due to metoclopramide, which is a dopamine D2 receptor blocker. Risperidone is a dopamine D2 receptor antagonist as well, so it should be avoided in this patient. Medications with anticholinergic properties, such as diphenhydramine or benztropine (Cogentin), can be used to treat acute dystonic reaction.

48. A

This patient has pantothenate kinase-associated neurodegeneration (PKAN), which is a type of neurodegeneration with brain iron accumulation (NBIA).

NBIA includes multiple disorders characterized by accumulation of iron in the basal ganglia, which results in symptoms such as parkinsonism, dystonia, and choreoathetosis.

PKAN is NBIA type 1, the most common form of NBIA. It is caused by mutations in *PANK2*, which encodes pantothenate kinase. Pantothenate kinase is involved in synthesis of coenzyme A. The classic form of PKAN begins in childhood. An abnormal gait may be the presenting symptom. Patients have rigidity, spasticity, and dystonia. Cognitive changes, seizures, and retinal degeneration may occur. Acanthocytosis may be present. PKAN is associated with the "eye of the tiger" sign, which results from decreased signal on T2-weighted MRI in the globus pallidus and substantia nigra with an area of hyperintensity in the center.

NBIA2B is caused by mutations in the *PLA2G6* gene. Mutations in this gene also cause infantile neuroaxonal dystrophy 1 and PARK14 (adult-onset dystonia-parkinsonism).

Neuroferritinopathy is a type of NBIA. It causes adult-onset of chorea, dystonia, parkinsonism, and orolingual dyskinesia.

49. D

The spinocerebellar ataxias are autosomal dominant. Historically, these have been divided into three types of autosomal dominant cerebellar ataxia (ADCA). Spinocerebellar ataxias with prominent extracerebellar abnormalities are classified as ADCA-I. Those with retinal degeneration are ADCA-II. Spinocerebellar ataxias with primarily cerebellar findings are categorized as ADCA-III.

SCA7 is the only disease listed that is in the category ADCA-II. SCA7 causes seizures and retinal degeneration. It demonstrates anticipation.

SCA3 (Machado-Joseph disease) is an autosomal dominant familial ataxia associated with bulged eyes, parkinsonism, facial fasciculations, and eye movement abnormalities. It is caused by mutations in the gene *ATXN3*.

SCA5 and SCA6 are pure cerebellar.

The most common genetic cause of ataxia in patients older than 40 years of age is SCA6. One of the earliest signs is positional downbeat nystagmus: When the head is straight back, the patient has downbeat nystagmus.

Dentatorubral-pallidoluysian atrophy (DRPLA) is considered to be one of the autosomal dominant cerebellar ataxias.

50. C

SCA5 demonstrates anticipation but is not caused by a repeat expansion mutation. It is caused by mutations in the gene *SPTBN2*.

Expanded CAG repeats are found in spinocerebellar ataxia types 1, 2, 3, 6, 7, 12, and 17.[3]

51. D

Some metabolic causes of recurrent ataxia include glucose transporter type 1 (GLUT-1) deficiency,, Hartnup disease, maple syrup urine disease, ornithine transcarbamylase deficiency, argininosuccinate synthase (ASS) deficiency, and pyruvate dehydrogenase deficiency.

52. A

Episodic ataxia type 1 (EA1) is associated with myokymia. This is seen between attacks, which are characterized by dysarthria and incoordination and last for minutes. EA1 is treated with carbonic anhydrase inhibitors, such as acetazolamide.

53. B

Episodic Ataxia type 2 (EA2) is caused by a mutation in the calcium channel. Attacks last hours to days. Between episodes of ataxia, patients have gaze-evoked nystagmus. EA2 is treated with acetazolamide. Caffeine, phenytoin, alcohol, exercise, and stress can trigger events. Some patients have an increased number of CAG repeats in the *CACNA1A* gene. This gene is also associated with SCA6 and with familial hemiplegic migraine.

Episodic ataxia type 1 is caused by a mutation in the potassium channel.

(Paroxysmal kinesigenic dyskinesia and paroxysmal non-kinesigenic dyskinesia are discussed later.)

54. B

This patient has FXTAS. His grandson has fragile X syndrome. FXTAS tends to affect men older than 50 years of age. It causes ataxia and tremor. Parkinsonism, peripheral neuropathy, and psychiatric symptoms can occur. Increased signal is seen in the middle cerebellar peduncles on T2-weighted MRI. It can also be seen in the splenium of the corpus callosum and the white matter. FXTAS is caused by a premutation in *FMR1*. Patients with FXTAS have an expanded number of CGG repeats but not sufficient to cause fragile X syndrome.

Dentatorubral-pallidoluysian atrophy causes ataxia, choreoathetosis, and dementia. It is caused by mutations in the gene *ATN1*.

Friedreich ataxia is caused by an expanded GAA trinucleotide repeat in the *FXN* gene on chromosome 9q. It is autosomal recessive.

Spinocerebellar ataxia type 2 is caused by mutations in *ATN2*.

55. A

This patient has alternating hemiplegia of childhood.

Alternating hemiplegia of childhood-1 (AHC1) is caused by a mutation in the sodium-potassium-ATPase, alpha-2 polypeptide (*ATP1A2*) gene on chromosome 1q. Mutations in the gene also cause familial basilar migraine and familial hemiplegic migraine-2 (FHM2).

Alternating hemiplegia of childhood-2 (AHC2) is caused by mutation in the sodium/potassium-transporting ATPase subunit alpha-3 (*ATP1A3*) gene on chromosome 19q. Mutation in the *ATP1A3* gene can also cause dystonia 12 (DYT12), which is rapid-onset dystonia-parkinsonism.

56. C

This patient has hypokalemic periodic paralysis.

The periodic paralyses are hereditary channelopathies characterized by flaccid weakness, often resulting from abnormal potassium levels. Carbonic anhydrase inhibitors, such as acetazolamide, may decrease attacks.

A carbohydrate-rich meal and rest after vigorous exercise are triggers for hypokalemic periodic paralysis. Hypokalemic periodic paralysis is caused by a mutation in *CACNA1S* (a calcium channel gene) or in the *SCN4A* (a sodium channel gene). Potassium is low during the attacks. Creatine kinase may be elevated.

Similar to hypokalemic periodic paralysis, hyperkalemic periodic paralysis can be caused by mutations in the *SCN4A* gene and can be triggered by rest after exercise; however, potassium tends to be elevated during the attacks. Fasting and potassium-rich foods are also triggers for hyperkalemic periodic paralysis. Some patients have myotonia or paramyotonia.

In addition to causing hypokalemic periodic paralysis and hyperkalemic periodic paralysis, mutations in the *SCN4A* gene on chromosome 17q also cause paramyotonia congenita, acetazolamide-responsive myotonia congenita, and a congenital myasthenic syndrome.

Mutations in the *KCNJ2* gene, which encodes a potassium inward rectifier, cause Anderson-Tawil syndrome, which is also associated with periods of flaccid weakness triggered by fluctuating potassium levels. These patients also have a prolonged QT interval, ventricular arrhythmias, syndactyly, and characteristic facial features.

Thyrotoxic periodic paralysis is caused by mutations in the *KCNJ18* gene, which also encodes a potassium channel rectifier. Weakness is triggered by thyrotoxicosis and hypokalemia. Glucose should be avoided. A low-carbohydrate diet is recommended. There is concern about malignant hyperthermia in patients with channelopathies, so depolarizing anesthetic agents should be avoided if the patient undergoes surgery.

Glycogen storage disease type V (GSD V), or McArdle disease, is the most common carbohydrate metabolism disorder. It is caused by defects in the gene that encodes myophosphorylase, which helps breakdown glycogen. GSD V causes exercise intolerance (e.g., muscle cramps, myoglobinuria). Patients do have a second-wind phenomenon. Warming up before exercise and a consuming a carbohydrate-rich diet may improve exercise tolerance.

Mitochondrial neurogastrointestinal encephalopathy (MNGIE) results in intolerance of large meals due to gastrointestinal dysmotility. Patients also have cachexia, leukoencephalopathy, weakness, ptosis, external ophthalmoplegia, and a sensorimotor polyneuropathy. Patients with MNGIE have mutations in *TYMP* that result in reduced thymidine phosphorylase levels and elevated levels of thymidine and deoxyuridine in the plasma. Muscle biopsy shows ragged red fibers.[4,5]

57. B

This patient has restless leg syndrome (RLS). Pregnancy is a risk factor for RLS. Iron deficiency can contribute to RLS. A ferritin level should be checked.

58. C

This patient has hemiballism, which is caused by lesions of the subthalamic nucleus.

59. C

This patient has paroxysmal kinesigenic dyskinesia (PKD). Patients with PKD have brief, frequent events triggered by movement. The events can occur multiple times per day. PKD is more common in males then in females, and it manifests in the first or second decade of life. Some cases of PKD are caused by mutations in proline-rich transmembrane protein 2 (*PRRT2*) on chromosome 16. PKD may improve with anti-epileptic medications such as carbamazepine or phenytoin. Some patients with PKD have benign convulsions in infancy. Infantile convulsions and choreoathetosis is the combination of convulsions and PKD.

Events are much less frequent in paroxysmal non-kinesigenic dyskinesia (PNKD), but they tend to last longer (minutes to hours). Triggers are alcohol, excitement, and caffeine. PNKD can be seen with mutations in the myofibrillogenesis regulator-1 gene (*MR-1*). PNKD is treated with benzodiazepines, but it does not respond to treatment as well as PKD.

Paroxysmal exercise-induced dyskinesia is triggered by prolonged exercise or hyperventilation. Acetazolamide and benzodiazepines have been used for treatment. Some patients have mutations in *SLC2A1*, which causes glucose transporter type 1 deficiency syndrome (GLUT-1 deficiency). These patients may respond to the ketogenic diet.

Mutations in the gene *NKX2.1*, which encodes thyroid transcription factor 1, cause benign hereditary chorea. Benign hereditary chorea is characterized by hypotonia, motor delay, and chorea beginning before 5 years of age. Hypotonia usually precedes chorea. Ataxia-telangiectasia can also cause chorea in this age group.

60. A

This child has hereditary hyperekplexia, which is most often caused by a mutation in the gene encoding the glycine receptor. Clonazepam has been used for treatment.

61. A

This patient has stiff-person syndrome, which is associated with antibodies to glutamic acid decarboxylase (GAD) and antibodies to amphiphysin. Antibodies to GAD 65 are associated with cerebellar degeneration, seizures, and type 1 diabetes mellitus as well. Antibodies to amphiphysin can be seen in certain patients with breast and lung cancers.

Breast and ovarian cancers are associated with Purkinje cell antibody-1 (PCA-1), which is also called anti-Yo. These antibodies cause cerebellar degeneration.

Antibodies to CRMP-5 are seen in patients with lung cancer and thymoma. They can cause a number of clinical syndromes.

Antibodies to the metabotropic glutamate receptor 5 (mGluR5) have been found in some patients with Hodgkin lymphoma and limbic encephalopathy. This is called Ophelia syndrome.

62. C

Tardive dyskinesia is caused by long-term use of dopamine receptor (D2) blockers, which include antipsychotics such as pimozide, risperidone, and ziprasidone. Metoclopramide, prochlorperazine (Compazine), and promethazine (Phenergan) are also D2 receptor blockers and can cause tardive dyskinesia.

Of the medications listed, tetrabenazine, which depletes monoamines from the nerve terminals, is the least likely to cause tardive dyskinesia.

REFERENCES

1. Armstrong MJ, Miyasaki JM. Evidence-based guideline: Pharmacologic treatment of chorea in Huntington disease. Report of the Guideline Development Subcommittee of the American Academy of Neurology. *Neurology* 2012;79:597–603.
2. Zesiewicz TA, Elble RJ, Louis ED, et al. Evidence-based guideline update: Treatment of essential tremor. Report of the Quality Standards Subcommittee of the American Academy of Neurology. *Neurology* 2011;77:1752–1755.
3. Ashizawa T. Common hereditary and sporadic degenerative ataxia. Presented at the annual meeting of the American Academy of Neurology, Washington, DC, 2015.
4. Statland JM, Barohn RJ. Muscle channelopathies: The nondystrophic myotonias and periodic paralyses. *Continuum (Minneap Minn)* 2013;19:1598–1614.
5. Tobon A. Metabolic myopathies. *Continuum (Minneap Minn)* 2013;19:1571–1597.

11.

NEUROANATOMY

QUESTIONS

CORTEX

1. **Which area of the cortex has a prominent layer V and contains the giant pyramidal cells of Betz?**
   A. Auditory cortex
   B. Frontal eye fields
   C. Primary motor cortex
   D. Visual cortex

2. **Which neurotransmitter is used by the pyramidal cells of the cerebral cortex?**
   A. Acetylcholine
   B. GABA
   C. Glutamate
   D. Glycine

3. **A patient describes a "pins and needles" sensation in his arm at the beginning of his seizures. It is thought that the seizures are arising from primary sensory cortex. Which Brodmann area or areas correspond to this region?**
   A. 3, 1, 2
   B. 6
   C. 22
   D. 44, 45

4. **Bilateral lesions of which area can cause ageusia (lack of taste)?**
   A. Insular cortex
   B. Pars triangularis
   C. Superior temporal gyrus
   D. Inferior temporal gyrus

5. **Stimulation of which area of the cortex in one hemisphere can produce bilateral movement?**
   A. Supplementary motor area
   B. Inferior frontal gyrus
   C. Prefrontal cortex
   D. Cingulate gyrus

6. **Which of the following gyri is primary auditory cortex?**
   A. Angular gyrus
   B. Inferior temporal gyrus
   C. Middle temporal gyrus
   D. Transverse gyrus of Heschl

7. **Which area of the cortex directs the activity of the primary motor cortex, assisting in reaching, grasping, and skilled movements?**
   A. Premotor cortex
   B. Orbitofrontal cortex

C. Dorsolateral prefrontal cortex
   D. Mesial frontal cortex

8. **Where are the frontal eye fields located?**
   A. Superior frontal gyrus
   B. Middle frontal gyrus
   C. Inferior fontal gyrus
   D. Precentral gyrus

CONNECTING SYSTEMS

9. **Which of the following structures most directly connects the hippocampi?**
   A. Stria terminalis
   B. Hippocampal commissure
   C. Ventral amygdalofugal pathway
   D. Medial forebrain bundle

10. **Which of the following is the largest commissure?**
    A. Anterior commissure
    B. Corpus callosum
    C. Posterior commissure
    D. Supraoptic commissure

11. **Which of the following structures connects the frontal lobe with the temporal and occipital lobes?**
    A. Cingulum
    B. Inferior longitudinal fasciculus
    C. Superior longitudinal fasciculus
    D. Projection fibers

LIMBIC SYSTEM

12. **In the Papez circuit, which structure carries information from the hippocampal formation to the mammillary bodies?**
    A. Anterior nucleus of the thalamus
    B. Entorhinal cortex
    C. Fornix
    D. Hippocampus

13. **Which of the following is the major input and output relay between vision, auditory, and somatosensory association cortex and the hippocampus?**
    A. Entorhinal cortex
    B. Fornix
    C. Piriform cortex
    D. Periamygdaloid cortex

14. **Which limbic structure is part of the ventral striatum and is involved in motivation, habits, and rewards?**
    A. Amygdala
    B. Cingulate gyrus

C. Nucleus accumbens

D. Subthalamic nucleus

BASAL GANGLIA

15. Fill in the blank: The main input to the basal ganglia is from the _____.
    A. Cerebral cortex
    B. Superior cerebellar peduncle
    C. Inferior cerebellar peduncle
    D. Thalamus

16. Which basal ganglia structures act as input nuclei to the basal ganglia?
    A. Caudate nucleus, putamen, and nucleus accumbens
    B. Globus pallidus externa and ventral pallidum
    C. Internal segment of the globus pallidus and substantia nigra pars reticulata
    D. Substantia nigra pars compacta and ventral tegmental area

17. Which of the following structures is part of the basal ganglia indirect pathway?
    A. Globus pallidus interna
    B. Globus pallidus externa
    C. Substantia nigra reticulata
    D. Substantia nigra pars compacta

18. Most of the output from the basal ganglia to the thalamus is to which of these structures?
    A. Medial dorsal, ventral lateral, and ventral anterior nuclei
    B. Pulvinar and centromedian nuclei
    C. Anterior and reticular nuclei
    D. Ventroposteromedial and ventroposterolateral nuclei

19. Which structure in the basal ganglia serves a motor function, projecting to primary motor cortex via the thalamus?
    A. Caudate
    B. Globus pallidus
    C. Pedunculopontine area
    D. Putamen

20. Fill in the blank: The portions of the striatum involved with emotion are called the _____.
    A. Ventral tegmental area
    B. Ventral striatum
    C. Ansa lenticularis
    D. Medial forebrain bundle

21. A lesion of which structure results in hemiballism?
    A. Globus pallidus internal segment
    B. Globus pallidus external segment
    C. Subthalamic nucleus
    D. Substantia nigra pars compacta

BRAINSTEM

22. Match the following lesion sites with its associated clinical findings:
    1) Lateral medulla
    2) Medial midbrain
    3) Medial medulla
    4) Ventral pons
    A. Contralateral hemiparesis, ipsilateral cranial nerve III (CN 3) palsy
    B. Contralateral hemiparesis, ipsilateral CN 6 palsy
    C. Ipsilateral hemiataxia, Horner syndrome, loss of pain and temperature of the ipsilateral face and contralateral body
    D. Ipsilateral CN 12 palsy, contralateral hemiparesis

23. Which of the following lesions is *least* likely to cause a pure motor hemiparesis?
    A. A lesion of the corticospinal tract in the basis pontis
    B. A lesion of the anterior limb of the internal capsule
    C. A cerebral peduncle lesion
    D. A lesion of the medullary pyramid

24. The "locked-in syndrome" is most likely to occur with bilateral lesions of which area?
    A. Lateral medulla
    B. Medial medulla
    C. Ventral pons
    D. Medial midbrain

25. Which of the following is most likely to be intact in a patient with locked-in syndrome?
    A. Vertical eye movements and blinking
    B. Horizontal eye movements
    C. Corticobulbar fibers

26. Lesions of the medulla can cause which of the following?
    A. Neurogenic pulmonary edema
    B. Early satiety
    C. Inability to sneeze
    D. Ondine's curse
    E. All of the above

THALAMUS

27. In the Papez circuit, which structure provides input to the anterior nucleus of the thalamus?
    A. Cingulate gyrus
    B. Mammillary bodies
    C. Entorhinal cortex
    D. Dentate nucleus

28. In the Papez circuit, to which structure does the anterior nucleus of the thalamus project?
    A. Cingulate gyrus
    B. Mammillary bodies
    C. Entorhinal cortex
    D. Dentate nucleus

29. Which nucleus is most likely to be injured in Wernicke-Korsakoff syndrome?
    A. Anterior nucleus
    B. Ventral anterior nucleus
    C. Mediodorsal nucleus
    D. Pulvinar

30. Match each thalamic nucleus with its description.

1) Centromedian nucleus
2) Mediodorsal nucleus
3) Pulvinar
4) Ventral lateral nucleus
5) Lateral geniculate nucleus (LGN)
6) Medial geniculate nucleus (MGN)
7) Reticular nucleus

A. This component of the extrageniculate visual pathway is involved in visual attention.
B. This component of the dentarubrothalamic tract receives input from the substantia nigra, globus pallidus, and cerebellum and projects to the motor cortex.
C. This nucleus is involved in a feedback loop between the cortex and striatum; it receives input from the globus pallidus and premotor cortex and projects to the caudate and putamen.
D. This nucleus receives input from limbic structures and has reciprocal connections with the prefrontal cortex.
E. This nucleus functions as a relay station in the auditory pathway.
F. This nucleus sends information to the visual cortex.
G. This nucleus forms a thin layer around the lateral thalamus.

31. **Which thalamic nucleus is involved in the generation of sleep spindles?**
    A. Anterior nucleus
    B. Mediodorsal nucleus
    C. Pulvinar
    D. Reticular nucleus

32. **True or False?**
    The thalamus integrates and relays information for all sensory modalities.

33. **Which thalamic nucleus is associated with taste sensation?**
    A. Anterior nucleus
    B. Centromedian nucleus
    C. Ventral posterolateral nucleus
    D. Ventral posteromedial nucleus

CEREBELLUM

34. **Which region of the cerebellum coordinates movement of the trunk?**
    A. Cerebellar hemispheres
    B. Paravermis
    C. Vermis

35. **Which lobe of the cerebellum is involved in eye movements and has connections with the vestibular system?**
    A. Anterior
    B. Flocculonodular
    C. Posterior

36. **Lesions of which lobe of the cerebellum cause the rostral vermis syndrome, which is characterized by a wide-based stance and gait ataxia?**
    A. Anterior
    B. Flocculonodular
    C. Posterior

37. **Lesions of which structure can cause head and trunk tremor, truncal imbalance, and nystagmus?**
    A. Cerebrocerebellum
    B. Spinocerebellum
    C. Vestibulocerebellum

38. **Which deep cerebellar nucleus is responsible for fine motor dexterity?**
    A. Dentate
    B. Emboliform
    C. Globose
    D. Fastigial

39. **Which peduncle carries most of the output from the cerebellum?**
    A. Inferior cerebellar peduncle
    B. Middle cerebellar peduncle
    C. Superior cerebellar peduncle

40. **Which type of cell is the major source of inhibitory output from the cerebellar cortex?**
    A. Purkinje cell
    B. Stellate cell
    C. Basket cell
    D. Granule cell

41. **Climbing fibers carry information from which of these structures into the cerebellum?**
    A. Inferior olive
    B. Reticular formation
    C. Trigeminal system
    D. Vestibular nuclei

CRANIAL NERVES

42. **Which of the following statements is *false*?**
    A. CN 4 is the smallest cranial nerve.
    B. CN 4 is the only cranial nerve that exits the brainstem on the dorsal aspect.
    C. CN 4 is the only cranial nerve that decussates.
    D. CN 6 has the longest intracranial course.

43. **Which nerve is responsible for the afferent limb of the corneal reflex?**
    A. The ophthalmic division of the trigeminal nerve (V1)
    B. The maxillary division of the trigeminal nerve (V2)
    C. The mandibular division of the trigeminal nerve (V3)
    D. Cranial nerve III

44. **A cavernous sinus thrombosis is least likely to involve which nerve?**
    A. The maxillary branch of the trigeminal nerve (V2)
    B. The mandibular division of the trigeminal nerve (V3)
    C. Cranial nerve IV
    D. Cranial nerve VI

45. **Which cranial nerve is responsible for general sensation from the anterior two thirds of the tongue?**
    A. The trigeminal nerve
    B. The facial nerve
    C. The glossopharyngeal nerve
    D. The vagus nerve

SPINAL CORD

46. A 55-year-old woman presents with falling and numbness. On examination, she has loss of vibration on the right up to T10 and loss of pain and temperature up to T10 on the left. What other finding would you expect on examination?
    A. Numbness of the right upper extremity
    B. Numbness of the left upper extremity
    C. Weakness of the right lower extremity
    D. Weakness of the left lower extremity

47. Which of the following are the most lateral tracts of the spinal cord and therefore the most vulnerable to extrinsic lateral insults?
    A. Dorsal and ventral spinocerebellar tracts
    B. Lateral corticospinal tract
    C. Lateral vestibulospinal tract
    D. Tectospinal tract

48. A patient presents with bilateral leg weakness, decreased pain sensation up to the level of the umbilicus, bowel and urinary incontinence, and intact proprioception and vibration. Which of the following is the most likely diagnosis?
    A. Anterior spinal artery infarct
    B. Cauda equina lesion
    C. Conus medullaris lesion
    D. Poliomyelitis

49. Which of the following disorders affect the posterior columns and corticospinal tracts of the spinal cord?
    A. Copper deficiency myelopathy after gastric bypass surgery
    B. Nitrous oxide myelopathy
    C. Vitamin B12 deficiency
    D. Human T-cell leukemia virus type 1 (HTLV-1)-associated myelopathy
    E. All of the above

50. Which of the following diseases is *least* likely to affect the posterior columns?
    A. AIDS-associated myelopathy
    B. Tabes dorsalis
    C. Posterior spinal artery infarct
    D. Poliomyelitis

51. A woman presents with bilateral hand weakness. On examination, she has muscle wasting in both hands. She has decreased pinprick and temperature sensation in the arms and shoulders, but light touch, vibration, and proprioception are intact. Reflexes in the arms are decreased. What is her diagnosis?
    A. Syringomyelia
    B. Vitamin E deficiency
    C. Primary lateral sclerosis
    D. Primary muscular atrophy

SPINAL ROOTS AND PERIPHERAL NERVES

52. Occipital neuralgia involves which nerve root?

    A. C1
    B. C2
    C. C3

53. Which of the following statements is *false*?
    A. C1 has no sensory roots.
    B. There is no C8 vertebra.
    C. A C5-6 disc herniation tends to affect the C5 nerve root.
    D. Batson's plexus may allow the spread of metastases and infections in the epidural space.

54. A 60-year-old woman presents with neck and right shoulder pain, weakness of her right hand, and numbness and tingling of her right fourth and fifth digits. She has decreased sensation in the fourth and fifth digits and weakness of the intrinsic hand muscles on the right. Reflexes are normal. Which of the following diagnoses is most likely?
    A. C5 radiculopathy
    B. C6 radiculopathy
    C. C7 radiculopathy
    D. C8 radiculopathy

55. Which nerve root exits above the T1 vertebral bone?
    A. C6
    B. C7
    C. C8
    D. T1

56. Which muscle above the knee is supplied by the peroneal division of the sciatic nerve?
    A. Gluteus minimus
    B. Small head of the biceps femoris
    C. Soleus
    D. Gracilis

57. True or False?
    Weakness of foot inversion suggests that a patient's foot drop is caused by a lesion proximal to the peroneal nerve at the fibular neck.

58. Which of the following nerves gives rise to the posterior interosseous nerve?
    A. Axillary
    B. Medial
    C. Radial
    D. Ulnar

CEREBROSPINAL FLUID AND
THE VENTRICULAR SYSTEM

59. What is the rate of cerebrospinal fluid (CSF) production?
    A. 5 mL/hr
    B. 10 mL/hr
    C. 20 mL/hr
    D. 35 mL/hr

60. Where is CSF absorbed into the blood?
    A. Arachnoid granulations
    B. Choroid plexus
    C. Foramina of Luschka and Magendie
    D. Foramen of Monro

BLOOD-BRAIN BARRIER

61. Fill in the blank: The blood-brain barrier results from the presence of _____ that link capillary endothelial cells in the brain.
    A. Cadherins
    B. Connexins
    C. Integrins
    D. Tight junctions

62. Fill in the blank: Areas of the brain where the blood-brain barrier is interrupted are called _____.
    A. Adherens junctions
    B. Circumventricular organs
    C. Desmosomes
    D. Gap junctions

63. Fill in the blank: The _____ is also known as the chemotactic trigger zone because it detects toxins that cause vomiting.

A. Median eminence
B. Area postrema
C. Organum vasculosum of the lamina terminalis
D. Subfornical organ

HYPOTHALAMUS

64. Which hypothalamic nucleus is most directly involved in regulating circadian rhythms?
    A. Anterior
    B. Arcuate
    C. Medial preoptic
    D. Suprachiasmatic

65. Which nucleus of the hypothalamus provides most of the innervation to preganglionic sympathetic neurons in the spinal cord?
    A. Anterior
    B. Lateral nucleus
    C. Paraventricular
    D. Supraoptic

NEUROANATOMY

ANSWERS

CORTEX

1. C

Primary motor cortex (Brodmann area 4) has a prominent layer V and contains the giant pyramidal cells of Betz.

The majority of the cortex is organized into six layers; together, they make up the neocortex. Layer V is called the large pyramidal layer or the internal pyramidal layer. The primary motor cortex has a relatively thicker layer V because of its projections to the brainstem, striatum, and spinal cord. Layers II and III are involved with cortical-cortical connections. Layer IV, the internal granular layer, receives information from the thalamus and is thickest in primary sensory cortices.

2. C

The pyramidal cells of the cerebral cortex use glutamate, which is excitatory.

Glycine, which is inhibitory, is predominantly found in the spinal cord.

3. A

Primary sensory cortex is Brodmann areas 3, 1, 2. This corresponds to the postcentral gyrus, which receives somatosensory input from the ventral posterolateral and ventral posteromedial nuclei of the thalamus.

Brodmann area 6 is premotor cortex.
Brodmann area 22 is Wernicke's area.
Brodmann areas 44 and 45 are Broca's area.

4. A

Bilateral lesions of the insular cortex can cause ageusia.

5. A

The supplementary motor area has its own smaller motor homunculus that is independent from primary motor cortex. Stimulation of the supplementary motor area can produce bilateral movement.

6. D

The transverse gyrus of Heschl is primary auditory cortex (Brodmann areas 41 and 42). Unilateral injury to the primary auditory cortex does *not* cause deafness.

7. A

The premotor cortex (Brodmann area 6) directs the activity of the primary motor cortex, assisting in reaching, grasping, and skilled movements. It lies anterior to the primary motor cortex (Brodmann area 4) on the lateral surface of the cerebral hemisphere. (The primary motor cortex is on the precentral gyrus.) Like the primary motor cortex, the premotor cortex contains a homunculus.

Orbitofrontal cortex is responsible for social behaviors, conscious perception of smell, and awareness of flavors. Lesions cause disinhibition and socially inappropriate behavior. Lesions can also cause poor olfactory discrimination.

The dorsolateral prefrontal cortex is involved in planning, judgment, problem-solving, and executive function.

The mesial frontal cortex and anterior cingulate gyrus are involved in motivation. Lesions cause abulia and reduced spontaneous movements. Patients may also have urinary incontinence and gait disturbance.

8. B

The frontal eye fields are located in the middle frontal gyrus.

CONNECTING SYSTEMS

9. B

The hippocampal commissure joins the hippocampi.

The stria terminalis and ventral amygdalofugal pathway connect the amygdala and hypothalamus.

The medial forebrain bundle connects the septal area and amygdala to the midbrain.

10. B

Commissures connect the two hemispheres, allowing information to travel from one hemisphere to the other. The largest commissure is the corpus callosum. Other commissures include the anterior, posterior, hippocampal, habenular, and supraoptic commissures.

11. C

The superior longitudinal fasciculus connects the frontal lobe with the temporal and occipital lobes.

Association fibers connect structures within one hemisphere. These fibers tend to arise from pyramidal cells in layers II and III of the cerebral cortex. The cingulum, inferior longitudinal fasciculus, superior longitudinal fasciculus, uncinate fasciculus, and occipitofrontal fasciculus are long association fibers (see Box 11.1).

Box 11.1 LONG ASSOCIATION FIBERS

- The uncinate fasciculus connects the inferior frontal lobe with the anterior temporal lobe.
- The cingulum, which is within the cingulate gyrus, connects the anterior perforated substance with the parahippocampal gyrus.
- The superior longitudinal fasciculus connects the frontal lobe with the temporal and occipital lobes.
- The inferior longitudinal fasciculus connects the temporal and occipital lobes.
- The occipitofrontal fasciculus connects the frontal lobe to the temporal and occipital lobes.

Projection fibers connect the cerebral cortex to subcortical structures, the brainstem, and the spinal cord.

U fibers are short association fibers that connect adjacent gyri.

LIMBIC SYSTEM

12. C

In the Papez circuit, the fornix carries information from the hippocampal formation to the mammillary bodies.

13. A

Input from vision, auditory, and somatosensory association cortex travels to the hippocampus by way of the entorhinal cortex. Also, olfactory input enters the hippocampus through the entorhinal cortex.

14. C

The nucleus accumbens, which is part of the ventral striatum, is involved in motivation, habits, and rewards. Dopamine is a key neurotransmitter in this process.

The amygdala is a limbic structure, but it is not part of the ventral striatum. In the amygdala, emotions are associated with stimuli. The amygdala has connections to the autonomic nervous system. Stimulation of the amygdala can cause fear.

The cingulate gyrus is a limbic structure, but it is not part of the ventral striatum.

The subthalamic nucleus is not a limbic structure.

BASAL GANGLIA

15. A

The main input to the basal ganglia is from the cerebral cortex, mainly the frontal lobe.

16. A

The caudate nucleus, putamen, and nucleus accumbens receive input to the basal ganglia.

The internal segment of the globus pallidus, ventral pallidum, and substantia nigra pars reticulata are output nuclei.

The substantia nigra pars compacta and ventral tegmental area are intrinsic nuclei, as are the external segment of the globus pallidus and intrinsic part of the ventral pallidum.

17. B

The basal ganglia direct pathway is the cortico-striato-pallidal pathway. In the direct pathway, the striatum sends projections to the globus pallidus internal segment and substantia nigra pars reticularis (GPi/SNr), which sends projections to the thalamus. The end result is excitation of the thalamus and ultimately the cortex.

The basal ganglia indirect pathway involves the globus pallidus externa (GPe) and then the subthalamic nucleus. This pathway is also known as the cortico-striato-GPe-subthalamo-GPi pathway.

18. A

Most of the output from the basal ganglia to the thalamus is to the medial dorsal, ventral lateral, and ventral anterior nuclei. The ventral lateral and ventral anterior nuclei send information to the motor cortex, premotor cortex, and supplementary motor area. Information from the medial dorsal nucleus travels to the prefrontal cortex.

19. B

The inner part of the globus pallidus (GPi) and the substantia nigra are the two major output nuclei of the basal ganglia. Motor information from the GPi travels to the ventral anterior and ventral lateral nuclei of the thalamus and then to the primary motor cortex.

20. B

The nucleus accumbens and adjacent portions of the caudate and putamen form the ventral striatum. These structures are involved in emotion.

The ansa lenticularis and the lenticular fasciculus are pathways between the internal segment of the globus pallidus and the thalamus.

Information travels from the ventral tegmental area to the striatum through the median forebrain bundle.

21. C

A lesion of the subthalamic nucleus can cause hemiballism.

BRAINSTEM

22.

1) C. Lesions of the lateral medulla cause ipsilateral hemiataxia, Horner syndrome, and loss of pain and temperature of the ipsilateral face and contralateral body.
2) A. Lesions of the medial midbrain cause contralateral hemiparesis and an ipsilateral CN 3 palsy.
3) D. Lesions of the medial medulla cause an ipsilateral CN 12 palsy and contralateral hemiparesis.

4) B. Lesions of the ventral pons cause a contralateral hemiparesis and an ipsilateral CN 6 palsy.

23. B

The corticospinal tract travels in the posterior limb of the internal capsule. A lesion here can cause a pure motor hemiparesis. Similarly, lesions of the corticospinal tract in the midbrain (cerebral peduncle), basis pontis, or medullary period can cause a pure motor hemiparesis.

24. C

Bilateral ventral pontine lesions, for instance those caused by basilar occlusion, are the most likely cause of locked-in syndrome.

25. A

Patients with locked-in syndrome have quadriplegia due to bilateral corticospinal tract lesions (secondary to involvement of the basis pontis). They also have inability to speak due to corticobulbar tract involvement and may have impaired horizontal eye movements due to CN 6 lesions. Vertical eye movements are intact, and the patient can blink. Somatosensory and reticular pathways are not affected.

26. E

Lesions of the medulla can cause neurogenic pulmonary edema, early satiety, inability to sneeze, and Ondine's curse.

Inability to sneeze is a rare finding in Wallenberg syndrome (lateral medullary syndrome) that is caused by involvement of the descending tract and spinal nucleus of the trigeminal nerve.

Lesions involving the nucleus ambiguus and reticular formation can cause Ondine' s curse, the lack of automatic breathing.

THALAMUS

27. B

In the Papez circuit, the mammillary bodies provide input to the anterior nucleus of the thalamus.

28. A

The anterior nucleus of the thalamus has input from the mammillary nucleus and projects to the cingulate gyrus in the Papez circuit.

In the Papez circuit, the fornix carries information from the hippocampal formation to the mammillary bodies, and the mammillothalamic tract connects the mammillary bodies and the anterior nucleus of the thalamus. Information then travels to the cingulate gyrus and finally back to the hippocampus via the entorhinal cortex.

29. C

The mediodorsal nucleus is injured in Wernicke-Korsakoff syndrome.

30.

1) C. The centromedian nucleus is involved in a feedback loop between the cortex and striatum. It receives input from the globus pallidus and premotor cortex and projects to the caudate and putamen.

2) D. The mediodorsal nucleus receives input from limbic structures and has reciprocal connections with the prefrontal cortex.

3) A. The pulvinar, which has reciprocal connections with parietal, temporal, and occipital cortex, is part of the extrageniculate visual pathway and is involved with visual attention.

4) B. The ventral lateral nucleus is a component of the dentarubrothalamic tract; it receives input from the substantia nigra, globus pallidus, and cerebellum and projects to the motor cortex.

5) F. The LGN sends information to the visual cortex.

6) E. The MGN is a relay station in the auditory pathway.

7) G. The reticular nucleus forms a thin layer around the lateral thalamus.

31. D

The reticular nucleus is involved in the generation of sleep spindles.

32. False

The thalamus integrates and relays information for all sensory modalities except olfaction.

33. D

The lateral geniculate nucleus (LGN), medial geniculate nucleus (MGN), ventral posterolateral (VPL) nucleus, and ventral posteromedial (VPM) nucleus are thalamic nuclei involved with sensation. The LGN is involved in vision, and the MGN is involved in hearing. The VPL nucleus is involved in limb sensation. The VPM nucleus is involved in taste sensation.

The ventral anterior and ventral lateral nuclei are involved with motor function.

The anterior and mediodorsal nuclei are involved with limbic functions.

CEREBELLUM

34. C

The cerebellum can be divided vertically into the vermis, paravermis, and cerebellar hemispheres.

The vermis coordinates truncal tone and movement.

The paravermis regulates limb movements. The paravermis is located just lateral to the vermis (in the medial cerebellar hemispheres).

The cerebellar hemispheres are involved in ipsilateral fine motor control.

35. B

The cerebellum can be divided horizontally into the anterior, posterior, and flocculonodular lobes.

The anterior lobe contains portions of the vermis and paravermis. It receives ipsilateral input from the spinal cord through the spinocerebellar pathways. (The cerebellum has ipsilateral connections with the body and spinal cord and contralateral connections with the cerebrum.)

The posterior lobe receives cerebrocortical information via the pons. The cerebellar hemispheres are in the posterior lobe.

The flocculonodular lobe, which consists of the flocculus and the nodulus (inferior vermis), receives vestibular input (see Table 11.1).

Table 11.1 CEREBELLAR ANATOMY

LOBE	ANATOMIC STRUCTURES IN THE LOBE	INPUT TO THE LOBE
Anterior	Vermis and paravermis	Spinocerebellar
Posterior	Cerebellar hemispheres	Cerebrocortical
Flocculonodular	Flocculus and nodulus (inferior vermis)	Vestibular

36. A

Patients with alcoholism tend to develop the rostral vermis syndrome, which affects the anterior lobe of the cerebellum. The syndrome is characterized by a wide-based gait and gait ataxia. The anterior lobe of the cerebellum receives the majority of the input from the spinocerebellar tracts.

The caudal vermis syndrome, which results from injury to the flocculonodular lobe, is characterized by truncal ataxia. Medulloblastoma is a cause of caudal vermis syndrome.

Cerebellar hemispheric syndrome is caused by lesions of the posterior lobe and is characterized by ataxia of ipsilateral appendicular movements (see Table 11.2).

37. C

The cerebellum has been divided into the spinocerebellum (also known as the paleocerebellum), the vestibulocerebellum (also known as the archicerebellum), and the

Table 11.2 CEREBELLAR LESIONS

LOBE	ANATOMIC STRUCTURES IN THE LOBE	SYNDROME CAUSED BY LESION OF THE LOBE
Anterior	Vermis and paravermis	Rostral vermis syndrome
Posterior	Cerebellar hemispheres	Cerebellar hemispheric syndrome
Flocculonodular	Flocculus and nodulus (inferior vermis)	Caudal vermis syndrome

cerebrocerebellum (also known as the neocerebellum or pontocerebellum).

The spinocerebellum/paleocerebellum corresponds to the anterior lobe. The vermis and paravermis are part of the spinocerebellum.

The vestibulocerebellum/archicerebellum corresponds to the flocculonodular lobe.

The cerebrocerebellum/neocerebellum corresponds to the posterior lobe. The lateral cerebellar hemispheres are part of the cerebrocerebellum. Due to its connections with the pons, it is also called the pontocerebellum. It is involved in planning and initiating movements and fine motor control.

The name of the vestibulocerebellum is derived from its vestibular connections. The flocculonodular lobe, which is in the vestibulocerebellum, receives information from and sends information to the vestibular nuclei. It is involved in maintaining body equilibrium and controlling eye movements. Lesions cause head and trunk tremor, truncal imbalance, and nystagmus (see Table 11.3).

38. A

The deep cerebellar nuclei of the cerebellum are the dentate, emboliform, globose, and fastigial nuclei.

The dentate nucleus, which is the most lateral of the deep nuclei, receives information from the cerebellar hemispheres and indirectly from the cortex. It sends information to ventral lateral and ventral anterior nuclei of the thalamus and impacts the corticobulbar and

Table 11.3 CLINICAL FINDINGS WITH CEREBELLAR LESIONS

LOBE	INPUT TO THE LOBE	ANATOMIC STRUCTURES IN THE LOBE	EFFECTS OF A LESION OF THE LOBE
Anterior (paleocerebellum, spinocerebellum)	Spinocerebellar tracts	Vermis and paravermis	Wide based gait, gait ataxia, dysmetria, dysdiadochokinesia, intention tremor
Posterior (neocerebellum, cerebrocerebellum, pPontocerebellum)	Cerebrocortical	Lateral cerebellar hemispheres	Delayed initiation or termination of movements, abnormal timing of movements, disturbance of skilled movements
Flocculonodular (archicerebellum, Vestibulocerebellum)	Vestibular	Flocculus and nodulus (inferior vermis)	Head and trunk tremor, truncal imbalance, nystagmus

corticospinal tracts. It is involved in motor planning and contributes to fine motor dexterity.

The dentate nucleus is part of the Guillain-Mollaret triangle, which is also known as the dentato-rubro-olivary pathway. Lesions in this pathway can cause palatal tremor.

The globose and emboliform nuclei, together known as the interposed nuclei, receive information from the paravermis. They send information to the red nucleus, the origin of the rubrospinal tract, which affects flexor tone.

The fastigial nucleus, which is the most medial of the deep nuclei, receives information from the vermis. It sends information to the reticular and vestibular nuclei and regulates the reticulospinal and vestibulospinal tracts (see Table 11.4).

Table 11.4 DEEP CEREBELLAR NUCLEI

NUCLEUS	STRUCTURE PROVIDING INPUT TO THE NUCLEUS	TRACTS REGULATED BY THE NUCLEUS
Fastigial	Vermis	Reticulospinal and vestibulospinal
Interposed (emboliform and globose)	Paravermis	Rubrospinal
Dentate	Lateral hemisphere	Corticospinal and corticobulbar

39. C

The superior cerebellar peduncle connects the cerebellum to the midbrain. The middle cerebellar peduncle connects the cerebellum to the pons. The inferior cerebellar peduncle connects the cerebellum to the medulla.

The superior cerebellar peduncle carries most of the output from the cerebellum. It contains fibers from the dentate, emboliform, and globose nuclei. Efferent fibers from the superior peduncle include the dentatorubral tract, the dentatothalamic tract, and the uncinate bundle of Russell.

40. A

Purkinje cells inhibit the deep cerebellar nuclei and are the major source of inhibitory output from the cerebellar cortex. Axons of some Purkinje cells project to vestibular nuclei.

41. A

Mossy fibers and climbing fibers provide input to the cerebellar cortex.

Climbing fibers travel from the inferior olive to the cerebellum. Climbing fibers, which are excitatory, make multiple synaptic contacts with a single Purkinje cell.

Mossy fibers excite granule cells which then excite multiple Purkinje cells.

Most types of cells (i.e., Purkinje, stellate, basket, and Golgi cells) in the cerebellar cortex are inhibitory. Granule cells are the exception.

CRANIAL NERVES

42. D

CN 4 has the longest intracranial course. It is the smallest cranial nerve. It is the only cranial nerve that decussates and the only one that exits the brainstem on the dorsal aspect. It innervates the superior oblique muscle, which is responsible for movement of the eye downward and inward.

43. A

V1 is the afferent limb of the corneal reflex. CN 7 is the efferent limb. The interneuron is the spinal nucleus of the trigeminal nerve.

The jaw-jerk reflex is mediated by the trigeminal nerve. When the lower jaw is tapped, the masseter and temporalis muscles contract. The 1a motor fibers in the mandibular division of the trigeminal nerve provide the afferent information. This information travels to the mesencephalic nucleus of the trigeminal nerve. The efferent limb is the mandibular fibers originating in the motor nucleus of the trigeminal nerve.

44. B

A cavernous sinus thrombosis is least likely to involve V3, which does not travel in the cavernous sinus.

The cavernous sinus syndrome can affect the abducens, trochlear, and oculomotor nerves as well as the V1 and V2 divisions of the trigeminal nerve (see Fig 11.1).

The abducens, trochlear, and oculomotor nerves and V1 travel through the superior orbital fissure.

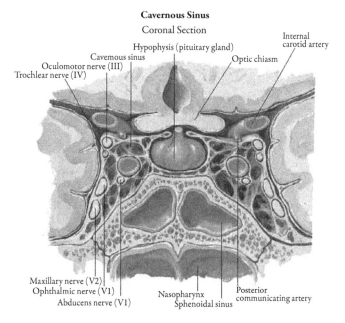

Figure 11.1 Relationship of cranial nerves within the cavernous sinus. (From Sundaram V, Barsam A, Alwitry A, Khaw P. *Training in Ophthalmology.* New York, Oxford University Press, 2009.)

45. A

The trigeminal nerve is responsible for *general sensation* from the anterior two thirds of the tongue. The facial nerve is responsible for *taste* from the anterior two thirds of the tongue.

The V3 division of the trigeminal nerve gives rise to the mandibular nerve, which exits the skull through the foramen ovale, and innervates the muscles of mastication. A branch of V3 becomes the lingual nerve, which provides tactile sensation to the lower gums and anterior two thirds of the tongue. V3 also gives rise to mental and inferior dental branches.

Taste sensation from the anterior two thirds of the tongue travels in the chorda tympani nerve to the geniculate ganglion.

The glossopharyngeal nerve provides taste and tactile sensation for the posterior one third of the tongue.

The vagus nerve is responsible for taste from the epiglottis and pharynx.

Information about taste travels through the cranial nerves (trigeminal, glossopharyngeal, and vagus) to the rostral solitary nucleus. Then it travels through the central tegmental tract to the ventral posteromedial (VPM) nucleus of the thalamus. Next, it travels to the insular cortex, posterior limb of the internal capsule, and operculum (gustatory cortex).

SPINAL CORD

46. C

This is Brown-Séquard syndrome, which results from hemicord lesions. Features of this syndrome include ipsilateral upper motor neuron-type weakness due to involvement of the corticospinal tract; ipsilateral loss of vibration sense and joint position due to involvement of the dorsal columns; and contralateral loss of pain and temperature sensation.

47. A

The dorsal and ventral spinocerebellar tracts are lateral within the spinal cord and are vulnerable to extrinsic lateral insults. They carry proprioceptive information from the lower extremities and trunk to the cerebellum.

The dorsal spinocerebellar tract arises from Clarke's nucleus, which extends from C8 to L2 in the spinal cord. It enters the cerebellum through the inferior cerebellar peduncle. It is an uncrossed tract.

The ventral spinocerebellar tract begins in the lumbar and sacral segments of the spinal cord. Most axons cross, but some do not. The tract enters the cerebellum through the superior cerebellar peduncle.

The lateral vestibulospinal tract provides extensor tone.

48. A

This patient has an anterior spinal artery infarct, which affects the anterior two thirds of the cord. The dorsal columns are spared, resulting in intact proprioception and vibration. There are multiple etiologies of anterior spinal artery infarction, one of which is aortic surgery. The anterior spinal artery, which arises from the vertebral arteries, receives blood from radicular arteries. The artery of Adamkiewicz, which is the largest radicular artery in the lower thoracic and upper lumbar region, can be injured during aortic surgery, resulting in anterior spinal artery infarction.

A cauda equina lesion involves the lumbosacral nerve roots below L2, not the spinal cord itself. The lesion causes radicular back pain and bilateral asymmetric leg weakness and sensory loss (all modalities). Later, there may be bladder involvement and impotence.

A conus medullaris lesion causes sensory loss in a saddle distribution. Bowel and bladder are involved early. (Poliomyelitis is discussed later.)

49. E

All of the conditions listed affect the posterior columns and corticospinal tracts, causing a posterolateral column syndrome. Patients have loss of vibration and proprioception, sensory ataxia, and a positive Romberg sign due to posterior column involvement and spastic paralysis due to involvement of the corticospinal tracts.

50. D

Poliomyelitis affects the anterior horn cells. It causes asymmetric weakness and muscle atrophy. Sensation is normal.

AIDS-associated myelopathy, tabes dorsalis, and posterior spinal infarcts affect the posterior columns.

51. A

This patient has syringomyelia, a cavity in the spinal cord, in the cervical region. A syrinx typically affects crossing spinothalamic fibers first, causing loss of pain and temperature in a cape-like distribution. (Loss of pain and temperature sensation with preservation of light touch, vibration, and proprioception is called dissociated sensory loss.) Anterior horn atrophy can cause weakness and muscle wasting. If the descending autonomic fibers are affected, the patient may have a Horner syndrome. Involvement of the corticospinal tracts results in spastic paraparesis with greater involvement of the legs than the arms.

Vitamin E deficiency affects the posterior columns, spinocerebellar tracts, and dorsal root ganglia.

Primary lateral sclerosis is an upper motor neuron disease. Sensation is normal.

Primary muscular atrophy is a lower motor neuron disease. Often, paraspinous or respiratory muscles are affected. Sensation is normal.

SPINAL ROOTS AND PERIPHERAL NERVES

52. B

C2 supplies sensation to the head through the greater and lesser occipital nerves.

53. C

A C5-C6 disc herniation usually affects the C6 nerve. The other statements are true.

54. D

This is a C8 radiculopathy. A C8 radiculopathy causes pain in the neck, shoulder, and ulnar part of the forearm. Sensory disturbance is in the fourth and fifth digits and the hypothenar eminence. Weakness is in the intrinsic hand muscles, finger extensors, and finger flexors. This could result from a C7-T1 disc herniation.

A C5 or C6 radiculopathy would affect the biceps and brachioradialis reflexes. A C7 radiculopathy would affect the triceps reflex.

55. C

The C8 nerve root exits above the T1 vertebral bone.

In the thoracic, lumbar, and sacral regions, the nerve roots exit below the same numbered vertebral bone (e.g., the T4 nerve root exits below the T4 vertebral bone).

In the cervical region, the nerve roots exit above the vertebral bone of the same number, except that C8 exits between the C7 and T1 vertebral bones. There is no C8 vertebral bone.

56. B

The small head of the biceps femoris is the muscle above the knee that is supplied by the peroneal division of the sciatic nerve.

57. True

In the peripheral nervous system, foot drop can be caused by lesions of the deep peroneal nerve, common peroneal nerve, sciatic nerve, lumbosacral plexus, or the L5 nerve root. Foot eversion and inversion are intact if the lesion involves only the deep peroneal nerve. Weakness of ankle inversion indicates that the lesion also affects the tibial nerve, which is a branch of the sciatic nerve with L5 innervation. If a patient has foot drop and ankle inversion weakness, the lesion involves the sciatic nerve, lumbosacral plexus, or the L5 nerve root.

(To accurately assess the strength of ankle inversion in a patient with foot drop, the foot should be dorsiflexed while testing inversion.)

58. C

The radial nerve gives rise to the posterior interosseus nerve. Lesions of the posterior interosseous nerve cause fingerdrop.

CEREBROSPINAL FLUID AND THE VENTRICULAR SYSTEM

59. C

The choroid plexus produces CSF at a rate of 20 mL/hr, which is about 500 mL/day.

60. A

CSF is absorbed from the subarachnoid space into the blood by arachnoid granulations.

CSF is produced by the choroid plexus. It then flows into the lateral ventricles. Next, it travels through the foramen of Monro into the third ventricle. CSF travels from the third ventricle to the fourth ventricle through the Sylvian aqueduct. It then exits the fourth ventricle through the foramina of Luschka and Magendie and travels into the subarachnoid space, where it is absorbed by arachnoid granulations.

BLOOD-BRAIN BARRIER

61. D

The blood-brain barrier results from the presence of tight junctions that link capillary endothelial cells in the brain.

62. B

Areas of the brain where the blood-brain barrier is interrupted are called circumventricular organs (see Box 11.2).

Box 11.2 CIRCUMVENTRICULAR ORGANS

- Subfornical organ
- Median eminence
- Neurohypophysis
- Vascular organ of lamina terminalis
- Pineal body
- Area postrema

63. B

The area postrema, which is one of the circumventricular organs, is known as the chemotactic trigger zone because it detects toxins that cause vomiting. It is located at the caudal aspect of the fourth ventricle. It has a high density of dopamine neurons, particularly D2 receptors. Medications that block dopamine D2 receptors prevent vomiting.

HYPOTHALAMUS

64. D

The suprachiasmatic nucleus, which is in the anterior hypothalamus, receives input from retinal ganglion cells via the retinohypothalamic tract. It acts as a circadian clock, regulating circadian rhythms. Release of γ-aminobutyric acid (GABA) from the suprachiasmatic nucleus inhibits melatonin release from the pineal gland.

Neurons in the arcuate nucleus secrete growth hormone-releasing hormone (GHRH). Neurons that secrete dopamine are also present in the arcuate nucleus.

Neurons in the medial preoptic nucleus secrete gonadotropin-releasing hormone.

(The anterior nucleus is discussed later.)

65. C

The anterior nucleus affects temperature and stimulates the parasympathetic nervous system.

The lateral nucleus affects appetite.

The paraventricular nucleus provides most of the innervation to preganglionic sympathetic neurons.

The supraoptic and paraventricular nuclei contain neurons that secrete oxytocin and vasopressin into the posterior pituitary.

12.

NEUROCHEMISTRY

QUESTIONS

1. **Which of the following structures provides most of the cortical cholinergic projections?**
   A. Basal nucleus of Meynert
   B. Pedunculopontine nucleus
   C. Substantia nigra pars compacta
   D. Substantia nigra pars reticulata

2. **What is the rate-limiting factor in acetylcholine synthesis?**
   A. Amount of choline
   B. Availability of choline acetyltransferase
   C. Availability of acetyl-CoA

3. **Which of the following causes increased acetylcholine release?**
   A. Botulism
   B. Lambert-Eaton syndrome
   C. Tick paralysis
   D. Black widow spider venom (latrotoxin)
   E. Curare

4. **True or False?**
   Muscarinic receptors are more common in the brain than nicotinic receptors.

5. **What is the result of depolarization of the nicotinic receptor?**
   A. Activation of adenyl cyclase
   B. Activation of phospholipase
   C. Increased chloride conductance
   D. Increased sodium conductance

6. **Monoamine oxidase (MAO) and catechol-*O*-methyltransferase (COMT) convert which of these neurotransmitters to homovanillic acid (HVA)?**
   A. Norepinephrine
   B. Epinephrine
   C. Dopamine
   D. Serotonin

7. **In the synthesis of dopamine, what is the rate-limiting enzyme?**
   A. Dopamine β-hydroxylase
   B. Dopa decarboxylase
   C. MAO types A and B
   D. Tyrosine hydroxylase

8. **In which structure is norepinephrine most prevalent?**
   A. Dorsal raphe nuclei
   B. Hypothalamus

C. Locus ceruleus
   D. Nucleus basalis of Meynert

9. **True or False?**
   There is no reuptake mechanism for epinephrine.

10. **Dopamine excess results in the positive symptoms of schizophrenia through which of these pathways?**
    A. Mesocortical pathway
    B. Mesolimbic pathway
    C. Nigrostriatal pathway
    D. Tuberoinfundibular pathway

11. **Dopamine excess results in tardive dyskinesia through which of these pathways?**
    A. Mesocortical pathway
    B. Mesolimbic pathway
    C. Nigrostriatal pathway
    D. Tuberoinfundibular pathway

12. **Which of the following is *not* derived from tyrosine?**
    A. Norepinephrine
    B. Epinephrine
    C. Dopamine
    D. Serotonin

13. **Where is serotonin produced?**
    A. Locus ceruleus
    B. Medial forebrain bundle
    C. Nucleus accumbens
    D. Raphe nuclei

14. **Where are serotonin receptors *least* likely to be found?**
    A. Heart
    B. Gastrointestinal tract
    C. Platelets
    D. Sexual organs

15. **At which serotonin receptor does ondansetron act?**
    A. 5-HT1a
    B. 5-HT1b/d
    C. 5-HT2a
    D. 5-HT3

16. **Fenfluramine, meperidine, and reserpine all can contribute to serotonin syndrome. What is the mechanism?**
    A. Increased serotonin release
    B. Decreased serotonin metabolism
    C. Inhibition of serotonin reuptake
    D. They are direct serotonin receptor agonists.

17. **γ-Aminobutyric acid (GABA) is synthesized from which of the following?**

A. Glutamate
B. Glycine
C. Tyrosine
D. Tryptophan

18. Which of the following is *not* a binding site on the GABA-A receptor?
   A. Barbiturate site
   B. Glycine site
   C. Steroid site
   D. Picrotoxin site

19. Which of the following is an agonist of the GABA-B receptor?
   A. Baclofen
   B. Clobazam
   C. Lorazepam
   D. Phenobarbital

20. Which of the following is synthesized from arginine?
   A. Adenosine
   B. Histamine
   C. Nitric oxide
   D. Taurine

21. Which of the following is an excitatory neurotransmitter?
   A. Aspartate
   B. GABA
   C. Glycine
   D. Taurine

22. What type of cell is responsible for most of the reuptake of glutamate?
   A. Astrocytes
   B. Ependymal cells
   C. Oligodendrocytes
   D. Neurons

23. Which receptor is ligand gated and voltage sensitive?
   A. α-Amino-3-hydroxyl-5-methyl-4-isoxazole-propionate (AMPA) receptor
   B. Histamine H1 receptor
   C. Kainate receptor
   D. *N*-methyl-D-aspartate (NMDA) receptor

24. Which of the following is an obligatory co-agonist to the NMDA receptor?
   A. Adenosine
   B. Calcium
   C. Glycine
   D. Magnesium

25. Fill in the blank: Activation of NMDA receptors requires removal of the _____ block.
   A. Calcium
   B. Magnesium
   C. Potassium
   D. Sodium

26. L-Aromatic amino acid decarboxylase, glutamic acid decarboxylase, and GABA transaminase require which of the following as a cofactor?
   A. Copper
   B. Oxygen
   C. Vitamin B6
   D. Vitamin C

27. Which of the following diseases is associated with reduced levels of glycine in the spinal cord and is treated with benzodiazepines?
   A. Hyperekplexia
   B. Stiff-person syndrome
   C. Paroxysmal kinesigenic dyskinesia
   D. Neuromyotonia

28. Which of the following is an antagonist of the glycine receptor?
   A. Bicuculline
   B. Picrotoxin
   C. Strychnine
   D. Succinic acid

29. Some patients with Rasmussen encephalitis have antibodies to which of these receptors?
   A. GABA-A
   B. GABA-B
   C. Glutamate
   D. Glycine

30. Long-term potentiation and long-term depression are dependent on which receptor?
   A. Acetylcholine
   B. GABA
   C. Glycine
   D. NMDA

31. Which of the following structures has the highest concentration of histamine?
   A. Locus ceruleus
   B. Dorsal raphe nuclei
   C. Nucleus basalis of Meynert
   D. Hypothalamus

32. Which of the following is *not* a function of astrocytes?
   A. Uptake glutamate and convert it to glutamine
   B. Maintain the normal concentration of potassium in the brain
   C. Guide migrating neurons during embryonic development
   D. Contribute to the blood-brain barrier
   E. React to injury by causing gliosis
   F. All of the above are functions of astrocytes

33. Which of the following is the precursor of cholesterol and fatty acids?
   A. Acetyl coenzyme A
   B. Mevalonic acid
   C. Phosphatidic acid

NEUROCHEMISTRY

ANSWERS

1. A

The basal nucleus of Meynert is the source of most cortical cholinergic projections. Patients with Alzheimer disease have loss of neurons in this region.

2. A

Acetylcholine (ACh) is synthesized from choline and acetyl-coenzyme A (acetyl-CoA) by choline acetyltransferase. The amount of choline is the rate-limiting factor.

ACh is degraded in the synaptic cleft by acetylcholinesterase. It is broken down into choline and acetate. Reuptake of choline occurs at the presynaptic terminal.

3. D

Black widow spider venom (latrotoxin) increases acetylcholine (ACh) release.

Curare blocks the ACh receptor. Quinine and procainamide also block or inactivate the ACh receptor.

Botulism, Lambert-Eaton syndrome, and tick paralysis are associated with decreased ACh release.

4. True

Muscarinic receptors are more common in the brain than nicotinic receptors. The M1 subtype of muscarinic receptors is the most common subtype in the central nervous system. It is found in the cerebral cortex, hippocampus, striatum, and thalamus at postsynaptic locations. In the peripheral nervous system, postganglionic parasympathetic terminals and postganglionic sympathetic sweat glands have muscarinic receptors.

The neuromuscular junction and adrenal medulla have nicotinic receptors.

5. D

Nicotinic receptors are ligand-gated ion channels. Depolarization of the nicotinic receptor results in increased sodium conductance.

Mutations in the nicotinic receptor have been found in patients with autosomal dominant nocturnal frontal lobe epilepsy (ADNFLE). These patients tend to respond well to oxcarbazepine and carbamazepine, which are sodium channel blockers.

The muscarinic acetylcholine receptor is a G protein-coupled receptor.

6. C

MAO and COMT convert dopamine to homovanillic acid.

Dopamine β-hydroxylase converts dopamine to norepinephrine (see Table 12.1).

Table 12.1 NEUROTRANSMITTER BREAKDOWN PRODUCTS

NEUROTRANSMITTER	BREAKDOWN PRODUCT
Dopamine	Homovanillic acid (HVA)
Serotonin	5-Hydroxyindoleacetic acid (5-HIAA)
Norepinephrine	Vanillylmandelic acid (VMA)

7. D

Conversion of tyrosine to L-dopa by tyrosine hydroxylase is the rate-limiting step in synthesis of dopamine. L-Dopa is then converted to dopamine by dopa decarboxylase.

Tyrosine hydroxylase deficiency causes a dopa-responsive dystonia (DYT5b).

8. C

Norepinephrine is most prevalent in the locus ceruleus.

9. True

Epinephrine is synthesized from norepinephrine by phenylethanolamine *N*-methyltransferase, which is found in certain neurons and in the adrenal medulla. There is no reuptake mechanism for epinephrine. It is broken down by MAO and COMT to vanillylmandelic acid (VMA).

10. B

There are four major dopamine pathways: mesolimbic, mesocortical, nigrostriatal, and tuberoinfundibular. It is thought that dopamine excess in the mesolimbic tract causes the positive symptoms of schizophrenia.

11. C

It is thought that dopamine excess in the nigrostriatal tract causes tardive dyskinesia.

Dopamine neurons in the tuberoinfundibular pathway prevent prolactin secretion. These neurons project from the hypothalamus to the anterior pituitary. Antipsychotics that block dopamine receptors can result in hyperprolactinemia because of this pathway.

12. D

Serotonin is derived from tryptophan.

Norepinephrine, epinephrine, and dopamine are derived from tyrosine.

13. D

Serotonin is produced in the raphe nuclei. Raphe neurons project through the medial forebrain bundle to multiple areas (i.e., frontal cortex, hippocampus, hypothalamus, striatum, and thalamus).

In the pineal gland, serotonin is converted to melatonin.

14. A

Serotonin receptors are least likely to be found in the heart. They are found in the gastrointestinal tract, platelets, and sexual organs.

15. D

Ondansetron is a 5-HT3 antagonist. The 5-HT3 receptor is in the area postrema/chemotactic trigger zone. Stimulation of this receptor causes projectile vomiting. Most serotonin receptors are G protein coupled; however, the 5HT-3 receptor is ligand gated.

Buspirone is a 5-HT1a receptor agonist.

Triptans are agonists at 5-HT1b/d receptors.

The 5-HT2a receptor is one of the receptors where hallucinogens such as lysergic acid diethylamide (LSD) act. Some atypical antipsychotics, such as risperidone, are antagonists to this receptor.

16. A

Fenfluramine, meperidine, and reserpine cause increased serotonin release.

17. A

GABA is synthesized from glutamate by glutamic acid decarboxylase (GAD). GABA is metabolized by GABA transaminase. Vigabatrin inhibits GABA transaminase, causing an increase in GABA.

18. B

There is no glycine binding site on the GABA A receptor. There is a glycine binding site on the NMDA receptor (see Box 12.1).

Muscimol is an agonist and bicuculline is an antagonist at the GABA binding site on the GABA-A receptor.

Picrotoxin, which is a chloride channel blocker, is a noncompetitive antagonist of GABA.

Bicuculline and picrotoxin are used in models of epilepsy.

Box 12.1 POSSIBLE BINDING SITES ON THE GABA-A RECEPTOR

- GABA
- Barbiturate
- Benzodiazepine
- Picrotoxin
- Steroid
- Volatile anesthetic

Benzodiazepines, barbiturates, anesthetics, and neurosteroids act at allosteric modulatory sites on the GABA-A receptor.

Zolpidem and zaleplon are nonbenzodiazepines that bind to the benzodiazepine site.

19. A

Baclofen is an agonist of the GABA-B receptor.

Clobazam, lorazepam, and phenobarbital all act at the GABA-A receptor.

20. C

Nitric oxide, a signaling molecule in the brain, is synthesized from arginine.

21. A

Aspartate is an excitatory neurotransmitter. GABA, glycine, and taurine are inhibitory neurotransmitters.

22. A

Astrocytes are responsible for glutamate reuptake. In the astrocyte, glutamate may be converted to glutamine, which may be exported to the extracellular space and then transferred to neurons.

23. D

The NMDA receptor is ligand gated and voltage sensitive.

24. C

The NMDA receptor has binding sites for glutamate and glycine. Glycine is an obligatory co-agonist to the NMDA receptor.

There is also a polyamine binding site on the NMDA receptor.

25. B

Activation of the NMDA receptor requires binding of glutamate and glycine, depolarization, and removal of the magnesium block. Magnesium is a voltage-dependent blocker. When depolarization occurs, the block is removed. Zinc also decreases flow through the NMDA receptor.

Calcium and sodium flow through the open NMDA receptor channel. Among the glutamate receptors (i.e.,

AMPA, kainate, and NMDA), the NMDA receptor is the most permeable to calcium.

The mushroom *Amanita muscaria* contains a NMDA receptor agonist. There are a number of NMDA receptor antagonists (see Box 12.2).

Box 12.2 NMDA RECEPTOR ANTAGONISTS

- Amantadine
- Dextromethorphan
- Felbamate
- Ketamine
- Memantine
- Phencyclidine (PCP)

---

26. C

L-Aromatic amino acid decarboxylase, glutamic acid decarboxylase (GAD), and GABA transaminase require vitamin B6 as a cofactor.

L-Aromatic amino acid decarboxylase deficiency manifests in infancy with developmental delay, abnormal tone (truncal hypotonia and limb hypertonia), choreoathetosis, and oculogyric crises. Patients may also have autonomic dysfunction.

GAD converts glutamic acid to GABA.

GABA transaminase metabolizes GABA (to succinic semialdehyde).

27. A

Hyperekplexia is associated with reduced glycine levels in the spinal cord.

Glutamic acid decarboxylase (GAD) antibodies are found in patients with stiff-person syndrome.

Paroxysmal kinesigenic dyskinesia can be caused by mutations in the *PRRT2* gene.

Potassium channel antibodies have been found in some patients with neuromyotonia.

28. C

Strychnine is an antagonist of the glycine receptor. It can be found in rat poison. It causes muscle spasms that can result in rhabdomyolysis.

29. C

Some patients with Rasmussen encephalitis have antibodies to the glutamate receptor.

30. D

Long-term potentiation and long-term depression are dependent on the NMDA receptor.

31. D

The highest concentration of histamine is in the hypothalamus. Specifically, histaminergic neurons are found in the lateral tuberomammillary nucleus of the hypothalamus. Histamine is synthesized from histidine.

Norepinephrine is found in the locus ceruleus.

Serotonin is found in the dorsal raphe nuclei.

Acetylcholine is found in the nucleus basalis of Meynert.

32. F

Astrocytes are important in potassium homeostasis. They are characterized by large negative membrane potentials which allow them to buffer extracellular potassium. Astrocytes also help to buffer extracellular pH.

33. A

Acetyl coenzyme A is the precursor of cholesterol and fatty acids. It is a two-carbon donor.

In cholesterol synthesis, two acetyl-CoA molecules are condensed to form acetoacetyl-CoA. This is condensed with another acetyl-CoA molecule to form 3-hydroxy-3-methylglutaryl-coenzyme A (HMG-CoA). HMG-CoA is converted to mevalonic acid by HMG-CoA reductase, which is the rate-limiting enzyme in cholesterol synthesis.

The rate-limiting step in fatty acid synthesis is conversion of acetyl-CoA into malonyl-CoA by acetyl-CoA carboxylase. Excess acetyl-CoA is converted into fatty acids.

Phosphatidic acid is the precursor of glycerolipids, which are derivatives of glycerol and fatty acids.

13.

NEUROGENETICS

QUESTIONS

1. A child is diagnosed with a disease. None of her three siblings have the disease, but two are found to be carriers. Neither of her parents has the disease. (Their carrier status was not tested.) What is the mode of inheritance?
   A. Autosomal dominant
   B. Autosomal recessive
   C. X-linked recessive
   D. X-linked dominant

2. Which of the following is *not* an autosomal dominant disorder?
   A. Achondroplasia
   B. Kennedy disease
   C. Neurofibromatosis type 2
   D. Tuberous sclerosis complex

3. Which of the following is *not* an X-linked recessive disorder?
   A. Duchenne muscular dystrophy
   B. Lesch-Nyhan disease
   C. Menkes disease
   D. Ornithine transcarbamoylase deficiency
   E. Phenylketonuria

4. What is the most common mode of inheritance of intellectual disability?
   A. Autosomal dominant
   B. Autosomal recessive
   C. X-linked

5. Which of the following diseases is *not* X-linked dominant?
   A. Aicardi syndrome
   B. Fabry disease
   C. Incontinentia pigmenti
   D. Rett syndrome

6. A child develops a disease at age 2 years and has severe symptoms. His father began having similar symptoms when he was 20 years old, and his symptoms are not severe. The child's grandfather was found to have the disease at age 75 years but has minimal symptoms. What is the term used for worsening symptoms with each generation?
   A. Anticipation
   B. Expressivity
   C. Imprinting
   D. Penetrance

7. What is the term for a disease that is caused by a combination of genetic and environmental factors?
   A. Complex trait
   B. Polygenic disease
   C. Pseudodominant inheritance
   D. Endophenotype
   E. Compound heterozygote

8. Which of the following is *not* a mitochondrial disease?
   A. Chronic progressive external ophthalmoplegia
   B. Leber hereditary optic neuropathy
   C. Neurogenic muscle weakness, ataxia, and retinitis pigmentosa
   D. Myoneuro-gastrointestinal encephalopathy
   E. Nonketotic hyperglycinemia

9. Which of the following statements is *false*?
   A. Mitochondrial diseases may demonstrate autosomal recessive inheritance.
   B. Heteroplasmy plays a role in mitochondrial disease.
   C. The same mitochondrial DNA (mtDNA) sequence may occur in patients with different diseases.
   D. Patients with the same mitochondrial disease may have different mtDNA mutations.
   E. Mitochondrial diseases often have strong penetrance.

10. Which of the following diseases is *not* caused by a trinucleotide repeat?
    A. Joubert syndrome
    B. Kennedy disease
    C. Fragile X syndrome
    D. Dentatorubral-pallidoluysian atrophy (DRPLA)

11. Which of the following diseases is caused by a GAA triplet repeat expansion?
    A. Friedreich ataxia
    B. Huntington disease
    C. Myotonic dystrophy type 1
    D. Oculopharyngeal muscular dystrophy

12. Which of the following diseases is caused by expansion of a tetranucleotide repeat?
    A. Facioscapulohumeral muscular dystrophy (FSHD)
    B. Machado-Joseph disease
    C. Myotonic dystrophy type 2
    D. Spinocerebellar ataxia type 10

13. Which of the following diseases is caused by expansion of a hexanucleotide repeat?
    A. Unverricht-Lundborg disease
    B. Chromosome 9p-linked frontotemporal dementia (FTD) and amyotrophic lateral sclerosis (ALS)

C. Spinocerebellar ataxia type 1

D. Spinocerebellar ataxia type 8

14. Which of the following diseases is *not* a channelopathy?

A. Cerebral autosomal dominant arteriopathy with subcortical infarcts and leukoencephalopathy (CADASIL)

B. Episodic ataxia type1

C. Episodic ataxia type 2

D. Familial hemiplegic migraine

E. Hyperekplexia

15. In a child with global developmental delay, which of the following should be performed first if no specific etiology is suspected?

A. Chromosomal microarray

B. Plasma amino acids and urine organic acids

C. Ammonia level

D. Karyotype

16. In which of the following diseases does imprinting *not* occur?

A. Prader-Willi syndrome

B. Myoclonus dystonia syndrome (dystonia 11)

C. Beckwith-Wiedemann syndrome

D. Russell-Silver syndrome

E. Huntington disease

17. In which of the following conditions is anticipation *least* likely to occur?

A. Dentatorubral-pallidoluysian atrophy

B. Fragile X syndrome

C. Spinocerebellar ataxia type 1

D. Spinocerebellar ataxia type 6

18a. A 2-year-old girl is brought to the clinic because of developmental delay. The family reports that she has no speech and does not sleep well but is very happy. On examination, she is laughing and drooling. She has a broad mouth with widely-spaced teeth. She is microcephalic, hypotonic, and ataxic. a. What other condition is common in this syndrome?

A. Epilepsy

B. Prolonged QT interval

C. Cardiac defects

D. Hypocalcemia

b. Where is the genetic defect in most patients with this syndrome?

A. Chromosome 5q

B. Chromosome 7q

C. Chromosome 15q

D. Chromosome 22q

19. A 7-year-old boy presents with school difficulties and behavior problems. The parents report temper tantrums and excessive eating. They say that he had difficulties feeding as a neonate but now he won't stop. They put a lock on the refrigerator at night to prevent him from eating. Although he's having learning difficulties, he is excellent at putting puzzles together. On examination, he is obese, has almond-shaped eyes, and has small hands and feet. Which test is most likely to yield the diagnosis?

A. Testing for expansion of CGG repeats on the X chromosome

B. Methylation analysis at 5′ *SNRPN* (small nuclear ribonucleoprotein polypeptide N)

C. Testing for expansion of CTG repeats in *DMPK*

D. Testing for Williams-Beuren syndrome critical region (WBSCR)

20. Which of the following disorders is *least* likely to occur in Down syndrome?

A. Moyamoya syndrome

B. Atlanto-axial subluxation

C. Obstructive sleep apnea

D. Infantile spasms

E. Peripheral neuropathy

21. An 8-year-old girl presents with school difficulties. The parents report no social problems. She is gregarious and empathetic. However, she's unable to do the work the other children are doing. She has a good short-term memory but significant problems with visuospatial skills. Her past medical history is remarkable for supravalvular aortic stenosis and hypercalcemia. What is the most likely diagnosis?

A. Angelman syndrome

B. DiGeorge syndrome

C. Turner syndrome

D. Williams syndrome

22. An 11-year-old boy is brought to the clinic because of difficulties in school. The teacher thinks he has autism. His mother states that she was diagnosed with a learning disability. The family history is remarkable for a maternal grandfather with intention tremor and gait unsteadiness. On examination, the boy has a long face and protuberant ears. What is the diagnosis?

A. Fragile X syndrome

B. Klinefelter syndrome

C. 47,XYY syndrome

D. Sotos syndrome

23. A 2-year-old girl presents with loss of developmental milestones. The parents said she was developing normally until 18 months of age. Then her speech decreased, and it is now nonexistent. She no longer plays with toys; instead, she wrings her hands. A defect in which of the following genes is most likely responsible?

A. *MECP2*

B. *UBE3A*

C. *ELN*

D. *CDKL5*

24. An infant with a submucosal cleft palate, hypotonia, and tetralogy of Fallot develops seizures. Laboratory studies show hypocalcemia. Which diagnosis is most likely?

A. Trisomy 21

B. DiGeorge syndrome

C. Prader-Willi syndrome

D. Congenital myotonic dystrophy

NEUROGENETICS

1. B

This disease is an autosomal recessive condition. Twenty-five percent of the children in this family have the disease, 50% are carriers, and 25% are healthy. If tested, both parents would be found to be carriers. In autosomal recessive conditions, genes from both parents at a particular locus must be mutated to cause the disease. Both genders are equally affected. Autosomal recessive conditions are more likely in consanguineous unions. A recessive trait that is common, such as blood type O, can result in what appears to be a dominant inheritance pattern.

If this were an autosomal dominant disease, one of the parents would have the disease, and 50% of the children would be affected. Only one copy of the mutation would be needed to express the trait. Both genders are equally affected in autosomal dominant diseases.

A mother carrying an X-linked recessive disease will pass the affected X chromosome to 50% of her sons; therefore, half of her sons will be affected by the disease. The mother is usually an asymptomatic carrier. A female may be affected due to non-random X-inactivation or if her father has the condition and her mother is a carrier.

X-linked dominant diseases usually affect males more severely than females. In some X-linked dominant diseases, affected males do not survive to birth. Each child of an affected female has a 50% chance of having the condition, regardless of gender. In the case of an affected male, all of his daughters but none of his sons will be affected.

In X-linked conditions, there is no male-to-male transmission. There can be an appearance of male-to-male transmission in the unusual circumstance in which an affected male has a child with a carrier female.

2. B

Spinobulbar muscular atrophy, also known as Kennedy disease, is X-linked recessive.

Tuberous sclerosis complex, neurofibromatosis type 1, neurofibromatosis type 2, and achondroplasia are autosomal dominant.

3. E

Phenylketonuria is autosomal recessive.

Lesch-Nyhan disease, Menkes disease, ornithine transcarbamoylase deficiency, and Duchenne muscular dystrophy are X-linked recessive. Adrenoleukodystrophy and Pelizaeus-Merzbacher disease are also X-linked recessive.

4. C

If inherited, intellectual disability most often is inherited in an X-linked pattern.

5. B

Fabry disease is X-linked recessive.

Aicardi disease, incontinentia pigmenti, and Rett syndrome are X-linked dominant.

6. A

This is anticipation, which occurs in some triplet repeat diseases, such as Huntington disease and myotonic dystrophy type 1. Subsequent generations have more copies of the triplet repeat, which is associated with more severe disease and an earlier presentation.

Oculopharyngeal muscular dystrophy is a triplet repeat disease that does *not* demonstrate anticipation. It is caused by mutations in the gene *PABPN1*. Originally, the disease was said to be a GCG triplet repeat disease. However, GCA, GCT, GCC, and GCG all encode alanine; therefore, it is now referred to as a GCN repeat ("N" indicates any base).

7. A

A disease that is caused by a combination of genetic and environmental factors is a complex trait. Examples include Alzheimer disease, Parkinson disease, stroke, migraine, multiple sclerosis (MS), amyotrophic lateral sclerosis (ALS), and restless leg syndrome (RLS).

Polygenic diseases are diseases caused by multiple genes. One example is cleft palate.

Pseudodominant inheritance is the term for a condition that gives the appearance of being an autosomal dominant disease but is not. For instance, an autosomal recessive condition that occurs in multiple generations can demonstrate pseudodominant inheritance. This may result from a high carrier frequency, or it may occur if the parents are genetically related.

An endophenotype is a characteristic that is associated with a condition but does not result from that condition.

A compound heterozygote is an individual who has two different abnormal alleles at a specific locus, one on each chromosome of a pair. This can be seen in autosomal recessive conditions.

8. E

Nonketotic hyperglycinemia is not a mitochondrial disease (see Box 13.1).

Box 13.1 MITOCHONDRIAL DISEASES

- Chronic progressive external ophthalmoplegia
- Kearns-Sayre syndrome
- Leber hereditary optic neuropathy (LHON)
- Leigh syndrome
- Myoclonic epilepsy and ragged red fibers
- Mitochondrial encephalomyopathy, lactic acidosis, and stroke-like episodes (MELAS)
- Neurogenic muscle weakness, ataxia, and retinitis pigmentosa (NARP)
- Myoneuro-gastrointestinal encephalopathy (MNGIE)

For unclear reasons, Leber hereditary optic neuropathy (LHON) affects males more than females.

Mutations in both nuclear- and mitochondrial-encoded genes can cause Leigh syndrome. The most common cause is a defect in complex IV (cytochrome *c* oxidase, also known as COX). The most common cause of COX-deficient Leigh syndrome is a mutation in *SURF1*.

Most cases of MELAS (mitochondrial encephalopathy, lactic acidosis, and stroke-like episodes) are caused by mutations in *MT-TL1* (transfer RNA mitochondrial, leucine 1).

9. E

Mitochondrial diseases often have reduced penetrance.

Heteroplasmy occurs when there are both normal mitochondria and mitochondria with mutant DNA within a cell. A mother passes on her mutant mtDNA, but her children have different amounts of the mutant mtDNA, and the amount also varies in different organs of the same individual. In addition, the proportion of mutant mitochondria can change with time.

If a disease results from a mutation in the mitochondrial genome, the disease demonstrates matrilineal inheritance because males do not pass mitochondria to their children. However, mitochondria also use some proteins that have been encoded by nuclear DNA. Defects in these proteins can cause diseases that follow nonmatrilineal inheritance patterns.

Genotype-phenotype correlations are poor with mitochondrial diseases. A mtDNA sequence may occur in patients with different diseases, and patients with the same mitochondrial disease may have different mtDNA mutations.

10. A

Joubert syndrome is not a trinucleotide disease.

In Kennedy disease, the triplet repeat is CAG. In fragile X syndrome, the triplet repeat is CGG. In dentatorubral-pallidoluysian atrophy (DRPLA), the triplet repeat is CAG (see Table 13.1).

Table 13.1 SELECTED TRIPLET REPEAT DISEASES

DISEASE	TRIPLET REPEAT
Dentatorubral-pallidoluysian atrophy (DRPLA)	CAG
Fragile X syndrome	CGG
Kennedy disease	CAG

11. A

Friedreich ataxia (FRDA) is caused by a GAA triplet repeat expansion. It results from mutations in the *FXN* (formerly *FRDA*) gene on chromosome 9q. Mutations in this gene cause decreased production of frataxin, which acts as a mitochondrial iron chaperone.

Huntington disease is caused by an expansion of the CAG triplet repeat in the gene *HTT* on chromosome 4. It is autosomal dominant.

Myotonic dystrophy type 1 is caused by expansion of the CTG repeat in the *DMPK* gene on chromosome 19. It is autosomal dominant.

Oculopharyngeal muscular dystrophy is caused by expansion of the triplet repeat GCN ("N" indicates any base) in the gene *PABPN1*, which encodes the polyadenylate binding protein nuclear 1.

12. C

Myotonic dystrophy type 2, which has also been called proximal myotonic myopathy (PROMM), is a tetranucleotide repeat disease. The repeat is CCTG. The mutated gene is *ZNF9* on chromosome 3, which encodes zinc finger protein 9. (This gene has also been called *CNBP*.)

Machado-Joseph disease, also known as spinocerebellar ataxia type 3 (SCA3), is due to an abnormal CAG repeat expansion in the gene *ATXN3*.

Spinocerebellar ataxia type 10 (SCA10) is a pentanucleotide repeat disease (ATTCT).

Most cases of FSHD result from a *contraction* mutation of *D4Z4* on chromosome 4, resulting in fewer repeats than normal. In addition, a permissive simple sequence length polymorphism and the 4qA variant at the terminus must be present for the disease to manifest clinically. The result of the combination of these genetic features is hypomethylation of the D4Z4 region. This region contains the *DUX4* gene, which encodes double homeobox protein 4 (DUX4). These mutations cause FSHD1. FSHD2 is caused by mutations in the *SMCHD1* gene. Mutations in the *SMCHD1* gene also affect DUX4 expression.[1]

13. B

Expansion of a hexanucleotide repeat (GGGGCC) in the gene *C9ORF72* is associated with autosomal dominant FTD and ALS linked to chromosome 9p.[2]

Spinocerebellar ataxia types 1 and 8 are triplet repeat diseases.

Unverricht-Lundborg Disease (EPM1) is most often caused by a dodecamer repeat expansion (CCCCGCCCCGCG) in the *CSTB* gene, which encodes cystatin B (see Tables 13.2 through 13.5).

Table 13.2 TRIPLET REPEAT DISEASES

DISEASE	TRIPLET REPEAT
Dentatorubral-pallidoluysian atrophy (DRPLA)	CAG
Fragile X syndrome	CGG
Friedreich ataxia	GAA
Huntington disease	CAG
Myotonic dystrophy type 1	CTG
Oculopharyngeal muscular dystrophy	GCN
Spinocerebellar ataxia type 1	CAG

Table 13.3 TETRANUCLEOTIDE REPEAT DISEASE

DISEASE	TETRANUCLEOTIDE REPEAT
Myotonic dystrophy type 2	CCTG

Table 13.4 PENTANUCLEOTIDE REPEAT DISEASE

DISEASE	PENTANUCLEOTIDE REPEAT
Spinocerebellar ataxia type 10	ATTCT

Table 13.5 HEXANUCLEOTIDE REPEAT DISEASE

DISEASE	HEXANUCLEOTIDE REPEAT
Amyotrophic lateral sclerosis (ALS) and frontotemporal dementia (FTD) (on chromosome 9p)	GGGGCC

14. A

CADASIL is not a channelopathy. It is caused by a mutation in *Notch 3* on chromosome 19p.

Episodic ataxia type 1 (EA1) is caused by a potassium channel defect. Patients with this condition have myokymia/neuromyotonia as well as ataxia.

Episodic ataxia type 2 (EA2) and familial hemiplegic migraine type 1 (FHM1) are caused by defects in calcium channels. In fact, EA2, FHM1, and spinocerebellar ataxia type 6 (SCA6) are all caused by mutations in *CACNA1A* on chromosome 19, which encodes the transmembrane pore-forming subunit of the P/Q-type voltage-gated calcium channel. SCA6 is associated with an expansion of CAG repeats within the *CACNA1A* coding region.

Whereas FHM1 is results from a calcium channel defect, FHM2 is caused by mutations in sodium-potassium adenosine triphosphatase (Na⁺,K⁺-ATPase) pumps, and FHM3 is caused by sodium channel mutations.

Hyperekplexia is caused by defects in the glycine receptor (see Box 13.2).

Box 13.2 NEUROLOGIC MANIFESTATIONS OF CHANNELOPATHIES

- Ataxia
- Congenital myasthenia syndrome
- Epilepsy
- Excessive pain, insensitivity to pain
- Hyperekplexia
- Migraine
- Myotonia
- Periodic paralysis

Defects in potassium channels can cause periodic paralysis. Potassium channel defects also cause benign neonatal convulsions and epilepsy with dyskinesia. Defects in sodium and chloride channels can cause myotonia. Defects in the *SCN9A* gene cause pain syndromes. Defects in nicotinic acetylcholine receptors can cause congenital myasthenic syndromes. Other nicotinic acetylcholine receptor defects are associated with frontal lobe epilepsy (Tables 13.6 and 13.7).[3]

Table 13.6 NEUROLOGIC CONDITIONS RESULTING FROM CHANNELOPATHIES

CONDITION	DEFECTIVE CHANNELS
Ataxia	Calcium, potassium
Congenital myasthenia syndrome	Nicotinic acetylcholine
Epilepsy	Calcium, GABA, nicotinic acetylcholine, potassium, sodium
Excessive pain, insensitivity to pain	Sodium
Hyperekplexia	Glycine
Migraine	Calcium, sodium
Myotonia	Chloride, sodium
Periodic paralysis	Calcium, potassium, sodium

Table 13.7 CHANNELOPATHIES THAT CAUSE NEUROLOGIC CONDITIONS

CHANNEL	CONDITIONS
Acetylcholine (nicotinic)	Epilepsy, congenital myasthenia
Calcium	Ataxia, epilepsy, migraine, periodic paralysis
Chloride	Myotonia
GABA	Epilepsy
Glycine	Hyperekplexia
Potassium	Ataxia, epilepsy, periodic paralysis
Sodium	Epilepsy, migraine, myotonia, pain syndromes, periodic paralysis

15. A

According to recommendations from the American Academy of Neurology, chromosomal microarray (CMA) should be performed before metabolic testing if no specific etiology for developmental delay is suspected. Karyotyping and subtelomeric fluorescence in situ hybridization (FISH) testing may be performed if CMA is not available.[4]

16. E

Imprinting occurs in Prader-Willi, Angelman, Beckwith-Wiedemann, and Russell-Silver syndromes. It also occurs with myoclonus-dystonia syndrome (DYT11 or DYT11-MD). It does not occur in Huntington disease.

Imprinting occurs when the expression of an allele depends on whether it is maternal or paternal in origin. For instance, in DYT11-MD, the maternal allele typically is methylated and expression is reduced. Consequently, if a mutation is inherited from the mother, it is less likely to cause disease. As a result, the disease is autosomal dominant with reduced penetrance. In DYT11-MD, the mutated gene is *SGCE*, which encodes epsilon-sarcoglycan.

Anticipation occurs in Huntington disease (i.e., subsequent generations have more severe disease and/or earlier onset of disease). Anticipation is seen in diseases caused by expanded triplet repeats. If a child has a greater number of repeats than the parent, the disease may manifest first in the child, in which case the autosomal dominant inheritance pattern is less evident.

In Huntington disease, anticipation is seen more often with paternal transmission than with maternal transmission because instability of the CAG repeat during spermatogenesis produces longer repeats.

17. D

Spinocerebellar ataxia type 6 (SCA6) and oculopharyngeal muscular dystrophy are triplet repeat diseases that do *not* demonstrate anticipation.

Anticipation is seen in dentatorubral-pallidoluysian atrophy, fragile X syndrome, and spinocerebellar ataxia type 1. It also occurs in Huntington disease and myotonic dystrophy type 1.

Spinocerebellar ataxia type 5 (SCA5) demonstrates anticipation, but it is not the result of a repeat expansion mutation. It is caused by mutations in the gene *SPTBN2*.

18a. A and 18b. C

This patient has Angelman syndrome, which is frequently associated with seizures.

Patients with Angelman syndrome appear normal at birth and initially have a normal head circumference. Developmental delay is noted at 6 to 12 months of age. There is no regression. They are clumsy and unsteady and usually have an ataxic gait. Speech is nonexistent or minimal. Receptive language is better than expressive. They seem happy and smile and/or laugh frequently. They have a short attention span. Magnetic resonance imaging results are normal. Patients with Angelman syndrome have a distinctive facial appearance. They have a prominent chin, a wide mouth, and widely spaced teeth. They often drool. Delayed head growth results in microcephaly, usually by 2 years of age. These patients tend to have problems sleeping, are often fascinated by water, and are sensitive to heat.

About 80% of patients with Angelman syndrome develop seizures, typically between 1 and 5 years of age. They may have seizures associated with fever in infancy. Multiple seizure types can be seen, including atypical absence and myoclonic seizures. There are specific electroencephalographic (EEG) findings in Angelman syndrome, including high-amplitude slow spike and wave discharges and waves with a triphasic morphology.

Angelman syndrome is caused by decreased expression of the *UBE3A* gene from the maternal chromosome. This can result from any of four mechanisms: deletion of 15q11-q13 from the maternal chromosome; paternal uniparental disomy; an imprinting defect resulting in decreased expression of the maternal copy of *UBE3A*; or mutations in the maternal copy of *UBE3A*. The most common cause is the first listed, deletion of 15q11-q13 from the maternal chromosome. Often, the evaluation begins with methylation studies.[5,6]

19. B

This patient has Prader-Willi syndrome (PWS). The first step in diagnosis is methylation studies. The small nuclear ribonucleoprotein polypeptide N gene (*SNRPN*) is located on chromosome 15q in the region associated with PWS. It is transcribed only from the paternally inherited chromosome. In patients with PWS, methylation studies demonstrate the absence of paternally imprinted genes at 15q11-13.

Prader-Willi syndrome may result from: deletion of 15q11-q13 from the paternal chromosome; maternal uniparental disomy; abnormal imprinting of the PWS region; or a balanced translocation involving chromosome 15. The most common cause is the first one listed, deletion of this region from the paternal chromosome.

Patients with PWS are hypotonic at birth and do not feed well. They have developmental delay. Between ages 6 and 12 years, they develop hyperphagia, which can result in significant obesity. They may develop obstructive sleep apnea. Children with PWS have cognitive impairment. Behavior problems such as temper tantrums, obsessive behaviors, skin picking, and difficulties with transitions may occur. Seizures occur in 10% to 20% of patients.

Patients with PWS tend to have a narrow bifrontal diameter, almond-shaped eyes, a thin upper vermillion, and genital hypoplasia. They also have an increased risk for strabismus and scoliosis.

Multiple endocrine problems can occur with PWS, including type 2 diabetes mellitus, growth hormone deficiency, central adrenal insufficiency, hypothyroidism, and hypogonadotropic hypogonadism.

Neonates with PWS resemble neonates with congenital myotonic dystrophy type I, which is associated with expansion of a CTG trinucleotide repeat in the *DMPK* gene on chromosome 19q, but the differentiation is easier as the child gets older.[7,8,9]

20. E

Newborns with Down syndrome (trisomy 21) are hypotonic. Cardiac anomalies are common, especially defects in the atrioventricular septum. Gastrointestinal anomalies are also common, including duodenal atresia, anal atresia, megacolon, and Hirschsprung disease. Polycythemia may occur in neonates. Cataracts, thyroid disease, and hearing defects are also concerns. Fontanelles are slow to close.

Patients with Down syndrome are at increased risk for moyamoya syndrome, atlanto-axial subluxation, obstructive sleep apnea (OSA), and infantile spasms. Due to the risk for OSA, a sleep study is recommended by 4 years of age.[10]

Cardiac abnormalities increase their risk for embolic strokes and brain abscesses.

Alzheimer disease is common in patients with Down syndrome by age 40 years. (The gene for amyloid precursor protein, a risk factor for Alzheimer disease, is on chromosome 21.)

21. D

This is Williams syndrome, which is caused by a mutation in the gene encoding elastin on chromosome 7q11. Children with Williams syndrome have supravalvular aortic stenosis and hypercalcemia. They often have a stellate iris and have elfin-facies. They are described as hypersocial and musically talented. They commonly have difficulties with visuospatial construction.

Diagnosis of Williams syndrome may be made with fluorescence in situ hybridization (FISH) or with deletion testing for the Williams-Beuren syndrome critical region on chromosome 7, which includes the elastin gene.

22. A

Fragile X is the most common inherited cause of mental retardation. It is associated with an increased number of CGG repeats in the *FMR1* gene on chromosome X.

Relatives of patients with Fragile X syndrome who have an *FMR1* premutation may develop late-onset cerebellar ataxia and intention tremor. This condition is referred to as fragile X-associated tremor/ataxia syndrome (FXTAS). On MRI, white matter lesions may be seen in the middle cerebellar peduncles or in the brainstem or both.

Patients with Klinefelter syndrome (XXY) have gynecomastia, small testicles, a wide arm span, and cognitive impairment (a relatively low verbal IQ and reading and writing disorders).

Patients with 47,XYY syndrome may have developmental delay and autism spectrum disorder but do not have atypical facial features.

Patients with Sotos syndrome have cerebral gigantism and are large for their size when young.

23. A

This patient has Rett syndrome. Most cases of Rett syndrome are caused by defects in *MECP2*, which encodes methyl-CpG-binding protein 2. It is X-linked dominant, so the vast majority of patients are female.

Initial development is normal but plateaus between 6 and 18 months. This is followed by regression, after which development finally stabilizes.

Deceleration of head growth, loss of purposeful use of the hands, gait apraxia, and loss of speech are characteristic. Patients develop stereotyped use of the hands, such as hand wringing.

Patients may have a prolonged QT interval, abnormal breathing, cold hands and feet, seizures, and scoliosis.

Mutations in *CDKL5*, which encodes cyclin dependent-like kinase 5, cause an early-onset seizure variant of Rett syndrome.

ELN encodes elastin. Defects in *ELN* are associated with Williams syndrome.

Defects in *UBE3A* are associated with Angelman syndrome.

24. B

Trisomy 21, DiGeorge syndrome, Prader-Willi syndrome, and congenital myotonic dystrophy all cause neonatal hypotonia. This patient has DiGeorge syndrome.

DiGeorge syndrome results from developmental defects of the third and fourth pharyngeal pouches and the fourth branchial arch. It is caused by a mutation at 22q11.2.

There are other conditions caused by deletions at 22q11.2, including velocardiofacial syndrome and Cayler cardiofacial syndrome. Deletions at 22q11.2 result in cardiac and palate anomalies, immunodeficiency due to thymic hypoplasia, distinctive facial features, and learning problems. Hypocalcemia and seizures also occur with this condition.

REFERENCES

1. Wicklund MP. The muscular dystrophies. *Continuum (Minneap Minn)* 2013;19:1535–1570.

2. DeJesus-Hernandez M, Mackenzie IR, Boeve BR, et al. Expanded GGGGCC hexanucleotide repeat in noncoding region of C9ORF72 causes chromosome 9p-linked FTD and ALS. *Neuron* 2011;72:245–256.

3. Kullmann DM, Waxman SG. Neurological channelopathies: New insights into disease mechanisms and ion channel function. *J Physiol* 2010;588:1823–1827.

4. Michelson DJ, Shevell MI, Sherr EH, et al. Evidence report: Genetic and metabolic testing on children with global developmental delay. Report of the Quality Standards Subcommittee of the American Academy of Neurology and the Practice Committee of the Child Neurology Society. *Neurology* 2011;77;1629–1635.

5. Williams CA, Beaudet AL, Clayton-Smith J, et al. Angelman syndrome 2005: Updated consensus for diagnostic criteria. *Am J Med Genet* 2006;140:413–418.

6. Clayton-Smith J, Laan L. Angelman syndrome: A review of the clinical and genetic aspects. *J Med Genet* 2003;40:87–95.

7. McCandless SE. Clinical report: Health supervision for children with Prader-Willi Syndrome. Committee on Genetics. *Pediatrics* 2011;127:195–204.

8. Cassidy SB, Schwartz S, Miller JL, Driscoll DJ. Prader-Willi syndrome. *Genet Med* 2012;14:10–26.

9. Driscoll DJ, Miller JL, Schwartz S, et al. Prader-Willi syndrome. In: Pagon RA, Adam MP, Bird TD, et al., editors. *GeneReviews* [Internet journal]. Seattle, Wash., University of Washington, October 6, 1998 (last revision: January 23, 2014). Available at http://www.ncbi.nlm.nih.gov/books/NBK1330/ (accessed January 20, 2016).

10. Bull MJ. Health supervision for children with Down syndrome. Committee on Genetics. *Pediatrics* 2011;128;393.

14.

NEUROINFECTIOUS DISEASES

1. **What is the most common cause of bacterial meningitis?**
   A. *Haemophilus influenzae*
   B. *Neisseria meningitidis*
   C. *Staphylococcus aureus*
   D. *Streptococcus pneumoniae*

2. **Which medications are used for empiric treatment of bacterial meningitis in patients younger than 50 years old who are otherwise healthy?**
   A. A second-generation cephalosporin and vancomycin
   B. Dexamethasone, a third-generation cephalosporin, and vancomycin
   C. Ceftriaxone alone
   D. Ampicillin and ceftriaxone

3. **True or False?**
   A person who has been vaccinated with the quadrivalent meningococcal vaccine is protected from meningococcal disease.

4. **Which of the following statements is *false*?**
   A. Chronic meningitis is meningitis lasting longer than 4 weeks.
   B. Fever is the most common clinical finding in acute meningitis.
   C. Some patients with meningitis need empiric treatment with vancomycin, ceftriaxone, ampicillin, dexamethasone, and acyclovir.
   D. Significantly elevated C-reactive protein and procalcitonin levels are more suggestive of viral meningitis than bacterial meningitis.

5. **Which of the following medications is added for coverage of anaerobic bacteria in patients who have otitis, sinusitis, or mastoiditis and suspected meningitis?**
   A. Ampicillin
   B. Doxycycline
   C. Linezolid
   D. Metronidazole

6. **True or False?**
   It is recommended that tube 1 from a lumbar puncture *not* be sent for Gram stain and culture.

7. **The neonatal intensive care unit requests a consultation on a newborn that they suspect has neonatal meningitis. If they are correct, which organism is most likely to be responsible?**

A. *Escherichia coli*
B. Group B *Streptococcus*
C. *Listeria monocytogenes*
D. *Streptococcus pneumoniae*

8. **Patients with defects in cell-mediated immunity are at increased risk for meningitis caused by which of the following organisms?**
   A. Enterobacteriaceae
   B. *Listeria monocytogenes*
   C. *Neisseria meningitidis*
   D. *Streptococcus pneumoniae*

9. **In the treatment of meningitis, ampicillin is added to antibiotic regimens to treat which of the following organisms?**
   A. Group B Streptococcus
   B. *Haemophilus influenzae*
   C. *Klebsiella pneumoniae*
   D. *Listeria monocytogenes*

10. **A 24-year-old nurse is exposed to meningococcal meningitis in the emergency department. What is the recommended treatment?**
    A. Ethambutol
    B. Rifampin
    C. Streptomycin
    D. Isoniazid (INH)

11. **Match the microscopic appearance with the bacterial species it describes.**
    1) Gram-positive coccus
    2) Gram-positive bacillus
    3) Gram-negative diplococcus
    4) Gram-negative coccobacillus
    5) Gram-negative bacillus
    A. *Streptococcus pneumoniae*
    B. *Neisseria meningitidis*
    C. *Haemophilus influenzae*
    D. *Listeria monocytogenes*
    E. *Klebsiella pneumoniae*

12. **Which of the following conditions is *least* likely to be associated with a brain abscess?**
    A. Lung abscess
    B. Cyanotic heart disease
    C. Osler-Weber-Rendu disease
    D. Angelman syndrome

13. **Which of the following diseases produces a central nervous system (CNS) toxin?**
    A. Diphtheria
    B. Shigellosis

C. Tetanus

D. All of the above produce a CNS toxin.

14. **True or False?**

The presence of immunoglobulin G (IgG) to a bacteria or virus in the cerebrospinal fluid (CSF) proves that the organism is the cause of the CNS infection.

15. A 20-year-old man presents with fever, headache, malaise, vomiting, and left leg weakness. On examination, his left leg is flaccid and areflexic. Sensation is intact. What is the most likely causative organism?

A. Cytomegalovirus (CMV)

B. Salmonella

C. Shigella

D. West Nile virus

16. What is the most common type of virus to cause meningitis?

A. Arthropod-borne viruses

B. Enteroviruses

C. Herpes simplex virus type 1 (HSV-1)

D. Herpes simplex virus type 2 (HSV-2)

17. A newborn develops seizures. Head computed tomography (CT) shows periventricular calcifications. What is the most likely diagnosis?

A. Congenital CMV infection

B. Congenital toxoplasmosis

C. Congenital syphilis

D. Congenital rubella

18. Which of the following viruses can cause tremor, myoclonus, parkinsonism, a poliomyelitis-like illness, and encephalitis?

A. Epstein-Barr virus (EBV)

B. Enterovirus

C. HSV-1

D. West Nile virus

19. Lymphocytic choriomeningitis virus is transmitted from which infected animals?

A. Birds

B. Cats

C. Hamsters or mice

D. Lizards

20. A 50-year-old woman presents with a blistering rash on her trunk and complains of pain and tingling in the area. What is the most likely diagnosis?

A. Recurrence of a latent varicella-zoster virus

B. CMV polyradiculopathy

C. HSV-1 infection

D. HSV-2 infection

21. Which of the following is most suggestive of an acute Epstein-Barr virus (EBV) infection?

A. IgM to the EBV viral capsid antigen (VCA)

B. IgG to the EBV viral capsid antigen (VCA)

C. IgM to Epstein-Barr nuclear antigen (EBNA)

D. IgG to Epstein-Barr nuclear antigen (EBNA)

22. What is the most sensitive test for diagnosing West Nile encephalitis?

A. CSF polymerase chain reaction (PCR)

B. Measurement of IgM antibodies in the CSF

C. CSF viral culture

23. A 30-year-old man with human immunodeficiency virus (HIV) infection presents with chronic headache, confusion, and fever. On examination, there is mild nuchal rigidity. Lumbar puncture shows an elevated opening pressure, 8 red blood cells (RBCs), 175 white blood cells (WBCs) with a lymphocytic predominance, a glucose level of 35 mg/dL, and a protein level of 100 mg/dL. Gram staining is negative. India ink staining reveals encapsulated fungi. What is the most likely diagnosis?

A. Aspergillosis

B. Cryptococcosis

C. Coccidioidomycosis

D. Histoplasmosis

24. CSF eosinophilic pleocytosis is most suggestive of which of the following infections?

A. Aspergillosis

B. Blastomycosis

C. Cryptococcosis

C. Coccidioidomycosis

E. Histoplasmosis

25. A 65-year-old man with renal failure develops meningitis. After his death, an autopsy is performed. He has thickened leptomeninges and soap bubble-like lesions in the basal ganglia. Which of the following infections is most likely?

A. Aspergillosis

B. *Cryptococcus neoformans*

C. Coccidioidomycosis

D. Histoplasmosis

26. Which of the following infections is most likely to occur in patients with poorly controlled diabetes and to cause black nasal mucosa?

A. Blastomycosis

B. Coccidioidomycosis

C. Histoplasmosis

D. Mucormycosis

27. A renal transplant recipient returns from the Mississippi River valley with weight loss, splenomegaly, anemia, fever, and altered mental status. He dies from the illness. On autopsy, he is found to have a diffuse meningitis with necrotizing granulomatous inflammation. Organisms resembling small dots are found in the cytoplasm of macrophages. Which of the following infections is most likely?

A. Aspergillosis

B. Coccidioidomycosis

C. Histoplasmosis

D. Mucormycosis

28. Which of the following statements is *false*?
    A. Tuberculomas can resemble posterior fossa tumors.
    B. Tuberculosis (TB) can be associated with plasma cells in the CSF.
    C. TB can cause stroke.
    D. TB usually causes noncaseating granulomas.
    E. TB can cause cranial nerve palsies and hydrocephalus.

29. What is the most common cause of sporadic viral encephalitis?
    A. EBV
    B. HSV-1
    C. HSV-2
    D. West Nile virus

30. A 20-year-old man presents with a 2-day history of headache, fever, and worsening confusion. In the emergency department, he has a focal seizure characterized by left-sided clonic activity of the face, arm, and leg. CSF analysis shows 300 RBCs, 120 WBCs (85% lymphocytes), glucose 60 mg/dL, and protein 100 mg/dL. CSF Gram staining is negative. Besides magnetic resonance imaging (MRI) of the brain, which test would be the most helpful in diagnosing this condition?
    A. Electroencephalography (EEG)
    B. Single-photon emission computed tomography (SPECT)
    C. Positron emission tomography (PET)
    D. Magnetic resonance angiogram (MRA)

31. A patient presenting shortly after onset of symptoms is thought to have HSV encephalitis. However, PCR analysis of the CSF is negative. What is the next step?
    A. Continue acyclovir and repeat the lumbar puncture.
    B. Discontinue acyclovir to prevent renal toxicity.
    C. Repeat the PCR on the same sample.
    D. Send CSF to an outside laboratory to verify that the PCR is negative.

32. A patient presents with new-onset seizures. MRI shows multiple cystic lesions. CT shows calcifications. What is the recommended treatment?
    A. Albendazole plus dexamethasone or prednisolone
    B. Dexamethasone
    C. Pyrimethamine
    D. Everolimus

33. Which of the following statements is *false*?
    A. Neurocysticercosis is the most common helminthic infection involving the CNS.
    B. MRI may miss some cases of neurocysticercosis: Patients can have brain parenchymal calcifications alone, which are missed on MRI but seen on CT.
    C. A patient with only calcifications does not need to be treated with cysticidal medications.
    D. Serum immune diagnostic tests for neurocysticercosis are both very sensitive and very specific.

34. An 18-year-old patient presents with fever, headache, confusion, and rash after a recent hiking trip. The rash started as macules at his wrists and ankles but now involves his trunk and face. CSF shows a mild pleocytosis. How is this treated?
    A. Augmentin
    B. Doxycycline
    C. Erythromycin
    D. Ceftriaxone

35. Which of the following statements is true?
    A. A brain lesion thought to be toxoplasmosis should be biopsied before treatment is begun.
    B. A negative CSF PCR result for toxoplasmosis excludes the diagnosis.
    C. Toxoplasmosis is the most common cause of a focal mass lesion in the brain of patients with HIV infection.
    D. Lack of antibodies to toxoplasmosis excludes the diagnosis.

36. Which of the following statements is *false*?
    A. Neurosyphilis can cause Heubner arteritis leading to stroke.
    B. When neurosyphilis involves the spinal cord, it is most often associated with degeneration of the anterior horn cells.
    C. Neurosyphilis is associated with microglial proliferation in the cortex and iron deposition.
    D. Plasma cells may be present in the CSF of patients with neurosyphilis.

37. Poliovirus has the greatest affinity for which type of cell?
    A. Cells in the dorsal root ganglion
    B. Cells in the pons
    C. Cells in the intermediolateral (IML) column
    D. Large motor cells in the ventral horn

38. CSF PCR analysis for which of the following viruses is often positive in patients with AIDS-associated primary CNS lymphoma and is a sensitive indicator of this tumor?
    A. CMV
    B. EBV
    C. Human herpesvirus type 6 (HHV-6)
    D. JC virus

39. Which of the following organisms infects the CNS via fast retrograde axonal transport from muscle and is associated with intracytoplasmic intraneuronal inclusions?
    A. CMV
    B. HIV
    C. Rabies virus
    D. *Bartonella*

40. A 24-year-old man with HIV infection who is taking highly active antiretroviral therapy (HAART) develops focal seizures. Which anti-epileptic medication should be started?
    A. Levetiracetam
    B. Carbamazepine
    C. Phenytoin
    D. Valproic acid

41. **Which of the following statements is *false*?**
    A. Doxycycline is the preferred treatment for post-treatment Lyme disease syndrome.
    B. Doxycycline is the preferred oral treatment for cranial neuropathy associated with Lyme disease.
    C. Encephalomyelitis and encephalopathy due to Lyme disease should be treated with parenteral antibiotics.
    D. Ceftriaxone, penicillin G, or cefotaxime may be used to treat Lyme disease when parenteral treatment is indicated.

42. **True or False?**
    JC virus and herpes virus can be found in normal brains.

43. **Which of the following diseases is associated with demyelination at the juxtacortical white matter, enlarged oligodendrocytes containing virions, and bizarre astrocytes?**
    A. EBV infection
    B. HIV infection
    C. Progressive multifocal leukoencephalopathy (PML)
    D. West Nile virus infection

44. **Subacute sclerosing panencephalitis is the name for a chronic infection with which of the following viruses?**
    A. Measles virus
    B. Mumps virus
    C. Rubella virus
    D. Varicella virus

45. **True or False?**
    CSF findings (cell count, protein, and glucose) are typically normal in patients with PML.

46. **Cowdry A bodies are *not* associated with which of the following diseases?**
    A. Herpes
    B. Subacute sclerosing panencephalitis (SSPE)
    C. CMV
    D. Polio

47. **Which type of inflammation is found in patients with prion infections?**
    A. Eosinophils
    B. Lymphocytes
    C. Polymorphonuclear lymphocytes
    D. Multinucleated giant cells
    E. None of the above

48. **Which of the following features is more characteristic of variant Creutzfeldt-Jakob disease than of sporadic Creutzfeldt-Jakob disease?**
    A. Florid plaques
    B. Increased signal in the basal ganglia and/or cortical ribbon
    C. Periodic sharp wave complexes on EEG
    D. Shorter clinical course

49. **Which of the following viruses causes T-cell leukemia and tropical spastic paraparesis?**
    A. CMV
    B. EBV
    C. HIV
    D. Human T-cell lymphotropic virus-1 (HTLV-1)

NEUROINFECTIOUS DISEASES

ANSWERS

1. D

The most common cause of bacterial meningitis is *S. pneumoniae.*

It is recommended that dexamethasone be added to the treatment of pneumococcal meningitis in adults. Due to antibiotic resistance, it is also recommended that these patients have a repeat lumbar puncture 48 hours after initiation of antibiotic therapy.

2. B

Dexamethasone, a third-generation cephalosporin, and vancomycin are recommended for empiric treatment of bacterial meningitis. Blood cultures should always be performed before antibiotics are administered.

Ampicillin is added to cover *Listeria* in patients older than 55 years of age and in those with decreased cell-mediated immunity.

Doxycycline is added if tick-borne illness is a possibility.

In neurosurgical patients, empiric therapy with vancomycin plus meropenem or ceftazidime is recommended for better gram-negative coverage.

3. False

The quadrivalent meningococcal vaccine does not contain serogroup B, so the vaccine does not completely prevent meningococcal disease.

4. D

Although fever, neck stiffness, altered mental status, and headache are classically associated with acute meningitis, they may not all be present. Fever is the sign most likely to be present. If there is altered level of consciousness, the patient is more likely to have bacterial meningitis than viral meningitis. Likewise, seizures and focal neurologic deficits are more common in patients with bacterial meningitis. Otitis media, sinusitis, or upper respiratory tract infection symptoms may precede bacterial meningitis.

Significantly elevated levels of C-reactive protein and procalcitonin are more suggestive of bacterial meningitis than viral meningitis (see Box 14.1).

5. D

If patients have otitis media, mastoiditis, or sinusitis and meningitis is suspected, metronidazole should be added.

Box 14.1 **POTENTIAL COMPLICATIONS DUE TO INFLAMMATION IN MENINGITIS**

- Cerebral edema
- Arteritis and infarctions (ischemic and hemorrhagic)
- Hydrocephalus (obstructive and communicating)
- Seizures
- Venous sinus thrombosis

Metronidazole is also added for head trauma and for neurosurgical patients. For instance, it is used for anaerobe coverage in patients undergoing ventriculostomy.

Linezolid helps to treat *Staphylococcus epidermidis* and *Staphylococcus aureus.*

Doxycycline is added for coverage of tick-borne bacterial infections.

Meropenem and ceftazidime cover gram-negative rods that cause nosocomial meningitis, such as *Pseudomonas aeruginosa*, *Escherichia coli*, and *Klebsiella pneumoniae.*

6. True

Due to the risk of contamination from skin flora (e.g., coagulase-negative *Staphylococcus*), it is recommended that tube 1 from a lumbar puncture not be sent for Gram stain and culture.

7. B

Group B *Streptococcus* is the most common cause of neonatal meningitis. *E. coli* is the second most common cause. *L. monocytogenes* is uncommon.

8. B

Women in the third trimester of pregnancy and patients with defective cell-mediated immunity are at increased risk for *Listeria monocytogenes* infection. As with group B *Streptococcus*, there is risk for maternal-fetal transmission of *Listeria*. Food-borne *Listeria* can cause outbreaks of listeriosis. The organism can be found in raw meat, raw milk, soft cheeses, and salads. *Listeria* grows in cold (refrigerator) temperatures. Pregnant women should avoid eating cold cuts unless they are heated first.

Patients with defects in the terminal common complement pathway, immunoglobulin deficiency, or asplenia are at increased risk for meningitis from *N. meningitidis* and *S. pneumoniae.*

9. D

Listeria is particularly a concern in patients older than 55 years of age and in patients with decreased cell-mediated immunity, such as those with hematologic malignancies, cancer, or HIV infection; organ transplant recipients; patients who chronically use corticosteroids; and pregnant women.

Gentamicin may be added to Ampicillin in patients with suspected *Listeria* infection who are obtunded or comatose.

10. B

Medical personnel exposed to meningococcal meningitis should be treated with rifampin.

Patients with asplenia, immunoglobulin deficiency, or defects in the terminal common complement pathway (C3, C5-C9) are at increased risk for *Neisseria meningitidis* and *Streptococcus pneumoniae* infection.

Meningococcemia is more likely to cause a rash involving the trunk and lower extremities than most viral causes of meningitis. The rash is petechial. Mucous membranes and conjunctiva may be involved. Viral exanthema tend to involve the face and chest initially.

11.

1) A
2) D
3) B
4) C
5) E

See Table 14.1, which provides a list of selected organisms and their descriptions.

Table 14.1 MICROSCOPIC APPEARANCE OF SELECTED ORGANISMS

ORGANISM	DESCRIPTION
Streptococcus pneumoniae	**Gram-positive coccus**
Listeria monocytogenes	**Gram-positive bacillus**
Neisseria meningitis	**Gram-negative diplococcus**
Haemophilus influenzae	**Gram-negative coccobacillus**
Klebsiella pneumoniae	**Gram-negative bacillus**

Escherichia coli and *Pseudomonas aeruginosa* are also gram-negative bacilli.

12. D

Lung abscesses and cyanotic heart disease are risk factors for brain abscesses. Osler-Weber-Rendu disease, also known as hereditary hemorrhagic telangiectasia, is associated with pulmonary arteriovenous malformations, which increase the risk for brain abscesses.

Brain abscesses can also occur with local spread, such as from otitis media or sinusitis.

13. D

Diphtheria, shigellosis, and tetanus all produce CNS toxins.

Shiga toxins produced by *Shigella dysenteriae* can cause altered mental status and seizures.

Tetanus toxin can cause trismus, rigidity, and opisthotonus.

Diphtheria toxin causes a palatal neuropathy and can cause a demyelinating polyneuropathy resembling Guillain-Barré syndrome.

14. False

IgG can be passively transferred to the CSF from the serum. The presence of *immunoglobulin M* (IgM) to an organism in the CSF indicates that the organism is responsible for the infection because IgM antibodies cannot be transferred across the blood-brain barrier. Their presence therefore indicates intrathecal production of antibodies. An elevated antibody index (i.e., the ratio of IgG to an organism in the CSF versus the serum compared to the ratio of the total IgG in the CSF versus the serum) can be helpful in determining whether there is intrathecal production of IgG.

15. D

This patient has West Nile myelitis. West Nile virus can cause a poliomyelitis-like syndrome (acute flaccid paralysis). Non-polio enteroviruses can as well.

16. B

Enteroviruses are the most common viral cause of meningitis.

HSV-2 is a common cause of recurrent meningitis.

17. A

(CMV is the most common congenital infection. The fetus is typically infected during maternal primary infection. Often the neonate is asymptomatic. Some patients present later with delayed speech due to hearing loss. CMV is the most common cause of acquired hearing loss in children. Neonates who are symptomatic may have meningoencephalitis, periventricular calcifications, microcephaly, migrational disturbances, or cerebellar hypoplasia. Non-neurologic complications present at birth include hepatitis with hyperbilirubinemia, thrombocytopenia, and coagulopathy.

Toxoplasma gondii causes congenital toxoplasmosis. Calcifications can be seen with toxoplasmosis, but they tend to be diffuse rather than limited to the periventricular area.

Symptoms of congenital syphilis include meningitis, mucocutaneous lesions, rashes, hepatosplenomegaly, lymphadenopathy, anemia, osteochondritis, and periostitis. Symptoms may not appear until 2 weeks after birth.

Congenital rubella is associated with intrauterine growth retardation, meningoencephalitis, chorioretinitis and cataracts, cardiovascular anomalies, hepatosplenomegaly, thrombocytopenia with or without purpura, bony radiolucencies, and dermal erythropoiesis.

18. D

West Nile virus can cause myoclonus, parkinsonism, a polio-like illness, and encephalitis.

Other flaviviruses, such as St. Louis encephalitis virus and Japanese encephalitis virus, can also cause encephalitis with parkinsonism. They can infect the basal ganglia, thalamus, and substantia nigra.

Encephalitis caused by arthropod-borne viruses may begin with flu-like symptoms such as myalgias, fever, and fatigue. Gastrointestinal symptoms may also be present in patients with West Nile virus infection.

19. C

Lymphocytic choriomeningitis virus is a cause of aseptic meningitis. It results from exposure to infected hamsters or mice.

20. A

This is herpes zoster (shingles), which is caused by reactivation of latent varicella-zoster virus (VZV). Both herpes simplex and VZV remain latent in sensory ganglia.

CMV polyradiculopathy is seen in patients with HIV infection.

HSV-2 is typically sexually transmitted.

21. A

First, patients have IgM to the EBV VCA. Next, they develop IgG to the VCA. IgG antibodies to EBNA develop after the virus establishes latency. EBNA antibody stays positive for life.

22. B

CSF IgM antibodies are most sensitive for diagnosing West Nile encephalitis.

23. B

This patient has meningitis due to infection by *Cryptococcus neoformans*, which is an encapsulated fungus. The capsule can be visualized with the use of India ink, but measurement of cryptococcal antigen is more sensitive. *Cryptococcus* infection leads to chronic meningitis characterized by an elevated opening pressure, decreased glucose, elevated protein, and a mild pleocytosis. Cryptococcal meningitis is most common in immunocompromised patients but can occur in immunocompetent individuals. *Cryptococcus* is the most common systemic fungal infection in immunocompromised patients with deficient cell-mediated immunity (e.g., HIV infection, organ transplantation).

In general, Grocott-Gomori methenamine silver (GMS) and periodic acid-Schiff (PAS) stains are useful for identifying fungi.

24. D

Coccidioidomycosis causes a CSF eosinophilic pleocytosis.

Coccidioidomycosis is caused by *Coccidioides immitis*, which is found in soil and dust in the Southwest. It results in a basal meningitis with small nodules. Acute hydrocephalus may occur.

The organism produces a necrotizing granulomatous inflammatory response with spherules. The spherules release endospores that cause inflammation.

25. B

C. neoformans infection causes soap bubble-like lesions in the basal ganglia.

26. D

Mucormycosis is an angioinvasive fungus that can cause thrombosis. It has nonseptate hyphae that branch at right angles. It tends to occur in patients with poorly controlled diabetes and in other immunocompromised patients. It can cause black nasal mucosa due to infarction. It spreads from the nose and sinuses to the brain and causes hemorrhagic lesions often involving the base of the frontal lobes or the deep gray nuclei.

Aspergillosis is also angioinvasive and occurs in immunocompromised hosts, but it has acutely branching septate hyphae. It forms fruiting bodies in culture or tissue section if the organism is exposed to air.

27. C

Histoplasma capsulatum is endemic in the Ohio and Mississippi River valleys. In infected persons, many *Histoplasma* organisms can be seen in the cytoplasm of macrophages; they look like small dots.

28. D

Tuberculosis produces caseating granulomas.

Tuberculosis is the most common mycobacterial infection of the CNS. It tends to cause basilar meningitis, which can lead to cranial nerve palsies and hydrocephalus. The affected basal meninges enhance with gadolinium. Tuberculous meningitis can also involve the Sylvian fissures, surround the spinal cord, and line the ventricles.

TB can cause arterial narrowing and stroke.

When TB causes vertebral disease (tuberculous spondylitis), it's called Pott's disease. It results in a gibbus deformity.

Granulomas in TB are composed of caseating necrosis with multinucleate giant cells, lymphocytes, and plasma cells. Granulomas occur along vessels in the meninges and in the parenchyma.

Sarcoidosis produces noncaseating granulomas, can cause hypothalamic dysfunction, often affects the base of the brain, and can produce cranial nerve palsies (See Box 14.2).

Box 14.2 CAUSES OF GRANULOMAS

- Mycobacteria
- Fungi
- Spirochetes
- Sarcoidosis
- Foreign material

29. B

HSV-1 is the most common cause of sporadic viral encephalitis.

In immunosuppressed patients with viral encephalitis, HSV-1, VZV, HHV-6, CMV, and EBV need to be considered. Clues that EBV is responsible are a sore throat, tonsillar enlargement, and lymphadenopathy.

30. A

This patient has HSV encephalitis and should be treated with acyclovir. HSV encephalitis is characterized by a triad of headache, fever, and altered mental status. Seizures are common. Patients may also have aphasia or hemiparesis. In addition to a lymphocytic pleocytosis and elevated protein, CSF RBCs are elevated. HSV encephalitis is associated with periodic lateralizing epileptiform discharges (PLEDs) on the EEG. In general, the most common cause of PLEDS is stroke.

31. A

The CSF PCR for herpes may be negative in the first 72 hours after symptom onset, so a spinal tap should be repeated and a second sample should be sent for PCR testing. Antibodies to HSV in the CSF may also be helpful. These can be detected in the second week after the onset of symptoms. IgM, IgG, and IgA antibodies to the N-methyl-D-aspartate (NMDA) receptor have been found in patients with HSV encephalitis.[1]

CSF IgM antibodies are also helpful in the diagnosis of VZV encephalitis.

VZV encephalitis causes demyelinating lesions and infarctions. VZV infects blood vessel endothelial cells and causes vasculitis.

32. A

This patient has neurocysticercosis, which is an infection of the CNS caused by ingestion of eggs from the pork tapeworm *Taenia solium*. American Academy of Neurology guidelines recommend consideration of albendazole plus dexamethasone or prednisone. Treatment with albendazole will hasten the death of the cysts and increase the inflammatory reaction. For this reason, steroids should be given with albendazole. In cases of cysticercotic encephalitis, in which there is a strong inflammatory reaction, there is concern that cysticidal drugs could worsen inflammation, leading to increased intracranial pressure.[2]

33. D

Serum immune diagnostic tests for neurocysticercosis are not ideal. The complement fixation test and serum enzyme-linked immunosorbent assay (ELISA) used historically are neither sensitive nor specific. Enzyme-linked immunoelectrotransfer blot using partially purified antigenic extracts has much better sensitivity and specificity if two or more lesions are present; however, it has a high false-negative rate when there is only one cysticercus.

CSF ELISA for anticysticercal antibodies has some usefulness. However, it also can give false-negative and false-positive findings.[3]

34. B

This patient has Rocky Mountain spotted fever (RMSF), which is a tickborne illness caused by the bacterium *Rickettsia rickettsii*. It is treated with doxycycline. RMSF causes a characteristic rash that begins on the wrists and ankles and spreads centripetally to the trunk. However, the rash is not always present.

Syphilis and meningococcemia also can cause a rash on the palms and soles.

35. C

A ring-enhancing lesion in a patient with AIDS is most likely toxoplasmosis, which is caused by the protozoa *Toxoplasma gondii*. An abscess caused by this organism is referred to as a "gold coin lesion" because of the discoloration from central coagulative or hemorrhagic necrosis. Patients may not have antibodies, and PCR of the spinal fluid may be negative. Lumbar puncture may not be safe if there is a focal mass lesion. If toxoplasmosis is suspected, one can begin with empiric treatment. It is not necessary to biopsy the lesion first. Pyrimethamine and sulfadiazine are often used to treat toxoplasmosis.

36. B

Syphilis is caused by the spirochete *Treponema pallidum*. Neurosyphilis has multiple forms, but it begins as meningitis.

Asymptomatic neurosyphilis is diagnosed by lumbar puncture.

Meningeal syphilis can occur at any time but is most common during the first 2 years after inoculation. The patient may have seizures, cranial nerve palsies, or hydrocephalus.

Meningovascular neurosyphilis is characterized by chronic meningitis and stroke. Infarctions occur because of inflammation and fibrosis affecting small arteries (Heubner arteritis). Branches of the middle cerebral artery are most commonly affected.

Paretic neurosyphilis results from chronic meningoencephalitis. It is characterized by dementia, psychiatric disturbances, seizures, tremor, dysarthria, hyperreflexia, and Argyll-Robertson pupils (pupils accommodate but do not react).

Tabetic neurosyphilis, or tabes dorsalis, develops many years after infection. The dorsal nerve roots and dorsal columns are affected. Symptoms and signs include lancinating pains, lower extremity areflexia, loss of vibration and position sense, sensory ataxia, a positive Romberg sign, and urinary incontinence. Charcot joints (neuropathic arthropathy) may develop.

In active neurosyphilis, the CSF shows pleocytosis with lymphocytes and some plasma cells, increased protein, increased gamma globulin with possible oligoclonal bands, normal glucose, and positive findings on serologic tests.

Neurosyphilis is treated with intravenous penicillin.

37. D

Poliovirus affects the anterior (ventral) horn cells. It is a classic cause of asymmetric flaccid paralysis. Patients also have fever and chills. CSF results are consistent with infection.

38. B

Patients with AIDS-associated primary CNS lymphoma tend to test positive for EBV in the CSF by PCR testing.

CMV can cause lumbosacral radiculitis in patients with HIV infection.

JC virus causes progressive multifocal leukoencephalopathy (PML).

HHV-6 causes roseola (sixth disease) in immunocompetent children. It also is a common cause of febrile seizures and can lead to febrile status epilepticus. Febrile status epilepticus is associated with damage to the hippocampi and later risk for temporal lobe epilepsy.[4]

39. C

Negri bodies are found in patients with rabies.

40. A

Levetiracetam has no drug interactions and should not affect this patient's medications for HIV. All of the others have a potential for interacting with antiretroviral agents.

Caution should be used when prescribing enzyme-inducing anti-epileptic drugs (AEDs) such as carbamazepine and phenytoin for patients who are using protease inhibitors or nonnucleoside reverse transcriptase inhibitors because these AEDs may reduce their levels and effectiveness. Similar caution should be paid when enzyme-inducing AEDs are prescribed to women taking oral contraceptives.[5]

41. A

Antibiotics are not recommended for post-treatment Lyme disease syndrome.

Lyme disease is caused by *Borrelia burgdorferi*, a spirochete that is transmitted by ticks. An infected tick must be attached for at least 24 hours to transmit the disease. Proper removal of a tick is with forceps.

The most common finding in Lyme disease is the characteristic rash. The rash is called erythema migrans, and it resembles a circular target.

Neurologic manifestations of Lyme disease include lymphocytic meningitis, cranial neuropathy, and radiculitis. Meningitis caused by Lyme disease typically manifests with fever, headache, meningismus, and photophobia. Also, the patient may have a painful radiculopathy or bilateral facial nerve palsies. HSV-2 can also cause radiculitis. Other causes of fever, headache, and cranial nerve abnormalities are fungal meningitis, HIV, syphilis, and tuberculosis. Sarcoidosis can also cause bilateral facial palsies.

Post-treatment Lyme disease syndrome is characterized by fatigue and joint pain. Antibiotics are not indicated.[6]

42. True

JC and herpes viruses can be found in normal brains.

43. C

In PML, JC virus infects oligodendrocytes and astrocytes. Most people carry JC virus. PML is caused by reactivation of the virus. It is an opportunistic infection that primarily affects patients with T-cell deficits, such as patients with AIDS or lymphoreticular malignancies. There is no specific treatment for PML in general. Antiretroviral therapy is the treatment for patients with PML due to HIV.

44. A

Subacute sclerosing panencephalitis (SSPE) is a degenerative disease that is seen in children and young adolescents who had measles at a young age. First, there is a change in personality and school performance. Then patients develop myoclonus, ataxia, and seizures, followed by rigidity and decreased responsiveness. SSPE causes demyelination that begins in the subcortical white matter. The EEG shows a periodic pattern. Discharges recur every 4 to 15 seconds. (In sporadic Creutzfeldt-Jakob disease, periodic discharges are seen every 0.5 to 1 second.) Elevated anti-measles antibody (IgG) in the serum and CSF is used to help diagnose the condition. CSF protein is increased, and oligoclonal bands can be seen.

45. True

CSF parameters are generally normal in PML. CSF PCR for JC virus may also be negative. Sometimes, brain biopsy is necessary for diagnosis.

46. D

Cowdry B bodies are intranuclear bodies associated with acute poliomyelitis.

Cowdry A bodies are intranuclear inclusions that occur in herpes, varicella zoster, SSPE, and CMV infection.

47. E

Prions do not cause an inflammatory reaction.

Eosinophils are associated with infection by metazoan parasites; lymphocytes are elevated in viral infections;

polymorphonuclear leukocytes are prominent in bacterial infections; and multinucleated giant cells are associated with infection by fungi or mycobacteria.

48. A

Creutzfeldt-Jakob disease (CJD) causes dementia, myoclonus, and motor abnormalities. Microscopically, spongiform encephalopathies such as CJD are characterized by spongiform change, loss of neurons, and gliosis.

Variant CJD (vCJD) is caused by exposure to transmissible bovine spongiform encephalopathy. Patients tend to be younger than in other forms of CJD and to have early psychiatric symptoms. The prion protein (PRNP) genotype is 129 MM. Hyperintense signal is seen in the pulvinar on diffusion-weighted imaging (DWI). Florid plaques, which consist of spongiform degeneration with an amyloid core, are found in vCJD.

Most cases of sporadic CJD occur in patients who are homozygotes at codon 129. The clinical course is shorter than in patients with variant CJD. Periodic sharp wave complexes may be seen on EEG. DWI shows signal changes in the basal ganglia and/or cortical ribbon (see Table 14.2 and Figure 14.1).

Table 14.2 COMPARISON OF SPORADIC AND VARIANT FORMS OF CREUTZFELDT-JAKOB DISEASE (CJD).

SPORADIC CJD	VARIANT CJD
No florid plaques	Florid plaques
Increased signal in basal ganglia and/or cortical ribbon	Increased signal in pulvinar
Periodic sharp wave complexes (PSWCs) on EEG	No PSWCs
Homozygotes at codon 129 (129 MM or 129 VV)	129 MM

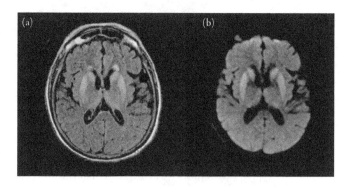

Figure 14.1 Sporadic Creutzfeldt-Jakob disease (CJD). FLAIR (A) and diffusion-weighted (B) images. (From Saba L. *Imaging in Neurodegenerative Disorders.* New York, Oxford University Press, 2015.)

49. D

HTLV-1 causes T-cell leukemia and HTLV-1-associated myelopathy, which is also known as tropical spastic paraparesis.

REFERENCES

1. Pruss H, Finke C, Höltje M, et al. *N*-Methyl-D-aspartate receptor antibodies in herpes simplex encephalitis. *Ann Neurol* 2012;72:902–911.
2. Baird RA, Wiebe S, Zunt JR, et al. Evidence-based guideline: Treatment of parenchymal neurocysticercosis. Report of the Guideline Development Subcommittee of the American Academy of Neurology. *Neurology* 2013;80:1424–1429.
3. Del Brutto OH. Neurocysticercosis. *Continuum Lifelong Learning Neurol* 2012;18:1392–1416.
4. Epstein LG, Shinnar S, Hesdorffer DC, et al. Human herpesvirus 6 and 7 in febrile status epilepticus: The FEBSTAT study. *Epilepsia* 2012;53:1481–1488.
5. Birbeck GL, French JA, Perucca E, et al. Evidence-based guideline: Antiepileptic drug selection for people with HIV/AIDS. Report of the Quality Standards Subcommittee of the American Academy of Neurology and the Ad Hoc Task Force of the Commission on Therapeutic Strategies of the International League Against Epilepsy. *Neurology* 2012;78:139–145.
6. Halperin JJ, Shapiro ED, Logigian E, et al. Practice parameter: Treatment of nervous system Lyme disease (an evidence-based review). Report of the Quality Standards Subcommittee of the American Academy of Neurology. *Neurology* 2007;69:91–102.

15.

NEUROLOGIC COMPLICATIONS OF SYSTEMIC DISEASES

QUESTIONS

1. Which of the following conditions is most likely to occur in a patient with tuberous sclerosis complex?
   A. Aortic regurgitation
   B. Mitral valve regurgitation
   C. Wolff-Parkinson-White syndrome
   D. Hypertrophic cardiomyopathy

2. A 50-year-old with cirrhosis becomes confused and develops asterixis. What is the classic electroencephalography (EEG) finding in hepatic encephalopathy?
   A. Alpha coma
   B. Beta coma
   C. Delta brushes
   D. Triphasic waves

3. Which of the following is *least* helpful in the treatment of hepatic encephalopathy?
   A. Antibiotics such as neomycin
   B. Decreasing ammonia production in the gastrointestinal tract
   C. Lorazepam
   D. Nonabsorbable disaccharides such as lactulose

4. What is the most common neurologic complication of inflammatory bowel disease?
   A. Encephalopathy
   B. Myopathy
   C. Peripheral neuropathy
   D. Stroke

5. Patients with chronic hepatitis C are at an increased risk for which of the following disorders?
   A. Cryoglobulinemia
   B. Idiopathic thrombocytopenic purpura
   C. Waldenstrom macroglobulinemia
   D. Monoclonal gammopathy of unknown significance

6. Wilson disease is caused by a defect in which of the following?
   A. A copper-transporting ATPase
   B. Ceruloplasmin production
   C. Cytochrome c oxidase
   D. Decreased urinary excretion of copper

7. Paraneoplastic gastroparesis is most likely to occur with which type of cancer?
   A. Breast
   B. Gastric
   C. Lung
   D. Prostate

8. What is the *least* common neurologic complication of bariatric surgery?
   A. Myelopathy
   B. Myopathy
   C. Peripheral neuropathy
   D. Subarachnoid hemorrhage

9. Which of the following diseases is most likely to cause fever, diarrhea, parkinsonism, and oculomasticatory myorhythmia?
   A. Celiac disease
   B. Crohn disease
   C. Ulcerative colitis
   D. Whipple disease

10. Which of the following diseases is most likely to cause a progressive myoclonic ataxia, occipital calcifications, and steatorrhea?
    A. Celiac disease
    B. Crohn disease
    C. Ulcerative colitis
    D. Whipple disease

11. A 30-year-old pregnant woman develops confusion and new-onset seizure activity. Vital signs show that she is afebrile but hypertensive. She seems to have difficulty focusing on objects. Which of the following features is most likely to be seen on magnetic resonance imaging (MRI)?
    A. Pituitary hemorrhage
    B. Increased T2 signal in both temporal lobes
    C. Mesial temporal sclerosis
    D. Symmetric vasogenic edema in the occipital and parietal lobes

12. An 18-year-old with polycystic kidney disease presents with severe headache, vomiting, and photophobia. Which diagnosis needs to be ruled out?
    A. Cluster headache
    B. Migraine
    C. Pituitary apoplexy
    D. Subarachnoid hemorrhage

13. Which of the following is *least* likely to occur in a patient with neurosarcoidosis?
    A. Cranial neuropathy
    B. Focal leptomeningeal disease

C. Periventricular white matter lesions

D. Stroke

14. Which of the following is the most common neurologic complication of polycythemia vera?

A. Peripheral neuropathy

B. Stroke

C. Seizure

D. Tremor

15. A 20-year-old woman presents with headache, altered mental status, seizures, and fever. The patient is found to have microangiopathic hemolytic anemia and thrombocytopenia. Schistocytes are seen on her peripheral blood smear. What is the most likely diagnosis?

A. Hemolytic uremic syndrome

B. Idiopathic thrombocytopenic purpura

C. Acute intermittent porphyria

D. Thrombotic thrombocytic purpura

16. Which nutritional deficiency is associated with acanthocytosis?

A. Folate deficiency

B. Vitamin A deficiency

C. Vitamin E deficiency

D. Vitamin K deficiency

17. In which of the following conditions is a "hung up" reflex (delayed relaxation) most likely to occur?

A. Liver disease

B. Kidney failure

C. Hypothyroidism

D. Myasthenia gravis

18. Which of the following conditions is *least* likely to be a result of hyperthyroidism?

A. Cerebellar ataxia

B. Stroke

C. Chorea

D. Periodic paralysis

19. In which of the following conditions is pheochromocytoma *least* likely to occur?

A. Neurofibromatosis type 1

B. Von Hippel-Lindau syndrome

C. Tuberous sclerosis complex

D. Multiple endocrine neoplasia type 2 (MEN 2)

20. A 20-year-old woman with central adrenal insufficiency is scheduled for appendectomy. Which medication should be given around the time of surgery?

A. Hydrocortisone

B. Fludrocortisone

C. Salt tablets

D. Desmopressin

21. A 20-year-old man is referred by his primary care physician for a pituitary mass that was found on MRI performed because of headaches. Which visual defect is most likely to be present?

A. Bitemporal hemianopsia

B. Binasal hemianopsia

C. Homonymous hemianopsia

D. An enlarged blind spot

22. A patient with a history of intellectual disability presents to the emergency department with muscle cramps and seizures. On examination, she is petite in height but has a stocky build with a round face. She has cataracts. Tetany is elicited. Which of the following is most likely to be present?

A. Polycystic kidney disease

B. A cherry red spot

C. Concentric cardiomyopathy

D. Shortening of the metacarpal and metatarsal bones

23. Which of the following is a medium-vessel vasculitis?

A. Giant cell arteritis

B. IgA vasculitis

C. Takayasu arteritis

D. Polyarteritis nodosa

24. PCA-2, ANNA-2, ANNA-3, amphiphysin, and GABA receptor paraneoplastic antibodies are all associated with which type of cancer?

A. Breast adenocarcinoma

B. Renal cell carcinoma

C. Small cell lung carcinoma

D. Thymoma

25. Which of the following syndromes is *not* typically associated with an increased risk for brain tumors?

A. Turcot syndrome

B. Gorlin syndrome

C. Li-Fraumeni syndrome

D. Peutz-Jeghers syndrome

NEUROLOGIC COMPLICATIONS
OF SYSTEMIC DISEASES

ANSWERS

1. C

Cardiac rhabdomyomas and Wolff-Parkinson-White (WPW) syndrome are cardiac complications of tuberous sclerosis complex. WPW syndrome can also occur in certain mitochondrial diseases and in some cases of hypokalemic periodic paralysis, Pompe disease (glycogen storage disease type 2), and Danon disease. (Danon disease is a rare, X-linked dominant disease associated with cardiomyopathy and intellectual disability. It is caused by mutations in the gene that encodes lysosomal associated membrane protein-2.)

2. D

Hepatic encephalopathy manifests with confusion and movement disorders such as asterixis, myoclonus, or tremor. Patients with fulminant liver failure can have increased intracranial pressure. Comatose patients with acute hepatic failure may have cerebral edema, which can be fatal. Grade 4 hepatic failure is associated with dilated pupils, loss of cranial nerve reflexes, posturing, and loss of deep tendon reflexes. An elevated ammonia level is seen in hepatic encephalopathy. Triphasic waves are the classic finding in hepatic encephalopathy, but they are not specific to liver disease.

Wilson disease and Niemann-Pick disease type C are diseases with neurologic manifestations that can cause cirrhosis.

3. C

Lorazepam is least helpful of the treatments listed in hepatic encephalopathy. Flumazenil, which is an antagonist of the benzodiazepine receptor, has been used in treatment. Lactulose helps lower ammonia. Antibiotics such as neomycin have been used to decrease intestinal bacteria that produce ammonia. A low-protein diet is also helpful.

4. C

Peripheral neuropathy is the most common neurologic complication of inflammatory bowel disease.

5. A

Patients with chronic hepatitis C often have cryoglobulinemia.

6. A

Wilson disease is caused by a defect in a copper-transporting adenosine triphosphatase (ATPase) that results from a mutation in the *ATP7B* gene on chromosome 13. Copper cannot be transported to the bile canaliculus to be excreted, so it accumulates in the liver. Excessive copper is then deposited in other tissues. Tremor is the most common neurologic manifestation. Urinary copper is increased. Serum copper and ceruloplasmin are reduced. Wilson disease is treated with copper chelation.

7. C

Anti-Hu antibodies (also known as antineuronal nuclear antibody type 1, or ANNA-1) antibodies are found in patients with lung cancer and can cause paraneoplastic gastroparesis.

8. D

Subarachnoid hemorrhage is not associated with bariatric surgery. Encephalopathy, myelopathy, myopathy, and peripheral neuropathy are possible complications of bariatric surgery.

9. D

Whipple disease is caused by the bacterium *Tropheryma whipplei*. It tends to affect middle-aged men. It causes systemic manifestations such as diarrhea, weight loss, fever, abdominal pain, and polyarthritis. Neurologic manifestations include changes in personality, cognitive decline, supranuclear gaze palsy, parkinsonism, and oculomasticatory myorhythmia. Intestinal biopsy aids in the diagnosis; periodic acid-Schiff (PAS)-positive bacteria are seen within macrophages.

10. A

Celiac disease is an immune-related reaction to gluten. Most patients have the HLA-DQ2 haplotype. Celiac disease can have numerous neurologic manifestations. Ataxia and neuropathy are among the most common. It can also cause seizures, progressive myoclonic ataxia, dementia, and myopathy. Occipital calcifications can be seen in patients with celiac disease. Blood tests for celiac disease included deamidated gliadin peptide antibodies (immunoglobulin A [IgA] and IgG), IgA anti-endomysial antibody, and anti-tissue transglutaminase antibodies (IgA and IgG). Duodenal biopsy can be done to confirm the diagnosis.

11. D

This patient has posterior reversible encephalopathy syndrome (PRES). Symptoms include headache, vision changes, seizures, and altered mental status. Symmetric vasogenic edema in the occipital and parietal lobes is expected. Sometimes, signal abnormality may extend more anteriorly as well. Hypertension and preeclampsia/eclampsia are risk factors for PRES. PRES can also occur in sepsis; in transplant recipients; in patients receiving cyclosporin or tacrolimus; and in autoimmune disease.

12. D

Subarachnoid hemorrhage needs to be ruled out. Patients with polycystic kidney disease are at a risk for cerebrovascular malformations such as saccular aneurysms and dolichoectasia. Some patients with tuberous sclerosis complex have polycystic kidney disease.

Pituitary apoplexy, which is caused by infarction or hemorrhage of the pituitary gland, is another cause of thunderclap headache. In addition to severe headache, the patient may have vision changes, ophthalmoplegia, altered mental status, and hormone dysfunction. Subarachnoid hemorrhage may be present. Risk factors include pituitary macroadenoma and postpartum status. Pituitary apoplexy needs to be treated with hydrocortisone.

13. D

The most common neurologic complications of sarcoid are cranial neuropathies (particularly of the facial nerve). Facial nerve palsy may be bilateral. Sarcoidosis can also cause meningitis, focal leptomeningeal disease, periventricular white matter lesions, myelopathy, neuropsychiatric symptoms, hypothalamic-pituitary dysfunction (e.g., diabetes insipidus), and hydrocephalus. Parenchymal lesions can cause headache, seizures, and cognitive changes. Stroke can occur but is rare. The patient may have an elevated concentration of angiotensin-converting enzyme (ACE). Hyercalcemia can occur. Lung involvement and conjunctival biopsy can aid in the diagnosis of neurosarcoidosis. Sarcoid is associated with noncaseating granulomas and multinucleated giant cells.

14. B

Polycythemia vera is a neoplastic condition in the marrow that causes overproduction of red blood cells. The most common neurologic complication of polycythemia vera is stroke.

15. D

This patient has thrombotic thrombocytopenic purpura (TTP). The classic findings in TTP are microangiopathic hemolytic anemia, thrombocytopenic purpura, neurologic abnormalities, fever, and kidney disease. It is treated with plasma exchange.

Hemolytic uremic syndrome (HUS) can also cause microangiopathic hemolytic anemia and thrombocytopenia. It tends to occur in children. Patients with HUS often have a gastrointestinal illness with fever and diarrhea. Then renal failure occurs, resulting in reduced urine output and edema. Anemia and thrombocytopenia cause paleness and petechiae. Neurologic symptoms are less prominent than in TTP, but headache, irritability, lethargy, and seizures can occur in HUS. *Escherichia coli* O157:H7 and *Shigella* infections can cause HUS.

HUS and TTP can be difficult to differentiate. Age helps to differentiate the two: HUS is primarily seen in children, whereas TTP is more likely to be seen in adults. Also, renal symptoms are more prominent in HUS, and neurologic symptoms are more prominent in TTP. In addition, TTP is associated with a deficiency of ADAMTS13, which is a metallopeptidase involved in processing von Willebrand factor.

Patients with idiopathic thrombocytopenia purpura (ITP) do not have anemia and are less ill appearing than patients with TTP. Intracranial hemorrhage can occur in ITP.

16. C

Vitamin E deficiency causes acanthocytosis. Acanthocytosis can be seen in many conditions.

Acanthocytosis occurs in abetalipoproteinemia and hypobetalipoproteinemia types I and II. A group of conditions involving acanthocytosis and neurologic symptoms, especially movement disorders, are called neuroacanthocytoses. Examples are chorea-acanthocytosis (choreoacanthocytosis), Huntington disease-like 2, McLeod syndrome, and pantothenate kinase-associated neurodegeneration (PKAN).

17. C

Hypothyroidism causes delayed relaxation during reflex testing.

18. A

Cerebellar ataxia can occur with hypothyroidism.

The most common movement disorder in hyperthyroidism is tremor. Usually, this is a postural tremor of the hands. It improves with beta-blockers. Chorea secondary to hyperthyroidism may also respond to beta-blockers.

Hyperthyroidism is associated with a number of neuromuscular disorders, including periodic paralysis, myasthenia gravis, neuropathy, and myopathy. Thyrotoxic periodic paralysis attacks are associated with hypokalemia and are treated with potassium and nonselective beta-blockers.

There is an increased risk for stroke in young patients with thyrotoxicosis.

19. C

Pheochromocytoma occurs in neurofibromatosis type 1, Von Hippel-Lindau (VHL) syndrome, and MEN 2. It is rare in tuberous sclerosis complex.

VHL syndrome is caused by mutations in the VHL tumor suppressor gene on chromosome 3. Hemangioblastoma is a common presentation. Patients with VHL syndrome are at risk for cerebellar and spinal cord hemangioblastomas, retinal angiomas, renal cell carcinoma, pheochromocytomas, epididymal cystadenomas, bilateral endolymphatic sac tumors, and kidney and pancreatic cysts.

Pheochromocytoma can be seen in patients with MEN type 2A and 2B. Patients with MEN 2 are at risked for medullary carcinoma of the thyroid. Patients with MEN 2A may develop parathyroid disease. A marfanoid habitus and mucosal neuromas are seen in patients with MEN 2B. (MEN 1 tends to affect the pituitary, pancreas, and parathyroid glands. Facial angiofibromas, meningioma, and ependymoma can also occur in MEN 1.)

20. A

Patients with adrenal insufficiency require stress dosing of steroids when they are ill or undergoing surgery. Glucocorticoids, such as prednisone and hydrocortisone, are typically used for replacement. Fludrocortisone is a mineralocorticoid. Mineralocorticoids are under control of the renin-angiotensin system and do not need replacement if a patient has central adrenal insufficiency.

21. A

Pituitary tumors typically cause bitemporal hemianopsia due to pressure on the optic chiasm.

Pituitary adenomas are a common type of pituitary tumor. They typically arise from the anterior pituitary. Prolactinoma is the most common pituitary adenoma. Bromocriptine, which is a dopamine agonist, can be used to treat prolactinomas. (Dopamine inhibits prolactin secretion.) Dopamine agonists can have psychiatric side effects.

Pituitary tumors that produce growth hormone can cause acromegaly. Neurologic complications of acromegaly include peripheral neuropathy, especially of the median nerve; proximal myopathy; and obstructive and central sleep apnea.

Pituitary tumors can also produce adrenocorticotropic hormone (ACTH), causing Cushing disease due to hypercortisolism. Patients have truncal obesity, hypertension, abdominal striae, hirsutum, glucose intolerance, and later osteoporosis. Neurologic complications include myopathy, headache, and possible cognitive and psychiatric changes.

22. D

Tetany can occur with hypocalcemia, hypomagnesemia, and respiratory alkalosis (as seen with hyperventilation). This patient has hypocalcemia due to pseudohypoparathyroidism. Specifically, she has Albright hereditary osteodystrophy. These patients can have seizures, tetany, intellectual disability, basal ganglia calcification, and cataracts. Shortening of the metacarpal and metatarsal bones can be seen.

23. D

Polyarteritis nodosa affects medium-sized vessels. It can cause neuropathy, including mononeuritis multiplex.

Small-vessel vasculitis is divided into anti-neutrophil cytoplasmic antibody (ANCA)-associated vasculitis and immune complex small-vessel vasculitis.

ANCA-associated vasculitis tends to cause granulomatosis. ANCA-associated small-vessel vasculitis includes granulomatosis with polyangiitis (formerly Wegener granulomatosis), eosinophilic granulomatosis with polyangiitis (formerly Churg-Strauss syndrome), and microscopic polyangiitis.

Immune complex systemic vasculitis includes IgA vasculitis (Henoch-Schönlein purpura). Immune complex systemic vasculitis tends to cause leukocytoclastic vasculitis.

Henoch-Schönlein purpura is more common in children than in adults. It manifests with systemic symptoms such as fever and anorexia. There may be an antecedent infection. Then the patient develops a rash (palpable purpura without thrombocytopenia), abdominal pain, and joint pain. Intussusception and glomerulonephritis can occur. The lungs may also be affected. Headache and behavioral changes can be seen, but significant central nervous system involvement is rare.

24. C

Purkinje cell antibody 2 (PCA-2), ANNA-1, ANNA-2, ANNA-3, amphiphysin, and γ-aminobutyric acid (GABA) receptor paraneoplastic antibodies are associated with small cell lung carcinoma.

25. D

Peutz-Jeghers syndrome is *not* usually associated with brain tumors. It is associated primarily with gastrointestinal, pancreatic, breast, gynecologic, or lung cancers.

Turcot syndrome is associated with gliomas and medulloblastomas in addition to adenomatous colon polyps and adenocarcinoma.

Gorlin syndrome, or basal cell nevus syndrome, is associated with basal cell carcinomas and medulloblastomas.

Li-Fraumeni syndrome is associated with gliomas, medulloblastomas, and primitive neuroectodermal tumors (PNETs) in addition to breast cancer, sarcomas, and leukemias.

16.

NEUROMUSCULAR DISEASES

QUESTIONS

1. Fill in the blank: The nerves proximal to the formation of the brachial plexus are the _____.
   - A. Nerve to the subclavius and lateral pectoral nerve
   - B. Suprascapular nerve and nerve to the subclavius
   - C. Dorsal scapular nerve and long thoracic nerves
   - D. Suprascapular nerve and lateral pectoral nerves

2. A 30-year-old woman undergoes radical mastectomy. Postoperatively, she has shoulder weakness and scapular winging. Which nerve was injured?
   - A. Axillary nerve
   - B. Long thoracic nerve
   - C. Subscapular nerve
   - D. Thoracodorsal nerve

3. A lesion of which of the following nerves is most likely to cause wrist drop?
   - A. Anterior interosseous nerve
   - B. Median nerve
   - C. Radial nerve
   - D. Ulnar nerve

4. Which of the following tests aids in differentiating posterior cord plexopathy from radial neuropathy?
   - A. Test shoulder abduction
   - B. Test finger extension
   - C. Test elbow extension
   - D. Test wrist extension

5. Which muscle abducts the shoulder through the first 15 degrees?
   - A. Deltoid
   - B. Serratus anterior
   - C. Supraspinatus
   - D. Trapezius

6. A patient presents with wrist drop, mild weakness of supination and elbow flexion, and sensory loss over the dorsum of the hand. Elbow extension is strong. A radial neuropathy is suspected. Where is the lesion most likely to be located?
   - A. In the axilla
   - B. In the spiral groove
   - C. Just above the elbow
   - D. In the forearm

7. A 24-year-old transcriptionist presents with wrist pain that is worse in her dominant hand. She has been awakening at night with paresthesias in her hands. It seems to improve when she shakes her hands. Tapping a reflex hammer to her wrist causes paresthesias in her hands. Which of the following is *least* likely to be present in this condition?
   - A. Numbness over the thenar eminence
   - B. Weakness of the thenar eminence
   - C. Decreased sensation in the first, second, third, and fourth digits with sparing of the medial side of the fourth digit
   - D. Paresthesias when the wrist is passively flexed

8. A lesion at which of the following locations causes ulnar palmar sensory loss and weakness of all the ulnar-innervated intrinsic hand muscles?
   - A. Carpal tunnel
   - B. Guyon's canal
   - C. Midpalm
   - D. Pisohamate hiatus

9. Which of the following muscles has innervation from the obturator nerve and the tibial division of the sciatic nerve?
   - A. Adductor magnus
   - B. Gluteus maximus
   - C. Pectineus
   - D. Short head of the biceps femoris

10. An obese patient presents with dysesthesia in the lateral aspect of the upper thigh. Compression of which nerve is most likely responsible?
    - A. Lateral femoral cutaneous nerve
    - B. Cutaneous branch of the obturator nerve
    - C. Intermediate cutaneous nerve of the thigh
    - D. Femoral nerve

11. A patient presents with pain in the buttock that radiates down the posterior aspect of his leg to the lateral aspect of his foot. He has decreased sensation in a similar distribution. Hip extension, knee flexion, plantar flexion, and toe flexion are weak, and his ankle jerk reflex is decreased. What is the diagnosis?
    - A. L4 radiculopathy
    - B. L5 radiculopathy
    - C. S1 radiculopathy
    - D. Peroneal lesion

12. What is the most common pattern of muscle weakness in myopathies?
    - A. Distal arm and distal leg weakness
    - B. Distal arm and proximal leg weakness
    - C. Proximal arm and distal leg weakness
    - D. Proximal arm and proximal leg weakness

13. Which of the following statements is *false*?
    A. Congenital myopathies tend to manifest with hypotonia and weakness.
    B. Congenital myopathies are often manifested at birth.
    C. Congenital myopathies tend to cause rapidly progressive clinical worsening.
    D. Historically, muscle biopsy was used to classify congenital myopathies.

14. A child is brought to the clinic for developmental delay. He is hypotonic and has proximal muscle weakness. He has a history of hip dislocation and was recently diagnosed with scoliosis. His mother states that the child's brother has similar symptoms and had an adverse reaction to halothane. The patient undergoes a muscle biopsy, which shows absence of mitochondria in the middle of the muscle fibers. What is the most likely diagnosis?
    A. Cap disease
    B. Central core disease
    C. Nemaline rod myopathy
    D. Zebra body myopathy

15. A newborn has a high-arched palate, hypotonia, and weakness. His creatine phosphokinase (CPK) level is slightly elevated. Muscle biopsy shows rods containing α-actinin that are in continuity with the Z lines. What is his diagnosis?
    A. Central core myopathy
    B. Nemaline myopathy
    C. Myotubular myopathy
    D. Congenital muscular dystrophy

16. A mutation in which of the following genes causes merosin-deficient congenital muscular dystrophy (CMD)?
    A. *POMT1*
    B. *POMGnT1*
    C. *LAMA2*
    D. *SEPN1*

17. True or False?
    Botulinum toxin should be used with caution in patients with a CMD.

18. Patients with which of the following conditions can have cardiac involvement?
    A. Merosin-deficient CMD
    B. Fukuyama CMD
    C. Rigid spine disease
    D. All of the above

19. Patients with which CMD may have seizures?
    A. Merosin-deficient CMD
    B. Fukuyama CMD
    C. Muscle-eye-brain disease
    D. All of the above

20. Which of the following diseases is associated with poor head control early in life, spinal stiffness and progressive restrictive respiratory failure later in life, and desmin positive inclusions?

    A. Alpha-dystroglycan-related dystrophies
    B. Collagen VI-related myopathies
    C. Laminin alpha$_2$-related CMD
    D. SEPN1-related myopathy

21. A 6-year-old boy presents with falls and difficulty running. His symptoms began at age 3 years. On examination, he has calf hypertrophy, mild lordosis, head lag when pulled to sitting from the supine position, and difficulty arising quickly from the floor. His CPK level is significantly elevated. Which treatment should be recommended?
    A. Carnitine
    B. Creatine
    C. Oral corticosteroids
    D. Coenzyme Q10

22. An 18-year-old competitive softball player presents with difficulty throwing a softball. On examination, she has a transverse smile, widened palpebral fissures, scapular winging, and reversal of the anterior axillary folds. Her deltoids are strong, but her biceps, triceps, and pectoral muscles are weak. She has no contractures. Which of the following is most likely to occur in this condition?
    A. Cardiomyopathy
    B. Dysphagia
    C. Hearing loss
    D. Respiratory insufficiency

23. A 50-year-old woman presents with difficulty swallowing. On examination, she has ptosis and ophthalmoplegia. She denies double vision. Her mother and sister have similar symptoms. What is the most likely diagnosis?
    A. Mitochondrial myopathy
    B. Myotonic dystrophy
    C. Fascioscapulohumeral dystrophy
    D. Oculopharyngeal dystrophy

24. Patients with which of the following conditions are most likely to have asymmetric facial weakness?
    A. Fascioscapulohumeral dystrophy
    B. Myasthenia gravis
    C. Myotonic dystrophy
    D. Oculopharyngeal dystrophy

25. A 10-year-old boy presents with toe walking. On examination, he has contractures at the elbows and ankles. An electrocardiogram (ECG) shows first-degree atrioventricular block. The creatine kinase (CK) level is mildly elevated. The patient's older brother had similar symptoms and later developed a rigid spine. A mutation in which of the following genes is most likely the cause?
    A. *LMNA*
    B. *SMN1*
    C. *SMN2*
    D. *ZNF9*

26. Which of the following is an autosomal dominant limb-girdle muscular dystrophy that often manifests with myalgia and is associated with rippling muscles and a very high CK level?
    A. LGMD1A (myotilinopathy)
    B. LGMD1B (laminopathy)
    C. LGMD1C (caveolinopathy)
    D. LGMD1E (desminopathy)

27. Which of the following is the most common limb-girdle muscular dystrophy?
    A. LGMD2A
    B. LGMD2B
    C. LGMD2C
    D. LGMD2I

28. Mutations in which of the following genes cause inclusion body myopathy with Paget disease and frontotemporal dementia?
    A. *JPH*
    B. *PRNP*
    C. *SLC52A3* (also known as *C20ORF54*)
    D. *VCP*

29. Which of the following is the *least* likely presentation of metabolic myopathy?
    A. Muscle cramps during brief exercise
    B. Muscle cramps during prolonged exercise
    C. Myoglobinuria when the patient is febrile
    D. Progressive lower extremity numbness

30. A 1-month-old presents with poor feeding. On examination, he is hypotonic and has macroglossia and hepatomegaly. He is found to be in congestive heart failure. What is the most likely diagnosis?
    A. Congenital myotonic dystrophy
    B. Central core disease
    C. Myotubular myopathy
    D. Pompe disease (acid maltase deficiency)

31. A 30-year-old man presents with progressive weakness of the hands and feet. He says he also has difficulty releasing objects. On examination, he has frontal balding, ptosis, bilateral cataracts, masseter wasting, facial weakness, and weak distal extremities. A mutation in which of the following genes is most likely?
    A. *DMPK*
    B. *GBE1*
    C. *MT-TK*
    D. *TIM*

32. Which of the following statements about differences between myotonic dystrophy type 1 (DM1) and myotonic dystrophy type 2 (DM2) is true?
    A. DM2 tends to cause proximal muscle weakness.
    B. DM2 tends to affect type 2 muscle fibers.
    C. Systemic manifestations are typically less severe in DM2.
    D. All of the above are true.

33. A child presents with muscle stiffness. On examination, his leg muscles appear hypertrophied. His stiffness improves with activity. On electromyography (EMG), a "dive bomber" sound is heard. During the short exercise test, a postexercise decrement in the compound muscle action potential is seen, followed by a rapid return to baseline. Which of the following is the most likely etiology?
    A. A calcium channel mutation
    B. A chloride channel mutation
    C. A sodium channel mutation
    D. A potassium channel mutation

34. A 20-year-old man presents with abnormal eye movements. On examination, he has bilateral ptosis with no fatigability and limited eye movement when tracking. He also has hearing loss and pigmentary retinopathy. He has mild weakness in the proximal upper extremities. Which of the following is most likely to occur in this condition?
    A. Glaucoma
    B. Pulmonary fibrosis
    C. Ragged red fibers
    D. Renal artery stenosis

35. A patient with Sjögren syndrome presents with fever, fatigue, and weakness. On examination, the patient has periorbital edema, a facial rash, and a rash on her hands (extensor surface). She has proximal muscle weakness. Anti-Jo 1 antibodies are present in the serum. Which of the following findings is expected on muscle biopsy?
    A. Infiltration of the muscle by CD8+ T lymphocytes
    B. Perifascicular atrophy
    C. Rimmed vacuoles
    D. Intranuclear inclusions

36. Humoral attacks on blood vessels and complement deposition occur in which inflammatory myopathy?
    A. Inclusion body myositis
    B. Dermatomyositis
    C. Polymyositis

37. A 60-year-old woman presents with difficulties walking downstairs. She also complains that she's not able to knit like she used to. On examination, she has quadriceps weakness and asymmetric atrophy of her wrist and finger flexors. What is the most likely diagnosis?
    A. Amyloidosis
    B. Inclusion body myositis
    C. Immune-mediated necrotizing myopathy
    D. Polymyositis

38. Which of the following conditions is *least* likely to respond to corticosteroids?
    A. Dermatomyositis
    B. Inclusion body myositis
    C. Polymyositis
    D. Immune-mediated necrotizing myopathy

39. Fill in the blank: Statin-induced myositis has been associated with reduced levels of _____?
    A. Coenzyme Q10
    B. Pyridoxine
    C. Vitamin B12
    D. Vitamin E

40. Which type of fibers are slow twitch and fatigue resistant and use oxidative metabolism?
    A. Type 1
    B. Type 2

41. What do "onion bulbs" represent?
    A. An inflammatory reaction
    B. A reaction to blunt trauma
    C. Demyelination and remyelination
    D. Ischemic injury to the nerve

42. Which of the following is most suggestive of a myopathic process on muscle biopsy?
    A. Atrophic angular fibers
    B. Group atrophy
    C. Fibrosis
    D. Target fibers

43. Which pathologic finding is *least* likely to be found in a myopathy?
    A. Central nuclei
    B. Fiber-type grouping
    C. Split fibers
    D. Small and large round fibers

44. Internal nuclei are most prominent in which of the following?
    A. Myotonic dystrophy
    B. Central core disease
    C. Nemaline rod myopathy

45. Which stain is most helpful for identifying glycogen storage diseases?
    A. Gomori trichrome stain
    B. Congo red stain
    C. Crystal violet stain
    D. Periodic acid–Schiff (PAS) stain

46. A 20-year-old woman presents with double vision. On examination, she has ptosis that worsens with prolonged upgaze. Myasthenia gravis is suspected. What is the most sensitive test for myasthenia gravis?
    A. Cooling test
    B. Repetitive nerve stimulation
    C. Single-fiber EMG of the frontalis muscle
    D. Inching

47. The majority of patients with myasthenia gravis have which type of antibody?
    A. Acetylcholine receptor binding antibodies
    B. Acetylcholine receptor modulating antibodies
    C. Acetylcholine receptor blocking antibodies

48. Which of the following statements regarding myasthenic crisis is *false*?

    A. It is more common early in the disease course than later.
    B. Initiation of steroids can trigger myasthenic crisis.
    C. Patients with acetylcholine receptor binding antibodies are at greater risk for myasthenic crisis than patients with muscle-specific tyrosine kinase (MuSK) antibodies.
    D. Anticholinesterase medications should be withheld while the patient is intubated.

49. A 50-year-old man presents with proximal leg weakness and dry mouth. Rapid repetitive nerve stimulation produces a significant increment. The patient most likely has which of the following cancers?
    A. Prostate cancer
    B. Small cell lung cancer
    C. Pancreatic cancer
    D. Multiple myeloma

50. Which of the following findings is more characteristic of myasthenia gravis than of Lambert-Eaton syndrome?
    A. Strength improves with repetition
    B. Ocular weakness
    C. Dry mouth
    D. Abnormal pupillary response

51. For each of the following, state whether it is usually a feature of an axonal neuropathy or a demyelinating neuropathy.
    1) Reduced compound muscle action potentials
    2) Significantly reduced conduction velocities

52. A woman presents with numbness in her feet. On examination, she has decreased sensations of pinprick and vibration. The results of a comprehensive metabolic profile, thyroid function tests, B12 level, and hemoglobin A1c are normal. Which of the following should be performed next?
    A. Glucose tolerance test
    B. Human immunodeficiency virus (HIV) testing
    C. Nerve biopsy
    D. Vitamin E level

53. A 20-year-old woman presents with wrist drop. She also had an episode of foot drop 3 months ago. Her mother and her sister have had similar experiences. A mutation in which of the following genes is responsible?
    A. *GDAP1*
    B. *GJ1B*
    C. *MPZ*
    D. *PMP22*

54. Which of the following is *not* an X-linked inherited neuropathy?
    A. Charcot-Marie-Tooth neuropathy X type 1 (*GJB1*-related Charcot-Marie-Tooth neuropathy)
    B. Fabry disease
    C. Kennedy disease
    D. Friedreich ataxia

55. A patient with leukemia develops foot drop after a single dose of vincristine. Nerve conduction studies show

a demyelinating polyneuropathy. A mutation in which of the following genes is most likely responsible?
- A. *HINT1*
- B. *MFN2*
- C. *PMP22*
- D. *RAB7A*

56. Which of the following is *not* consistent with Friedreich ataxia?
- A. Abnormal sensory nerve conduction studies
- B. GAA triplet repeat expansion
- C. Reduced compound muscle action potentials
- D. Square-wave jerks

57. A patient presents with difficulty walking, which has been worsening over the past few days. He states that his legs initially became weak, but now his arms seem weak as well. Sensation is intact. He has areflexia. The cerebrospinal fluid (CSF) protein level is high, but the CSF white blood cell count is normal. Which of the following diagnoses should be considered?
- A. Spinal cord compression
- B. Cervical spondylosis
- C. Transverse myelitis
- D. Acute inflammatory demyelinating polyradiculoneuropathy (AIDP)

58. Which of the following is often the first abnormal finding in nerve conduction studies in acute AIDP?
- A. Prolonged F-wave latencies
- B. Conduction block
- C. Temporal dispersion
- D. Significantly decreased amplitude of the compound muscle action potential (CMAP)

59. Which Guillain-Barré syndrome (GBS) variant is characterized by ophthalmoparesis, areflexia and ataxia and tends to be associated with GQ1b antibodies?
- A. Acute motor-sensory axonal neuropathy (AMSAN)
- B. Bickerstaff brainstem encephalitis
- C. Miller-Fisher variant
- D. Sensory Guillain-Barré syndrome

60. Which of the following causes a descending paralysis?
- A. Botulism
- B. Diphtheria
- C. Tick paralysis
- D. Porphyria

61. True or False?
Sensory disturbances are more common in chronic inflammatory demyelinating neuropathy (CIDP) than in AIDP.

62. Which of the following disorders is most likely to be symmetric?
- A. Subacute inflammatory demyelinating polyneuropathy (SIDP)
- B. Multifocal motor neuropathy (MMN)
- C. Multifocal acquired demyelinating sensory and motor neuropathy (MADSAM)

63. Which of the following conditions is most likely to respond to steroids?
- A. Acute inflammatory demyelinating polyradiculoneuropathy (AIDP)
- B. Acute motor axonal neuropathy (AMAN)
- C. Multifocal motor neuropathy (MMN)
- D. Multifocal acquired demyelinating sensory and motor neuropathy (MADSAM)

64. Which of the following is most consistent with immunoglobulin M-monoclonal gammopathy of undetermined significance (IgM-MGUS)?
- A. Asymmetric distal polyneuropathy
- B. Symmetric proximal polyneuropathy
- C. Slowed conduction velocities consistent with demyelination
- D. Decreased amplitudes of compound muscle action potentials

65. Which of the following systemic diseases is most closely associated with the syndrome of polyneuropathy, organomegaly, endocrinopathy, M protein, and skin changes (POEMS)?
- A. Lymphoma
- B. Osteosclerotic myeloma
- C. Small-cell lung cancer
- D. Thymoma

66. A 50-year-old man presents with hand weakness. On examination, he has atrophy and fasciculations in his left hand, brisk reflexes in all four extremities, a brisk jaw jerk, and a normal sensory examination. Which of the following is the most likely diagnosis?
- A. Amyotrophic lateral sclerosis
- B. Primary lateral sclerosis
- C. Progressive muscular atrophy
- D. Spinal muscular atrophy

67. Which of the following conditions is most likely to be present in a patient with early ALS?
- A. Autonomic disturbance
- B. Incontinence
- C. Ophthalmoplegia
- D. Spasticity

68. What is the mechanism of action of riluzole?
- A. It is a GABA antagonist.
- B. It inhibits glutamate release.
- C. It is a glycine agonist.
- D. It is an NMDA antagonist.

69. A 40-year-old man with a history of diabetes mellitus presents with difficulty swallowing. On examination, he has perioral and tongue fasciculations, proximal weakness, and gynecomastia. Which of the following genes is most likely responsible?
- A. Androgen receptor gene
- B. Estrogen receptor gene
- C. Insulin receptor gene
- D. Testosterone receptor gene

NEUROMUSCULAR DISEASES

ANSWERS

1. C

The dorsal scapular nerve and the long thoracic nerve are proximal to the formation of the brachial plexus. The dorsal scapular nerve (C4, C5) supplies the major and minor rhomboid muscles. The long thoracic nerve (C5, C6, C7) supplies the serratus anterior.

The suprascapular nerve and nerve to the subclavius arise from the upper trunk.

The lateral pectoral nerve is a branch of the lateral cord, which is derived from the anterior branches of the upper and middle trunks of the brachial plexus.

2. B

The long thoracic nerve, which innervates the serratus anterior, can be injured during mastectomy. This results in scapular winging. Pressure on the shoulder from heavy objects can also injure the long thoracic nerve. In addition, the long thoracic nerve is often affected in Parsonage-Turner syndrome.

Parsonage-Turner syndrome, which is also known as neuralgic amyotrophy, tends to occur after a viral infection, immunization, or surgery. The patient has sudden, severe pain in the shoulder that often begins at night. This is followed by weakness of the shoulder and proximal arm. The phrenic nerve or anterior interosseous nerve may also be affected. There is a hereditary form of neuralgic amyotrophy.

Serratus anterior weakness causes medial winging of the scapula. Lateral winging of the scapula can be caused by weakness of rhomboid or trapezius muscles. The rhomboid muscles are innervated by the dorsal scapular nerve. The trapezius muscle is innervated by the spinal accessory nerve, C3, and C4. The spinal accessory nerve can be injured during cervical lymph node biopsy or other surgery in the cervical region. Trapezius weakness causes shoulder drop as well scapular winging.

Scapular winging can also occur in myopathies. Sarcoglycanopathies and limb-girdle muscular dystrophy 2A (LGMD2A) are associated with scapular winging.

3. C

Wrist drop can occur with central nervous system lesions and with lesions of the C7 root, posterior cord of the brachial plexus, radial nerve in the axilla, radial nerve at the spiral groove, or posterior interosseous nerve.

4. A

The branches of the posterior cord are the radial nerve, the axillary nerve, the thoracodorsal nerve, and the subscapular nerve. To differentiate a posterior cord plexopathy from a radial neuropathy, a muscle innervated by the axillary, thoracodorsal, or subscapular nerve should be tested.

The radial nerve is responsible for elbow and wrist extension. One of its branches, the posterior interosseous nerve, is responsible for finger extension.

Testing shoulder abduction may help to differentiate posterior cord plexopathy from radial neuropathy. The deltoid, which is innervated by the axillary nerve, is one of the muscles responsible for shoulder abduction. Weakness of shoulder abduction would make a posterior cord plexopathy lesion more likely than a radial neuropathy. Loss of sensation in the upper arm is also seen with axillary nerve injury.

5. C

The supraspinatus muscle, which is innervated by the suprascapular nerve (C5, C6), abducts the shoulder through the first 15 degrees. The deltoid muscle, which is innervated by the axillary nerve (C5, C6), abducts the arm from 15 to 90 degrees. The trapezius and serratus anterior muscles are involved in abduction of the arm from 90 to 180 degrees.

6. B

This patient has injury of the radial nerve in the spiral groove, which is the most common site of radial nerve injury. The radial nerve can be injured at the spiral groove as a result of fracture of the humerus. "Saturday night palsy" is caused by injury of the radial nerve in the spiral groove.

The radial nerve can be injured at multiple locations. Knowledge of radial nerve anatomy allows prediction of the site of injury (see Box 16.1).

When the radial nerve is injured in the spiral groove, the patient has finger drop, wrist drop, and sensory changes in the distribution of the superficial radial sensory nerve. Supination is mildly weak. Weakness of the brachioradialis causes weakened elbow flexion. Elbow extension is spared because the triceps is not affected by a radial neuropathy at the spiral groove. The triceps is affected by radial nerve injury in the axilla, such as from crutches. Patients with radial neuropathy in the axilla also have decreased sensation in the posterior arm and forearm.

Box 16.1 RADIAL NERVE ANATOMY

- The radial nerve is a branch of the posterior cord of the brachial plexus.
- In the upper arm, the radial nerve gives off cutaneous branches and innervates the triceps and anconeus muscles.
- The radial nerve then travels through the spiral groove of the humerus.
- Distal to the spiral groove but above the elbow, the radial nerve innervates the brachioradialis and extensor carpi radialis longus.
- Distal to the elbow, the radial nerve divides into the superficial radial sensory nerve and the deep radial motor branch.
- The superficial radial sensory nerve is typically a pure cutaneous sensory nerve. It supplies the lateral dorsum of the hand and part of the thumb.
- The deep radial motor branch supplies the extensor carpi radialis brevis and the supinator before traveling under the arcade of Frohse through the supinator muscle.
- When it travels into the supinator, the nerve becomes the posterior interosseous nerve, which is a pure motor nerve. The posterior interosseous nerve supplies the extensors of the wrist, thumb, and fingers.

7. A

This patient has carpal tunnel syndrome, which is caused by median nerve compression. It is the most common entrapment neuropathy. It is a clinical diagnosis. In idiopathic cases, the dominant hand is usually affected more than the nondominant hand. Nocturnal hand paresthesias are a common symptom. Sensory changes occur before motor changes. Patients have decreased sensation in the first, second, third, and fourth digits with sparing of the medial side of the fourth digit. Sensation over the thenar eminence should be normal because it is innervated by the palmar cutaneous sensory branch of the median nerve, which arises before the carpal tunnel. Weakness of thumb abduction and opposition occur late.

A cervical radiculopathy is in the differential diagnosis of carpal tunnel syndrome. Pain in the neck, paresthesias from the neck or shoulder down the arm, weak arm muscles, sensory disturbances in the arm or forearm, and reduced biceps or triceps reflexes raise concern for a radiculopathy.

8. B

Ulnar nerve lesions do not cause sensory symptoms proximal to the wrist. The ulnar nerve provides no sensation proximal to the wrist.

The ulnar nerve does not travel through the carpal tunnel. It travels through Guyon's canal at the wrist. A proximal canal lesion causes ulnar palmar sensory loss and weakness of the all the ulnar-innervated intrinsic hand muscles.

In Guyon's canal, the ulnar nerve splits into the superficial and deep branches. The superficial branch exits the canal, supplies the palmaris brevis (a hypothenar muscle), and provides sensation to the fourth and fifth digits. Fibers from the deep branch exit Guyon's canal to supply the other hypothenar muscles: the abductor digiti minimi, the flexor digiti minimi, and the opponens digiti minimi. After exiting Guyon's canal via the pisohamate hiatus, the deep branch supplies the rest of the ulnar-innervated muscles in the hand (the third and fourth lumbricals, the palmar interossei, the adductor pollicis, and the deep head of the flexor pollicus brevis). Therefore, a lesion at the pisohamate hiatus causes weakness of ulnar intrinsic hand muscles but spares the hypothenar muscles.

Ulnar neuropathy at the elbow can cause atrophy of hypothenar and thenar muscles, but thumb abduction is spared. Weakness of the flexor digitorum profundus can cause difficulty making a fist; the patient is unable to tuck in the fourth and fifth digits. The patient may demonstrate a benediction posture of the hands. Froment's sign and Wartenberg's sign may be seen. (Froment's sign is characterized by flexion of the thumb and index finger when pinching paper. Wartenberg's sign is caused by difficulty adducting the little finger: The little finger is abducted when the patient tries to hold the fingers together.)

9. A

The adductor magnus has innervation from the obturator nerve and the tibial division of the sciatic nerve.

The gluteus maximus is supplied by the inferior gluteal nerve.

The short head of the biceps femoris is the only muscle above the knee supplied by the peroneal division of the sciatic nerve.

The pectineus is innervated by the obturator and femoral nerves. It is an adductor of the thigh.

10. A

This patient has meralgia paresthetica, which is caused by compression of the lateral femoral cutaneous nerve. This nerve can be compressed under the inguinal ligament. Common risk factors include diabetes, obesity, pregnancy, constricting clothing, and trauma.

11. C

This patient has an S1 radiculopathy. S1 provides sensation to the sole and the lateral aspect of the foot. S1 also provides innervation to the hip extensors (gluteus maximus), knee flexors (hamstrings), plantar flexors (gastrocnemius and soleus muscles), toe flexors (flexor digitorum longus), and intrinsic foot muscles. The patient's ankle jerk reflex is reduced because the gastrocnemius muscle is affected.

An L4 radiculopathy would cause a decreased knee jerk. The quadriceps muscle is responsible for the knee jerk.

12. D

The most common pattern of muscle weakness in myopathies is symmetric weakness in the proximal arms and legs.

13. C

Causes of hypotonia and weakness in the newborn include congenital myopathies, congenital muscular dystrophies, congenital myotonic dystrophy, congenital myasthenic syndromes, spinal muscular atrophy, acid maltase deficiency (Pompe disease), and Prader-Willi syndrome.

Congenital myopathies tend to be manifested at birth with hypotonia, weakness, and hyporeflexia. Facial, bulbar, extraocular, or respiratory weakness may be present. Ptosis occurs in many types of congenital myopathy. Orthopedic abnormalities may be present. Mental status and sensation are normal. The serum CK level is normal or slightly elevated; significant elevations are more consistent with muscular dystrophy. If progression occurs in a congenital myopathy, it is slow, not rapid.

In an older child, congenital myopathy may manifest with scoliosis, a rigid spine, cardiomyopathy, pes cavus or foot drop, malignant hyperthermia, or respiratory weakness.

Historically, muscle biopsy was used to help diagnose and classify congenital myopathies (see Table 16.1).

Table 16.1 CLASSIFICATION OF CONGENITAL MYOPATHIES BY MUSCLE BIOPSY FINDINGS

MUSCLE BIOPSY FINDINGS	DISEASES
Rods	Nemaline myopathy
Cores	Central core disease, multi-minicore disease
Central nuclei	Centronuclear/myotubular myopathy
Hypotrophy of type 1 fibers	Congenital fiber type disproportion

Currently, genetics, muscle magnetic resonance imaging (MRI), and muscle ultrasound also aid in diagnosis. Genetic testing is complicated by the fact that multiple genes can cause a similar phenotype and a genetic mutation can cause variable phenotypes. For instance, multiple genes have been found to cause nemaline myopathy. Mutations in *ACTA1*, which encodes α-skeletal actin (also known as skeletal muscle α-actin), can cause multiple types of congenital myopathy.[1]

14. B

This patient has central core disease, which is often caused by mutations in the *RYR1* gene on chromosome 19q. This gene can also cause multi-minicore disease, centronuclear myopathies, and cone-rod disease. *RYR1* mutations are also associated with hip dislocation, club feet, scoliosis,

and rigid spine. The *RYR1* gene encodes the ryanodine receptor that is found in muscle. This is a calcium channel receptor. Mutations in the *RYR1* gene are associated with malignant hyperthermia. Patients with other core myopathies are also at risk.

Inhalational agents, such as halothane, and the muscle relaxant succinylcholine can cause malignant hyperthermia in susceptible individuals. In the operating room, a rising end-tidal carbon dioxide level is an early sign of malignant hyperthermia. Other signs of malignant hyperthermia are hyperthermia, muscle rigidity, tachycardia, metabolic acidosis, hyperkalemia, and myoglobinuria due to rhabdomyolysis. Malignant hyperthermia is treated with cooling, fluids, and dantrolene. Dantrolene inhibits intracellular calcium release. It should not be given with calcium channel antagonists.

Mutations in *RYR1* and *SEPN1* both can cause congenital myopathy and a phenotype resembling congenital muscular dystrophies.[1,2]

15. B

This patient has nemaline myopathy. Defects in multiple genes cause nemaline myopathy, most commonly mutations in *NEB*, which encodes nebulin. Severe cases of nemaline myopathy are often the result of mutations in *ACTA1*.[1]

16. C

The CMDs include collagenopathies, merosinopathies, dystroglycanopathies, and unclassified muscular dystrophies.

Merosin-deficient CMD is the most common CMD in the European population. It is also referred to as MDC1A. It manifests with weakness, hypotonia, respiratory insufficiency, and feeding difficulties. Contractures may be present at birth. Central nervous system abnormalities such as seizures, dysmyelination, and intellectual disability can occur. Merosin-deficient CMD is caused by mutations in *LAMA2*, which encodes laminin-α2.[2,3]

17. True

Botulinum toxin should be used with caution in patients with CMD because of the risk for prolonged weakness.[3]

18. D

Merosin-deficient CMD, Fukuyama CMD, and rigid spine disease all have cardiac involvement.

In a patient with muscle disease, an elevated level of creatine kinase-MB (CK-MB) does not necessarily indicate cardiac involvement.

19. D

Ocular involvement and seizures are most common in the dystroglycanopathies but can also occur in patients with merosin-deficient CMD. Lissencephaly type II/pachygyria can be seen in Fukuyama CMD, muscle-eye-brain disease, and Walker-Warburg syndrome, which are dystroglycanopathies. An occipital encephalocele can occur in patients with Walker-Warburg syndrome, which is the most severe of the dystroglycanopathies. Cerebellar cysts are seen in some dystroglycanopathies.[2,3]

20. D

This is SEPN1-related myopathy, which is caused by mutations in *SEPN1*, which encodes selenoprotein N. SEPN1-related myopathy often manifests with poor head control.

Both SEPN1-related myopathy and collagen VI-related dystrophies can cause unexpected respiratory failure and cor pulmonale.

Collagen VI-related dystrophies are also associated with congenital contractures and excessive laxity. Examples of collagen VI-related dystrophies are Ullrich CMD and Bethlem myopathy. Both are associated with hyperkeratosis and keloid formation.

Head drop and spinal rigidity also occur in LMNA-related dystrophy, but the CPK level is higher in these patients than in those with SEPN1-related myopathy. LMNA-related dystrophy is caused by mutations in lamin A/C, which is encoded by *LMNA*. Lamin A/C mutations can also cause Emery-Dreifuss muscular dystrophy.[2]

21. C

This patient most likely has Duchenne muscular dystrophy (DMD). Corticosteroids prolong ambulation.

DMD is one of the dystrophinopathies. It is usually caused by out-of-frame mutations in *DMD*, which encodes for the protein dystrophin. In-frame mutations cause Becker muscular dystrophy (BMD). Both DMD and BMD are X-linked recessive.

Patients with DMD gradually lose motor milestones and become wheelchair bound. Patients develop joint contractures and scoliosis. DMD is associated with decreased pulmonary function, cardiac arrhythmias and dilated cardiomyopathy, and cognitive impairment. Female carriers of DMD can also develop dilated cardiomyopathy.

BMD is less severe, and intellect is typically normal.

22. C

This patient has facioscapulohumeral dystrophy (FSHD). The first sign is usually facial weakness, but arm weakness with difficulty performing overhead activities is more likely to bring the patient to medical attention. The pectoral muscles are particularly weak, resulting in reversal of the anterior axillary folds. A "triple hump" sign can be seen because of preserved deltoid strength and scapular winging. (The humps are the deltoid, the shoulder bones, and the winged scapula.) Surgery may be required to fix the scapula in place. Weak abdominal muscles can cause abdominal protuberance. Cardiomyopathy, respiratory insufficiency, and bulbar weakness are not common in FSHD; although some patients have cardiac arrhythmia. Life expectancy is typically normal. Hearing loss and retinal vascular abnormalities are common in FSHD. Patients can have Coat syndrome, which refers to an exudative retinopathy.

23. D

This patient most likely has oculopharyngeal muscular dystrophy (OPMD), which causes ptosis and dysphagia. Patients often have ophthalmoparesis as well, but diplopia is rare. OPMD usually manifests in the fifth or sixth decade of life with ptosis. It is associated with expansion of the GCN trinucleotide repeat in the gene *PABPN1*, which encodes for polyadenylation-binding protein nuclear 1. OPMD is autosomal dominant. Anticipation does *not* occur in OPMD.

Facioscapulohumeral dystrophy and myotonic dystrophy usually do not cause ophthalmoplegia.

Mitochondrial myopathy tends to cause ptosis and ophthalmoplegia without pharyngeal involvement.

The combination of ptosis and ophthalmoparesis can occur in other myopathies and in neuromuscular junction disorders such as myasthenia gravis. Certain congenital myopathies, such as nemaline myopathy and central core myopathy, cause ptosis without ophthalmoparesis.

24. A

Facial weakness is most likely to be asymmetric in facioscapulohumeral dystrophy (FSHD). In FSHD, weakness begins in the face and spreads in a rostrocaudal pattern. Limb muscle involvement may also be asymmetric. There may be highly variable clinical phenotypes among different family members with FSHD.

Most cases of FSHD are classified as FSHD1, which has multiple specific genetic features. Patients with FSHD1 have a contraction mutation of *D4Z4* on chromosome 4 that results in fewer repeats than normal. In addition, a permissive simple sequence length polymorphism and the 4qA variant at the terminus must be present for the disease to manifest clinically. The combination of these genetic features leads to hypomethylation of D4Z4 region. This region contains the *DUX4* gene, which encodes double homeobox protein 4 (DUX4). Type 2 FSHD is caused by mutations in the *SMCHD1* gene. Mutations in the *SMCHD1* gene also affect DUX4 expression. Both FSHD1 and FSHD2 are autosomal dominant.[4]

In myotonic dystrophy, facial weakness causes ptosis and a "hatchet-face" or "fish-mouth" look. The mastication muscles are particularly affected.

25. A

This patient has Emery-Dreifuss muscular dystrophy (EDMD). Early contractures of the elbow flexors and ankle plantar flexors are characteristic findings. Contractures of the spine also occur early. Patients have a humeroperoneal pattern of weakness and cardiac disease. Patients with EDMD are at risk for sudden death. They may require a pacemaker with an internal cardiac defibrillator.

Most patients with EDMD have mutations in the gene *LMNA*, which encodes lamin A/C. This mutation is autosomal dominant. Other patients with EDMD have mutations in *EMD*, which encodes emerin. This is X-linked recessive. There are other, less common genetic mutations that can cause EDMD. Female carriers of X-linked EDMD are at risk for cardiac disease.

Mutations in *SMN1* on chromosome 5q are the most common cause of spinal muscular atrophy. *SMN1* and *SMN2* encode for survival motor neuron protein, but *SMN1* produces more functional protein. *SMN2* is adjacent to *SMN1* and modifies the severity of spinal muscular atrophy; more copies of *SMN2* result in less severe disease.

Mutations in the gene *ZNF9* (also known as *CNBP*) cause myotonic dystrophy type 2 (DM2).

26. C

Typically, but not always, limb-girdle muscular dystrophies (LGMDs) affect the proximal muscles in the upper and lower extremities and have autosomal inheritance. Historically, autosomal dominant LGMDs were classified as type 1 and autosomal recessive LGMDs were classified as type 2. The autosomal recessive LGMDs are more common than those inherited in an autosomal dominant manner and are usually associated with a higher CK level. An exception is LGMD1C, which causes a significantly elevated CK.

In addition to a significantly elevated CK, LGMD1C is associated with rippling muscles. Percussion with a reflex hammer causes rippling of the muscle. Hypertrophic cardiomyopathy and cardiac arrhythmias can also occur in LGMD1C.

LGMD1A is caused by mutations in *MYOT*, which are also the cause of myotilin-associated myofibrillar myopathy. Dysarthria is a characteristic finding.

LGMD1B is caused by mutations in LMNA and is allelic with Emery-Dreifuss muscular dystrophy (EDMD). Limb contractures occur in both conditions. Patients with LGMD1B can have significant cardiac disease; life-threatening arrhythmias and cardiomyopathy can occur.

LGMD1E is associated with myofibrillar myopathy and cardiomyopathy.[5,6]

27. A

LGMD2A (calpainopathy), which is associated with mutations in *CAPN3*, is the most common LGMD. Most patients develop symptoms before adulthood. The proximal lower extremities are weaker than the upper extremities, but scapular winging is present. LGMD2A is usually not associated with cardiac disease.

LGMD2B (dysferlinopathy) is also a common type of LGMD. It is associated with very high CK levels. It is caused by mutations in *DYSF*. Mutations in *DYSF* also cause Miyoshi myopathy. Miyoshi myopathy is characterized by distal weakness primarily affecting the calf muscles.

LGMD2I is caused by mutations in *FKRP*. LGMD2I is one of the dystroglycanopathies. It is associated with scapular winging, calf hypertrophy, and early cardiorespiratory involvement.

Sarcoglycanopathies (LGMD2C through 2F) resemble dystrophinopathies. However, Duchenne muscular dystrophy and Becker muscular dystrophy are more common than LGMD. In sarcoglycanopathies, symptoms begin in childhood and progressive proximal weakness occurs. Calf hypertrophy and lumbar hyperlordosis are seen. Respiratory failure and cardiomyopathy are common.[5]

28. D

Mutations in the gene *VCP* cause inclusion body myopathy with Paget disease and frontotemporal dementia (IBMPFD1), which is also called multisystem proteinopathy 1. This disorder can also be associated with motor neuron disease. The gene *VCP* encodes valosin-containing protein, which is a type of adenosine triphosphatase (ATPase).

Mutations in *SLC52A3* (previously called *C20ORF54*) are responsible for some cases of Fazio-Londe syndrome, which is also known as progressive bulbar palsy of childhood. *SLC52A3* encodes a riboflavin transporter, and there have been attempts to treat Fazio-Londe syndrome with riboflavin.

Mutations in *PRNP* and *JPH* cause Huntington disease-like 1 and Huntington disease like-2, respectively.

29. D

Metabolic myopathy can manifest with progressive weakness or exercise intolerance, such as cramps and myalgia. Myoglobinuria may occur with exercise or when the patient is febrile.

Metabolic causes of exercise intolerance include fatty acid oxidation disorders, defects of glycogenolysis, mitochondrial disorders, and myoadenylate deaminase deficiency. Brief exercise uses glycogen. Therefore, symptoms manifesting during a short amount of exercise suggest a glycogen storage disorder. Prolonged exercise requires free fatty acids. Symptoms that develop with prolonged exercise suggest a lipid storage disease.

Carnitine palmitoyl transferase II deficiency is the most common cause of recurrent myoglobinuria in adults. Triggers include fever, exercise, fasting, and valproic acid. The CK level is usually normal or mildly elevated between episodes.

Glycogen storage disease type V, or McArdle disease, also causes episodes of myoglobinuria. CK is elevated during and between episodes. Patients with McArdle disease may experience a second wind with exercise. Warming up before exercise and consuming a carbohydrate-rich diet may help with exercise tolerance. McArdle disease is caused by mutations in the gene that encodes myophosphorylase.

Patients with glycogen storage disease type VII, or Tarui disease, have some similarities to those with McArdle disease. For example, patients with Tarui disease have exercise intolerance but worsen if given glucose before exercise. Tarui disease is caused by deficiency of phosphofructokinase.[7]

30. D

This patient has Pompe disease, which is glycogen storage disease type II (GSD II). This is a lyosomal storage disease caused by acid maltase deficiency. The gene responsible for GSD II is *GAA*. GSD II can manifest in the newborn period with macroglossia, hypotonia, weakness, congestive heart failure, and hepatomegaly. It can manifest later in life with progressive proximal weakness. It can resemble a limb-girdle muscular dystrophy or polymyositis. GSD II can also manifest with respiratory failure. Myotonic discharges may be seen in the paraspinal muscles. Enzyme replacement is available.

31. A

This patient has myotonic dystrophy type 1 (DM1), which is caused by an expanded CTG repeat in the *DMPK* (dystrophia myotonica protein kinase) gene on chromosome 19. Patients with adult-onset DM1 have a distinctive facial appearance, grip myotonia, and distal weakness. Patients have frontal balding, ptosis, and wasting of the temporalis and masseter muscles. "Christmas tree" cataracts are characteristic of DM1. Myotonia, which causes a crescendo-decrescendo pattern (described as a "dive bomber" sound) on EMG, has been treated with mexiletine. Respiratory muscle weakness leads to pneumonia. Obstructive sleep apnea and sleep hypoventilation can occur. Modafinil has been used for hypersomnia. Arrhythmias may result in sudden death. Endocrine dysfunction is common (e.g., diabetes mellitus, hypogonadism, hyperlipidemia). Cholelithiasis, constipation, and dysphagia can occur in DM1. Patients have been described as apathetic or may have an avoidant personality. Mild cognitive impairment may be present. Subcortical white matter changes can be seen on MRI. DM1 is autosomal dominant. Anticipation occurs.

Congenital myotonic dystrophy is more severe than adult-onset DM1 and is usually inherited from the mother. Patients are hypotonic at birth and may have arthrogryposis. The mouth is often tent-shaped. Facial weakness causes poor suck. Reflexes are decreased or absent. Myotonia is *not* present in infancy. Respiratory distress is common. Patients with congenital myotonic dystrophy have delayed milestones and cognitive impairment.

Mutations in *GBE1* cause glycogen storage disease type IV (GSD IV), which results in glycogen branching enzyme deficiency. This is also known as Anderson disease. Some patients with this condition have adult polyglucosan body disease, which is associated with dementia, upper and lower motor symptoms, and cerebellar ataxia.

Mutations in *TIM* cause triosephosphate isomerase deficiency, which leads to hemolytic anemia and neurologic deterioration in early childhood.

Mutations in the gene *MT-TK* are associated with myoclonic epilepsy with ragged red fibers.

32. D

DM2 causes muscle pain, stiffness, and weakness. DM1 tends to cause distal muscle weakness, whereas DM2 causes proximal muscle weakness. (DM2 has been called proximal myotonic myopathy.) Patients with DM2 are less likely to have facial weakness than patients with DM1. Calf hypertrophy can be seen in DM2. Systemic manifestations are less common in DM2 than in DM1, but patients with DM2 can have arrhythmia, endocrine dysfunction, cataracts, and white matter changes.

In both DM1 and DM2, muscle biopsy shows increased internal nuclei, and pyknotic nuclear clumps can be seen. In DM1, type 1 fibers tend to be more affected. In DM2, type 2 fibers tend to be more affected.

DM2 is autosomal dominant, like DM1, but it does *not* demonstrate anticipation. DM2 is caused by a quadruple nucleotide repeat (CCTG) in the *ZNF9* gene, which has also been called *CNBP*.

33. B

This is myotonia congenita, which is caused by a chloride channel mutation. The mutation is in the gene *CLCN1* on chromosome 7q35. Patients with myotonia congenita have muscle hypertrophy, especially in the legs, and myotonia. Clinically, myotonia improves with exercise, as in patients with myotonic dystrophy. Patients with myotonia congenita have characteristic findings on the short exercise test during electrodiagnostic testing. The compound muscle action potential decreases after brief exercise and then rapidly returns to normal.

Myotonia worsens with exercise in patients with paramyotonia congenita, which is caused by a sodium channel mutation. Mutations in the gene *SCN4A* on chromosome 17q23 cause paramyotonia congenita, hyperkalemic periodic paralysis, hypokalemic periodic paralysis, and potassium-aggravated myotonias (myotonia fluctuans, myotonia permanens, and acetazolamide-sensitive myotonia).

Andersen-Tawil syndrome and thyrotoxic periodic paralysis are caused by mutations in the potassium channel. Anderson-Tawil syndrome is characterized by distinctive facial features, ventricular arrhythmias, and episodic weakness. Flaccid weakness can occur in patients with Anderson-Tawil syndrome with high, low, or normal potassium levels. Hypokalemia can cause weakness in patients with thyrotoxic periodic paralysis.

34. C

This patient has Kearns-Sayre syndrome, which is caused by a deletion in mitochondrial DNA. Progressive external ophthalmoplegia and pigmentary retinopathy are characteristic.

Patients with Kearns-Sayre syndrome can have heart block and may require pacemakers. Patients also tend to have sensorineural deafness, a proximal myopathy, cerebellar ataxia, high CSF protein, and short stature. Endocrinopathies may be present. Patients may benefit from treatment with coenzyme Q10 and L-carnitine. Some patients have low CSF folic acid and have been given folinic acid.

Pearson syndrome is also caused by a mitochondrial DNA deletion and is associated with progressive external ophthalmoplegia. However, patients with Pearson syndrome also tend to have sideroblastic anemia and pancreatic dysfunction.

35. B

This patient has dermatomyositis, which is an inflammatory myopathy. Dermatomyositis occurs in both children and adults. It is more common in women than in men. Typical features are a heliotrope rash on the eyelids, Gottron papules on the knuckles, a sun-sensitive rash on the face and upper body, and subcutaneous calcifications over pressure points such as the elbows. Patients have symmetric proximal weakness in the upper and lower extremities. On muscle biopsy, perifascicular atrophy is seen.

Interstitial lung disease and myocarditis are possible complications of dermatomyositis. Anti-Jo 1 antibodies are often present in the serum of patients with inflammatory myopathy and interstitial lung disease. Gastrointestinal hemorrhage can occur from vasculopathy in dermatomyositis.

Adults with dermatomyositis are at increased risk for cancer. Patients with juvenile dermatomyositis do not have this risk. Anti-TIF1 antibodies may be found in patients with dermatomyositis and cancer.

Dermatomyositis is associated with autoimmune conditions such as systemic lupus erythematosus, Raynaud syndrome, and Sjögren syndrome. Anti-nuclear antibodies (ANA) may be present in patients with dermatomyositis.

Sjögren syndrome is characterized by xerophthalmia (dry eyes) and xerostomia (dry mouth). Patients may have a small-fiber neuropathy. Salivary gland biopsy and the presence of anti-Ro (SSA) and anti-LA (SSB) antibodies help to confirm the diagnosis of Sjögren syndrome.[8]

36. B

In addition to perifascicular atrophy, muscle biopsy in patients with dermatomyositis may demonstrate humoral attacks on blood vessels and complement deposition.

Infiltration of the muscle by CD8+ T lymphocytes is seen in polymyositis.

Rimmed vacuoles, intranuclear inclusions, and intracytoplasmic inclusions are found in inclusion body myositis. Rimmed vacuoles can also occur in patients with certain types of muscular dystrophies (see Table 16.2).

Table 16.2 COMPARISON OF PATHOLOGIC FINDINGS IN INFLAMMATORY MYOPATHIES

DISEASE	MUSCLE BIOPSY FINDINGS
Dermatomyositis	Perifascicular atrophy
Inclusion body myositis	Red-rimmed vacuoles on Gomori trichrome stain
Polymyositis	CD8+ lymphocytes infiltrating the muscle

37. B

This patient has inclusion body myositis (IBM). IBM affects the finger flexors, wrist flexors, and quadriceps.

The weakness tends to be asymmetric, which is unusual in autoimmune myopathies. Patients may have dysphagia. Red-rimmed vacuoles are seen on Gomori trichrome stain. Antibodies to cytosolic 5′-nucleotidase 1A may be present in patients with IBM.

Immune-mediated necrotizing myopathy can occur in autoimmune conditions or malignancies. In some patients, it follows statin use. These patients may have antibodies to 3-hydroxy-3-methylglutaryl-coenzyme A (HMG-CoA) reductase. Some patients with immune-mediated necrotizing myopathy have anti-signal recognition particle (SRP) antibody, which can be associated with dilated cardiomyopathy (see Table 16.3).[8]

Table 16.3 ANTIBODIES IN INFLAMMATORY MYOPATHIES

DISEASE	ANTIBODIES
Dermatomyositis	Anti-transcription intermediary factor 1γ (anti-TIF1 γ)
Inclusion body myositis	Cytosolic 5′-nucleotidase 1A (anti-cN1A)
Immune-mediated necrotizing myopathy	Signal recognition particle (SRP)

38. B

Corticosteroids are used to treat dermatomyositis, polymyositis, and immune-mediated necrotizing myopathy. Inclusion body myositis does not respond to corticosteroids.

Methotrexate has also been used for dermatomyositis, polymyositis, and immune-mediated necrotizing myopathy. It does carry a risk for pulmonary fibrosis, so some recommend avoiding it in patients with dermatomyositis who have interstitial lung disease or anti-Jo 1 antibodies.[8]

39. A

Statin-induced myositis has been associated with reduced levels of coenzyme Q10. Certain mutations in the gene *SLCO1B1* indicate predisposition to statin myopathy. The *SLCO1B1* gene encodes for an organic anion transporter in the liver.

Other medications that cause myopathy include zidovudine (AZT) and steroids.

AZT can cause a mitochondrial myopathy associated with ragged red fibers.

Steroid myopathy can occur in patients who are receiving steroids for other myopathies, such as inflammatory myopathies. EMG and muscle biopsy help to differentiate steroid myopathy from inflammatory myopathies. Insertional activity is normal in steroid myopathy and may be abnormal in inflammatory myopathies. Steroid myopathy tends to affect type 2 muscle fibers.

40. A

Type 1 fibers are slow twitch and fatigue resistant; they use oxidative metabolism.

Type 2 fibers are fast twitch and fatigue prone; they use glycolytic metabolism. Usually, there are twice as many type 2 fibers as type 1 fibers.

41. C

Onion bulbs indicate demyelination and remyelination. They are seen in Charcot-Marie-Tooth disease (e.g., CMT1A). They are also seen in chronic inflammatory demyelinating neuropathy (CIDP).

Tomaculi (focal hypermyelination) are seen in hereditary neuropathy with liability to pressure palsies (HNPP).

42. C

Of the features listed, fibrosis is most suggestive of a myopathic process. Atrophic angular fibers, group atrophy, and target fibers are more suggestive of a neurogenic process. Target fibers, which indicate active denervation and reinnervation, can be seen in amyotrophic lateral sclerosis (ALS).

43. B

Fiber-type grouping occurs in neuropathy. Muscle fibers that are reinnervated by an anterior horn cell assume the properties of that cell.

Central nuclei, split fibers, and the combination of small and large round fibers are more consistent with myopathy.

44. A

Internal nuclei are most prominent in myotonic dystrophy.

45. D

PAS stain identifies glycogen storage diseases.

Crystal violet and Congo red stains identify amyloid.

Oil red O identifies lipid and is helpful in the diagnosis of lipid storage diseases.

46. C

Fatigable weakness is characteristic of neuromuscular junction disorders such as myasthenia gravis (MG).

Single fiber EMG of the frontalis muscle is the most sensitive test for MG. It shows increased jitter and blocking in MG. However, this is not specific for MG.

Cooling improves weakness in MG because of improved neuromuscular transmission.

Repetitive nerve stimulation (RNS) is used to help diagnose MG. RNS causes a compound muscle action potential (CMAP) decrement in MG. However, RNS may be normal in ocular MG.

Inching is a nerve conduction study technique for detecting focal demyelination.

47. A

Patients with myasthenia gravis (MG) can have binding, modulating, or blocking antibodies to the acetylcholine receptor.

Most patients with MG have acetylcholine receptor binding antibodies. These antibodies can also be found in other diseases at lower levels, such as in patients with systemic lupus erythematosus and in relatives of patients with MG.

Acetylcholine receptor modulating antibodies are often seen in MG patients with thymoma. Also, striated muscle antibodies are associated with an increased risk for thymoma.

Children with MG are less likely to be seropositive than adults with MG. The absence of antibodies does not rule out MG. Lack of decrease in antibody levels with immunosuppressive therapy suggests that the therapy is not effective.

Patients with MG who are negative for acetylcholine receptor antibodies may have muscle-specific tyrosine kinase (MuSK) antibodies. MuSK is involved in the formation of clusters of acetylcholine receptors at the endplate.

Both MuSK-related MG and MG associated with acetylcholine receptor antibodies tend to occur in females and can manifest in adolescence. Patients with MuSK-related MG tend to have less ocular involvement then MG patients with acetylcholine receptor antibodies. Patients with MuSK-related MG may present with isolated head drop, facial weakness and atrophy, tongue weakness and atrophy, or weakness of the neck or shoulders. Patients with MuSK-related MG may worsen with edrophonium or develop fasciculations. They may require more aggressive therapy. Rituximab has been used.[9]

48. C

Myasthenic crisis is more common during the first few years after diagnosis. Infection, initiation of steroids, a rapid steroid taper, surgery, pregnancy, stress, and aminoglycosides can trigger myasthenic crisis. Patients who are anti-MuSK antibody positive are at higher risk for myasthenic crisis than patients with acetylcholine binding receptor antibodies.

When a patient is intubated for myasthenic crisis, anticholinesterase medications are withheld to prevent secretions and aspiration.

Myasthenic crisis can be treated with intravenous immunoglobulin (IVIG) or plasmapheresis.

49. B

This patient has Lambert-Eaton syndrome (LEMS), which is associated with small cell lung cancers. Patients with LEMS often have antibodies to P/Q-type voltage-gated calcium channels.

50. B

Both myasthenia gravis (MG) and Lambert-Eaton syndrome (LEMS) are neuromuscular junction disorders. Patients with MG are more likely to present with ocular weakness than patients with LEMS. Patients with LEMS may have an abnormal pupillary response, which is not typical of MG. Patients with LEMS have autonomic dysfunction. Dry mouth is a symptom in LEMS. Patients with LEMS have worse leg weakness than arm weakness, whereas arm weakness is usually worse than leg weakness in MG. Reduced deep tendon reflexes are more likely in LEMS than in MG. Both MG and LEMS show a decrement with 3 Hz repetitive nerve stimulation. However, LEMS shows a significant increment with rapid repetitive nerve stimulation or brief intense exercise that does not occur in MG.

51.

1) Axonal
2) Demyelinating

Reduced compound muscle action potentials (CMAPs) tend to occur in conditions affecting the axon. However, conduction block, which occurs in acquired demyelinating conditions, can cause a decrease in amplitude of the CMAP.

Significantly reduced conduction velocities tend to occur in demyelinating conditions.

52. A

A normal hemoglobin A1c level does not rule out diabetes mellitus (DM), which is the most common cause of peripheral neuropathy. A glucose tolerance test is more sensitive.

DM can cause multiple types of neuropathy. A distal symmetric polyneuropathy is common in patients with DM. DM can also cause a small-fiber neuropathy, autonomic neuropathy, oculomotor palsy, mononeuropathies, diabetic amyotrophy, and diabetic neuropathic cachexia.

Diabetic lumbosacral radiculoplexus neuropathy, which is a type of diabetic amyotrophy, can cause significant atrophy of the thigh muscles. It tends to occur in male patients older than 50 years of age. It manifests with acute pain in the back, hip, or thigh. This is followed by weakness and atrophy. It is typically asymmetric.

Diabetic neuropathic cachexia also tends to occur in older men with poor glycemic control. Patients have weight loss, truncal dysesthesia, and depression.[10]

53. D

This patient has hereditary neuropathy with liability to pressure palsies (HNPP), which is characterized by focal compression neuropathies. Tomacula are seen on nerve biopsy. HNPP is caused by deletion of the *PMP22* gene on chromosome 17. *PMP22* encodes peripheral myelin protein-22.

Mutations in *GDAP1* cause Charcot-Marie-Tooth neuropathy type 4A (CMT4A), which is associated with diaphragm paralysis.

54. D

Friedreich ataxia is autosomal recessive. Fabry disease, Kennedy disease, and Charcot-Marie-Tooth neuropathy X (CMTX) are X-linked neuropathies.

55. C

This patient has Charcot-Marie-Tooth neuropathy type 1A (CMT1A), which usually manifests with leg weakness

and atrophy in the second decade of life. Deep tendon reflexes are decreased, and patients develop foot deformities. Patients with CMT1A who are asymptomatic may develop symptoms when given vincristine. CMT1A is caused by duplication of *PMP22*, whereas hereditary neuropathy with liability to pressure palsies is caused by a deletion in this gene. Both conditions are autosomal dominant.

If patient has CMT1A phenotype but is negative for *PMP22*, then CMTX may be the diagnosis if there is no male-to-male transmission. CMTX is the X-linked type of CMT. CMT1X is the most common type of CMTX. It is caused by mutations in *GJ1B*, which encodes connexin 32, a gap junction protein.

If patient has CMT1A phenotype and is negative for *PMP22* but there is male-to-male transmission, then the patient may have CMT1B, which is caused by a mutation in the *MPZ* gene.

Mutations in the gene *HINT1* cause neuromyotonia and axonal neuropathy.

Mutations in the gene *RAB7A* cause hereditary sensory and autonomic neuropathy type 1B and CMT2B.

Mutations in *MFN2* cause CMT2A, which is an axonal form of CMT. (CMT type 1 is demyelinating; CMT type 2 is axonal; CMT type 4 is autosomal recessive.) CMT2A is usually severe. It manifests in early childhood and is associated with postural tremor and optic atrophy.[11]

56. C

Friedreich ataxia usually manifests before age 20 years with gait ataxia. Eventually, the cerebellum, corticospinal tracts, posterior columns, spinocerebellar tracts, dorsal root ganglia, and peripheral nerves are all affected. Patients with Friedreich ataxia develop limb and trunk ataxia and dysarthria. The lower extremities become weak, and there is wasting in the hands and feet. Vibration and position sense are lost, and reflexes are reduced. Plantar responses are extensor. Square-wave jerks are a common ocular finding. Sensorineural deafness, diabetes, and cardiac conduction defects may be present.

Large myelinated sensory axons are affected in Friedrich ataxia. Patients with Friedreich ataxia have abnormal sensory nerve conduction studies and normal compound muscle action potentials. Reinnervated motor units result in decreased recruitment and prolonged, polyphasic, high-amplitude motor unit action potentials on EMG.

Friedreich ataxia is caused by a mutation in the gene *FXN*, which encodes frataxin. Frataxin is an iron-binding protein found in mitochondria. Patients with Friedreich ataxia have an expanded GAA trinucleotide repeat in the *FXN* gene. The gene is on chromosome 9q.

57. D

This patient has AIDP, which is the most common form of Guillain-Barré syndrome (GBS). AIDP is characterized by symmetric, ascending weakness with areflexia. This can progress to quadriparesis and respiratory failure. Measurement of the forced vital capacity and negative inspiratory force can help to predict whether the patient is at risk for respiratory failure. Patients can have cardiac arrhythmias and autonomic dysfunction (e.g., sinus tachycardia). Albuminocytologic dissociation is a classic finding in AIDP.

AIDP is immune mediated. T cells target peripheral nervous system myelin in AIDP. AIDP is usually a postinfectious (or post-vaccination) process.

Campylobacter jejuni is the illness that most commonly precedes GBS. It is associated with the axonal form of GBS, anti-GM1 antibodies, and a worse prognosis.

Findings that suggest a diagnosis other than GBS include asymmetric weakness, bowel and bladder dysfunction at the onset of symptoms, and a sensory level.[12]

58. A

Prolonged F-wave latencies are often the first sign of AIDP on nerve conduction studies.

Conduction block and temporal dispersion do occur in acquired demyelinating neuropathies, but prolongation of F-wave latencies usually occurs first.

The sural nerve may be spared in some patients with Guillain-Barré syndrome (GBS).

59. C

Acute motor axonal neuropathy (AMAN) is an axonal variant of GBS. Facial weakness is less common in AMAN than in AIDP. *Campylobacter jejuni* infection commonly precedes AMAN. The target in AMAN is the nodal and paranodal axolemma, whereas in AIDP it is myelin.

Acute motor-sensory axonal neuropathy (AMSAN) is also an axonal variant of GBS. It has a worse prognosis than AMAN or AIDP. There is axonal damage to the ventral and dorsal roots in AMSAN.

Sensory GBS may be associated with antibodies to GD1b.

Bickerstaff brainstem encephalitis is another GBS variant. It is characterized by encephalopathy, ophthalmoparesis, and ataxia.

In Miller-Fisher syndrome and Bickerstaff brainstem encephalitis, patients may have antibodies to GQ1b.

Antibodies to GT1a are seen in GBS patients who present with bulbar palsy.[12,13]

60. A

Botulism, diphtheria, tick paralysis, and porphyria are in the differential diagnosis of GBS.

Botulism causes a descending paralysis.

Diphtheria can cause an ascending paralysis. It is caused by an exotoxin produced by *Corynebacterium diphtheriae*. It results from a distal polyneuropathy involving the limbs (a symmetric sensorimotor peripheral neuropathy). An exudate of the throat and trachea is characteristic. Diphtheria causes a palatal neuropathy. In addition to palatal paralysis, other cranial nerves may become involved. Patients may have lack of accommodation with preservation of the light reflex.

Tick paralysis and porphyria also cause an ascending flaccid paralysis.

61. True

CIDP causes symmetric proximal and distal weakness. Sensory disturbance is more common in CIDP than in AIDP. Decreased reflexes and albuminocytologic association are seen in CIDP, as in AIDP. Increased CSF white blood cells should raise suspicion for an infectious etiology.

Patients with CIDP have evidence of acquired demyelination similar to that seen in patients with AIDP, such as temporal dispersion, conduction block, increased distal CMAP duration, and prolonged or absent F waves. As in AIDP, T-cell activation is thought to play role in the pathogenesis of CIDP.

Patients with CIDP should be evaluated for lymphoproliferative disease.

62. A

SIDP is an intermediate condition between AIDP and CIDP. (SIDP patients are those who progress for longer than 4 weeks but less than 8 weeks.) AIDP, SIDP, and CIDP are usually symmetric. CSF protein is elevated in SIDP, as in AIDP and CIDP.

Types of chronic acquired demyelinating polyneuropathy include CIDP, distal acquired demyelinating symmetric neuropathy (DADS), MMN, and MADSAM.

Distal acquired demyelinating symmetric neuropathy can cause motor or sensory symptoms. Often it is associated with a monoclonal protein.

Multifocal motor neuropathy causes asymmetric weakness. It tends to begin in the upper extremities in the territory of a specific peripheral nerve. Evidence of demyelination is seen on motor nerve conduction studies. Anti-GM1 antibodies may be present.

MADSAM causes asymmetric weakness and sensory loss. Similar to MMN, MADSAM tends to involve the upper extremities first. CSF protein is elevated in MADSAM.[13]

63. D

MADSAM is most likely to respond to steroids. It also responds to intravenous immunoglobulin (IVIG).

MMN, AMAN, and AIDP do not respond well to steroids. GBS can be treated with IVIG or plasmapheresis. MMN can be treated with IVIG.

Chronic inflammatory demyelinating polyneuropathy (CIDP) and subacute inflammatory demyelinating polyneuropathy (SIDP) respond to steroids.

64. C

IgM-MGUS is typically associated with a distal large-fiber, sensory-predominant neuropathy with sensory ataxia. Nerve conduction studies are consistent with demyelination.

Neuropathy in patients with IgM monoclonal gammopathy is called distal acquired demyelinating symmetric neuropathy with M protein (DADS-M). This is considered a variant of CIDP. However, these patients have more sensory loss and less weakness than most patients with CIDP and are less likely to respond to treatment than those with typical CIDP. Often patients with DADS-M have antibodies to myelin-associated glycoprotein (MAG).

65. B

POEMS is a paraneoplastic sensorimotor neuropathy. It is associated with osteosclerotic myeloma.

An elevated level of serum vascular endothelial growth factor (VEGF) may be helpful in the diagnosis of POEMS.

Small-cell lung cancer can be associated with a sensory neuronopathy (sensory ganglionopathy).

66. A

This patient has upper and lower motor neuron signs. Amyotrophic lateral sclerosis (ALS) is the most likely diagnosis. It may begin with weakness and atrophy in a limb or with bulbar signs such as dysphagia.

The El Escorial World Federation of Neurology criteria are used to diagnose ALS. Definite ALS requires upper motor neuron and lower motor neuron signs in three of four regions (bulbar, cervical, thoracic, and lumbosacral regions).[14]

Primary lateral sclerosis only affects the upper motor neurons.

Progressive muscular atrophy and spinal muscular atrophies affect the lower motor neurons. Other motor neuron diseases include X-linked spinal bulbar muscular atrophy, monomelic amyotrophy, poliomyelitis, and West Nile virus poliomyelitis.

67. D

Spasticity is the condition most likely to be seen in early ALS. Autonomic disturbance, incontinence, ophthalmoplegia, movement disorders, and sensory abnormalities should raise concern for a diagnosis other than ALS.

ALS is the most common acquired motor neuron disease. However, there are familial forms. The most common genetic cause of ALS is mutations in *C9orf72*. An expansion of a hexanucleotide repeat in the gene *C9orf72* causes familial ALS and familial frontotemporal dementia. Mutations in the gene encoding superoxide dismutase also cause familial ALS. Mutations in *TARDP* and *FUS* are less common causes of familial ALS (see Box 16.2).

***Box 16.2* GENES THAT ARE MUTATED IN FAMILIAL AMYOTROPHIC LATERAL SCLEROSIS**

- *C9orf72*
- *SOD1*
- *TARDP*
- *FUS*

---

68. B

American Academy of Neurology guidelines indicate that riluzole should be offered to patients with ALS. The goal is to slow disease progression. Riluzole inhibits glutamate release. It can decrease appetite and raise liver function tests.

Percutaneous endoscopic gastrostomy (PEG) and noninvasive ventilation (NIV) may prolong survival in patients with ALS.[15]

69. A

This patient has Kennedy disease, which is also known as X-linked spinobulbar muscular atrophy. It is a motor neuron disease caused by mutations in the gene *AR*, which encodes the androgen receptor. There is an expanded number of CAG repeats in the gene. Patients have progressive bulbar and extremity weakness. Tongue and perioral fasciculations are characteristic features. Androgen insensitivity causes gynecomastia, infertility, and impotence. Patients are at increased risk for diabetes mellitus.

REFERENCES

1. North KN, Wang CH, Clarke N, et al. Approach to the diagnosis of congenital myopathies. *Neuromuscul Disord* 2014;24:97–116.
2. Bönnemann CG, Wang CH, Quijano-Roy S, et al. Diagnostic approach to the congenital muscular dystrophies. *Neuromuscul Disord* 2014;24:289–311.
3. Kang PB, Morrison L, Iannaccone S, et al. Evidence-based guideline summary: Evaluation, diagnosis, and management of congenital muscular dystrophy. Report of the Guideline Development Subcommittee of the American Academy of Neurology and the Practice Issues Review Panel of the American Association of Neuromuscular and Electrodiagnostic Medicine. *Neurology* 2015;13:1369–1378.
4. Wicklund MP. The muscular dystrophies. *Continuum (Minneap Minn)* 2013;19:1535–1570.
5. Narayanaswami P, Weiss M, Selcen D, et al. Evidence-based guideline summary: Diagnosis and treatment of limb-girdle and distal dystrophies. Report of the Guideline Development Subcommittee of the American Academy of Neurology and the Practice Issues Review Panel of the American Association of Neuromuscular and Electrodiagnostic Medicine. *Neurology* 2014;83:1453–1463.
6. Murphy AP, Straub V. The classification, natural history and treatment of the limb girdle muscular dystrophies. *J Neuromuscul Dis* 2015;2:S7–S19.
7. Tobon A. Metabolic myopathies. *Continuum (Minneap Minn)* 2013;19:1571–1597.
8. Amato AA, Greenberg SA. Inflammatory myopathies. *Continuum (Minneap Minn)* 2013;19:1615–1633.
9. Sanders DB, Guptill JF. Myasthenia gravis and Lambert-Eaton myasthenic syndrome. *Continuum (Minneap Minn)* 2014;20:1413–1425.
10. Russell JW, Zilliox LA. Diabetic neuropathies. *Continuum (Minneap Minn)* 2014;20:1226–1240.
11. Saporta MA. Charcot-Marie-Tooth disease and other inherited neuropathies. *Continuum (Minneap Minn)* 2014;20:1208–1225.
12. Dimachkie MM, Saperstein DS. Acquired immune demyelinating neuropathies. *Continuum (Minneap Minn)* 2014;20:1241–1260.
13. Bril V, Katzberg HD. Acquired immune axonal neuropathies. *Continuum (Minneap Minn)* 2014;20:1261–1273.
14. Brooks BR, Miller RG, Swash M, et al. El Escorial revisited: Revised criteria for the diagnosis of amyotrophic lateral sclerosis. *Amyotroph Lateral Scler Other Motor Neuron Disord* 2000; 1:293–299.
15. Miller RG, Jackson CE, Kasarskis EJ, et al. Practice parameter update. The care of the patient with amyotrophic lateral sclerosis: Drug, nutritional, and respiratory therapies (an evidence-based review). Report of the Quality Standards Subcommittee of the American Academy of Neurology. *Neurology* 2009;73:1218–1226.

17.

NEURO-ONCOLOGY

Please note: The World Health Organization 2007 central nervous system tumor classification system was used for this chapter. A new classification is under development.

QUESTIONS

1. Which of the following statements is *false*?
   A. Most primary brain tumors are glial tumors.
   B. Brain metastases are less common than primary brain tumors.
   C. Seizures are a common presenting symptom of low-grade gliomas.
   D. Risk factors for primary brain tumors include ionizing radiation and immunosuppression.

2. Which of the following statements is *false*?
   A. Oligodendrogliomas are characterized by cells with a "fried egg" appearance, microcalcifications, and branching capillaries.
   B. Oligodendrogliomas have a tendency to bleed.
   C. Patients with oligodendrogliomas frequently present with seizures.
   D. Oligodendrogliomas most commonly occur in the temporal lobe.

3. Which of the following tumors arises from small nests of cells in the sacrum and clivus?
   A. Chordoma
   B. Choriocarcinoma
   C. Craniopharyngioma
   D. Atypical teratoid/rhabdoid tumor

4. Which of the following cancers is *least* likely to spread to the brain?
   A. Breast
   B. Gastrointestinal
   C. Melanoma
   D. Prostate
   E. Renal

5. Which of the following cancers is *least* likely to cause hemorrhagic metastases?
   A. Choriocarcinoma
   B. Gastrointestinal
   C. Melanoma
   D. Renal

6. Which of the following inherited cancer syndromes is *least* likely to be associated with medulloblastoma?
   A. Li-Fraumeni syndrome
   B. Turcot syndrome
   C. Gorlin syndrome
   D. Cowden syndrome

7. Which of the following is the most common intracranial primitive neuroectodermal tumor (PNET)?
   A. Pineoblastoma
   B. Ependymoblastoma
   C. Medulloblastoma
   D. Cerebral neuroblastoma

8. Which of the following is *least* likely to be the cause of an intraventricular tumor?
   A. Subependymal giant cell astrocytoma
   B. Central neurocytoma
   C. Subependymoma
   D. Paraganglioma

9. Which of the following is *least* likely to be found in the lumbar cistern?
   A. Schwannoma
   B. Meningioma
   C. Central neurocytoma
   D. Myxopapillary ependymoma
   E. Paraganglioma of the filum

10. Fill in the blank: Meningiomas arise from _____ _____.
    A. Dura cells
    B. Arachnoid cells
    C. Pia cells

11. Which of the following is *not* a characteristic of meningiomas?
    A. Whorls are present.
    B. Psammoma bodies are present.
    C. Desmosomes are present.
    D. They stain with epithelial membrane antigen (EMA).
    E. They stain with Congo red.

12. A large number of patients with dysplastic gangliocytoma of the cerebellum (Lhermitte-Duclos disease) have which of the following syndromes?
    A. Cowden syndrome (multiple hamartoma syndrome)
    B. Gorlin syndrome
    C. Von Hippel-Lindau disease
    D. Von Recklinghausen disease

13. Which of the following is an infiltrating malignant glial tumor that spreads to involve multiple areas of the brain but does not have a clear epicenter?
    A. Astroblastoma
    B. Chordoid glioma

C. Gliomatosis cerebri

D. Glioblastoma multiforme

14. A 28-year-old woman who presents with headache and vomiting is diagnosed with a brain tumor in the emergency department. Computed tomography (CT) indicates a mass effect. What is recommended to be done first?

A. Start an anti-epileptic medication, preferably one that is not an enzyme inducer.

B. Start Decadron.

C. Start temozolomide.

D. Order a magnetoencephalography (MEG) scan.

15. A 20-year-old man presents with an intraventricular tumor, which is resected. On light microscopy, it resembles an oligodendroglioma but stains positively for synaptophysin. Which of the following tumors fits this description?

A. Central neurocytoma

B. Gangliocytoma

C. Ganglioneuroblastoma

D. Ganglioglioma

16. Which of the following is a tumor of the filum terminale that mimics an ependymoma with pseudorosettes but is positive for synaptophysin and chromogranin?

A. Astroblastoma

B. Paraganglioma of the filum terminale

C. Gangliocytoma

D. Ganglioneuroblastoma

17. A 7-year-old boy undergoes surgery for a medulloblastoma in the cerebellum. On postoperative day 2, dysarthria is noted. This worsens, and then he stops speaking altogether. What is this syndrome?

A. Posterior fossa syndrome

B. Broca aphasia

C. Transcortical motor aphasia

D. Selective mutism

18. A 23-year-old woman presents with a mass that appears to be a cyst with an enhancing mural nodule. The mass is *least* likely to be which of the following tumors?

A. Ganglioglioma

B. Hemangioblastoma

C. Meningioma

D. Pilocytic astrocytoma

E. Pleomorphic xanthoastrocytoma

19. What is the most common pineal tumor?

A. Germinoma

B. Pineoblastoma

C. Pineocytoma

D. Astrocytoma

20. True or False?

To be diagnosed as a pituitary adenocarcinoma, the tumor must have metastasized.

21. One type of tumor manifests with seizures in children, often in the temporal lobe. It is low grade and resembles an oligodendroglioma microscopically but has a mucinous component in which neurons seem to float. There may be accompanying cortical dysplasia. This tumor is which of the following?

A. Central neurocytoma

B. Craniopharyngioma—adamantinomatous type

C. Desmoplastic infantile astrocytoma

D. Dysembryoplastic neuroepithelial tumor

E. Ganglioglioma

22. An 18-year-old woman presents with seizures. Magnetic resonance imaging (MRI) shows a cyst with an enhancing nodule in the temporal lobe. Eosinophilic granular bodies and pilocytic cells are seen on histopathology. What is the diagnosis?

A. Craniopharyngioma—adamantinomatous type

B. Dysembryoplastic neuroepithelial tumor

C. Ganglioglioma

D. Meningioma

23. A 30-year-old receiving chemotherapy develops vomiting, headache, and seizures. She is found to have a sagittal sinus thrombosis. Which of the following medications is most likely responsible?

A. L-Asparaginase

B. Busulfan

C. Chlorambucil

D. Cytarabine

E. Ifosfamide

24. Which of the following statements is *false*?

A. Most primary central nervous system (CNS) lymphomas are B-cell lymphomas.

B. Primary CNS lymphoma responds well to steroids but recurs.

C. Primary CNS lymphoma can resemble glioblastoma multiforme on MRI.

D. Primary CNS lymphoma occurs as a single, localized lesion.

E. Primary CNS lymphoma is characterized by perivascular cuffing, which can be seen with reticulin stain.

25. Which of the following is *least* likely to be seen in a patient with a hypothalamic hamartoma?

A. Behavioral problems

B. Gelastic seizures

C. Precocious puberty

D. Metastases

26. Chemical meningitis can occur if there is leakage from which type of cyst?

A. Colloid cyst

B. Epidermoid cyst

C. Neurenteric cyst

D. Rathke's cleft cyst

27. Which of the following cysts is associated with sudden death.

A. Colloid cyst

B. Epidermoid cyst

C. Neurenteric cyst

D. Rathke's cleft cyst

28. Which of the following findings predicts a better prognosis in oligodendrogliomas and grade III astrocytomas?

A. Epidermal growth factor receptor amplification

B. Deletion of phosphatase and tensin homolog (PTEN)

C. Mutation in isocitrate dehydrogenase 1 and 2

D. *N-Myc* gene amplification

29. A 24-year-old man is referred by his primary care physician for a pituitary mass found on MRI. Which visual field defect might be present?

A. Bitemporal hemianopsia

B. Binasal hemianopsia

C. Homonymous hemianopsia

30. Which of the following is the most common pituitary lesion?

A. Pituitary adenoma

B. Pituitary carcinoma

C. Lymphocytic hypophysitis

D. Metastasis

31. Which of the following is the most common type of pituitary adenoma?

A. Adrenocorticotropic hormone-secreting tumor

B. Growth hormone-secreting tumor

C. Prolactinoma

D. Thyroid-stimulating hormone-secreting tumor

32. A 25-year-old man is found to have a prolactinoma. On examination, he has a visual field defect. Which of the following is the first-line treatment?

A. Surgery

B. Radiation

C. Chemotherapy

D. Bromocriptine

33. What are the two most common brain tumors of childhood?

A. Medulloblastoma and pilocytic astrocytoma

B. Ependymoma and germinoma

C. Oligodendroglioma and ganglioglioma

D. Schwannoma and meningioma

34. A 2-year-old presents with chaotic eye movements and quick jerks of the extremities. Which of the following tumors should be considered?

A. Ependymoma

B. Germinoma

C. Medulloblastoma

D. Neuroblastoma

35. A 2-year-old is found to have a brain tumor, which is resected. The tumor has small blue cells, similar to medulloblastoma, and stains positive for vimentin. There is a mutation of *INI1/hSNF5* on chromosome 22. Which of the following tumors is most likely?

A. Atypical teratoid/rhabdoid tumor

B. Desmoplastic cerebral astrocytoma of infancy

C. Neuroblastoma

D. Rhabdomyosarcoma

36. A 55-year-old woman presents with seizures. MRI shows an enhancing lesion involving the corpus callosum in a butterfly pattern. Biopsy shows necrosis with pseudopalisading and microvascular proliferation. What is the diagnosis?

A. Glioblastoma multiforme

B. Anaplastic astrocytoma

C. Lymphoma

D. Atypical teratoid/rhabdoid tumor

37. Which of the following is *not* associated with prominent numbers of eosinophilic granular bodies?

A. Ganglioglioma

B. Pilocytic astrocytoma

C. Pleomorphic xanthoastrocytoma

D. Subependymoma

38. Subependymal giant cell astrocytomas (SEGAs) are associated with which disease?

A. Ataxia-telangiectasia

B. Neurofibromatosis type 1

C. Tuberous sclerosis complex

D. Von Hippel-Lindau disease

39. Loss of heterozygosity (LOH) for 1p and 19q predicts sensitivity to chemotherapy with PCV (procarbazine, lomustine, and vincristine) in which type of tumor?

A. Ependymomas

B. Medulloblastomas

C. Oligodendrogliomas

D. Retinoblastomas

40. True or False?
Areas of necrosis can be seen in low-grade ependymomas.

41. A 16-year-old boy presents with difficulties riding his skateboard. MRI shows a cyst with a mural nodule in the cerebellum. The tumor is resected, and Rosenthal fibers, eosinophilic granular bodies, microcysts, and long bipolar cytoplasmic cell processes are seen. What is the most likely diagnosis?

A. Ependymoma

B. Hemangioblastoma

C. Medulloblastoma

D. Pilocytic astrocytoma

42. True or False?
Carcinomatous meningitis and lymphomatous meningitis can be associated with very low glucose levels, similar to bacterial meningitis.

43. Which of the following statements is *false*?

A. In the familial form of retinoblastoma, one copy of the tumor suppressor *Rb* gene is inactivated in the germ line.

B. Patients with familial retinoblastoma are at increased risk for melanoma.

C. A patient with bilateral retinoblastomas and an osteosarcoma has trilateral retinoblastoma.

D. Flexner-Wintersteiner rosettes are seen in retinoblastoma.

44. A 30-year-old woman presents with seizures and altered mental status. She is eventually diagnosed with anti-NMDA receptor encephalitis. Which of the following tumors is most closely associated with this diagnosis?
    A. Breast cancer
    B. Pituitary adenoma
    C. Cervical cancer
    D. Ovarian teratoma

45. Which of the following antibodies can cause pseudo-obstruction syndrome?
    A. Anti-Hu
    B. Anti-Ri/ANNA-2
    C. Anti-Yo
    D. Anti-Tr

46. Which of the following types of antibodies cause Lambert-Eaton myasthenic syndrome?
    A. Antibodies to the AMPA receptor
    B. Antibodies to P/Q-type voltage-gated calcium channels
    C. Antibodies to voltage-gated potassium channels
    D. Antibodies to the metabotropic glutamate receptor mGluR1
    E. Antibodies to leucine-rich, glioma-inactivated 1 (LGI1) protein

47. A 20-year-old man presents with decreased hearing and unsteadiness. MRI shows mass lesions in the internal auditory canals bilaterally. Pathology shows Antoni A and Antoni B patterns and Verocay bodies.

    a. What are these lesions?
       A. Ependymomas
       B. Schwannomas

    C. Meningiomas
    D. Central neurocytomas

    b. Which of the following diagnoses should be considered?
       A. Tuberous sclerosis complex
       B. Neurofibromatosis type 1
       C. Neurofibromatosis type 2
       D. Ménière disease

48. Which of the following medications is most likely to cause chronic encephalopathy?
    A. Cyclosporin
    B. Etoposide
    C. Ifosfamide
    D. Methotrexate
    E. Tamoxifen

49. A patient develops severe weakness after one dose of vincristine. Which of the following is the most likely cause?
    A. The patient has Charcot-Marie-Tooth disease.
    B. The patient is a child.
    C. The patient is taking carbamazepine.
    D. The patient is taking phenytoin.

50. Mutations in which chromosome are associated with neurofibromas, schwannomas, meningiomas, and atypical teratoid/rhabdoid tumor (AT/RT).
    A. Chromosome 3
    B. Chromosome 11
    C. Chromosome 17
    D. Chromosome 22

NEURO-ONCOLOGY

ANSWERS

1. B

Brain metastases are more common than primary brain tumors. Brain metastases are most often found at the cerebral gray-white junction.

2. D

Oligodendrogliomas are diffusely infiltrating gliomas. They typically occur in the cerebral hemispheres, most often in the frontal lobe.

3. A

Chordomas are invasive tumors that arise from notochord remnants in the clivus and sacrum.

Choriocarcinomas are a type of germ cell tumor.

Craniopharyngioma is an epithelial tumor in the sellar region that is thought to arise from Rathke's pouch epithelium.

Atypical teratoid/rhabdoid tumors are most commonly found in the cerebellum but can occur in the cerebrum.

4. D

Of the cancers listed, prostate cancer is least likely to metastasize to the brain. Similarly, cervical cancer rarely metastasizes to the brain. Breast, gastrointestinal, lung, and renal cancers, as well as melanoma, are more likely to spread to the brain.

5. B

Of those listed, gastrointestinal cancers are least likely to cause hemorrhagic metastases. Choriocarcinoma, melanoma, and renal cancers are more likely to cause hemorrhagic metastases. Metastases with the highest risk of bleeding include lung, melanoma, renal, choriocarcinoma, and thyroid cancer. Lung cancer causes the highest proportion of hemorrhagic metastases, but melanoma and choriocarcinoma have the highest relative incidence. Eighty percent of melanoma brain metastases are associated with hemorrhage.

6. D

Cowden syndrome is characterized by multiple hamartomas. The CNS finding is dysplastic gangliocytoma of the cerebellum, which is known as Lhermitte-Duclos disease. It is autosomal dominant, and there is also a high risk of developing breast cancer or thyroid cancer. There is a germline mutation in the tumor suppressor gene *PTEN* on chromosome 10q23.

Li-Fraumeni syndrome is caused by a TP53 (a tumor suppressor) germline mutation, which results in multiple neoplasms such as breast cancer, sarcoma, and brain tumors including astrocytoma, medulloblastoma, PNET, choroid plexus carcinoma, and ependymoma.

Turcot syndrome is associated with a familial adenomatous polyposis mutation on the *APC* tumor suppressor gene (chromosome 5q21). Patients can have many polyps in the colon and are at risk for brain tumors such as medulloblastoma, malignant glioma, and ependymoma.

Gorlin syndrome is nevoid basal cell carcinoma syndrome, which is caused by a germline mutation in the Patched gene (*PTCH*) on chromosome 9q22. It is autosomal dominant and manifests with developmental anomalies such as jaw cysts, rib abnormalities, macrocephaly, facial appearance, dural calcifications, and increased risk of medulloblastomas and meningiomas.

7. C

Medulloblastoma is the most common intracranial PNET.

8. D

The differential diagnosis of an intraventricular tumor includes subependymal giant cell astrocytomas, which are found in tuberous sclerosis complex, central neurocytoma, choroid plexus papilloma and carcinoma, ependymoma, and subependymoma. Intraventricular meningiomas are rare but can occur.

Paragangliomas are neuroendocrine tumors that are thought to arise from neural crest cells associated with autonomic ganglia. It is uncommon for paragangliomas to occur in the CNS, but when they are present, they tend to occur in the cauda equina region and are intradural.

9. C

Schwannomas, meningiomas, myxopapillary ependymomas, and paragangliomas of the filum terminale can be found in the lumbar cistern.

Central neurocytoma is an intraventricular tumor.

10. B

Meningiomas arise from arachnoid cells. In general, they are more common in women than in men and tend to occur in older patients. Risk factors include ionizing radiation and hereditary tumor syndromes. Meningiomas may enlarge during pregnancy.

11. E

Congo red stains amyloid.

Meningiomas typically stain positive for vimentin and epithelial membrane antigen (EMA). On light microscopy, whorls or psammoma bodies may be seen. There may be calcification or cysts. Desmosomal intercellular junctions are seen on electron microscopy.

Meningiomas are dural-based tumors. A "dural tail" may be seen on MRI. Most meningiomas are circumscribed, are isodense on MRI, and homogenously enhance with contrast. There may be hyperostosis of the overlying bone. Seizure is a common presenting symptom in approximately 30% of patients, and angiography shows a "sunburst effect" or "blushing" with large dural arteries.

Most meningiomas are World Health Organization (WHO) grade I, but there are more aggressive variants. The aggressive variants tend to be more common in men. Papillary, rhabdoid, and anaplastic meningiomas are World Health Organization (WHO) grade III.

12. A

A significant number of patients with dysplastic gangliocytoma of the cerebellum (Lhermitte-Duclos disease) have Cowden syndrome (multiple hamartoma syndrome), which is caused by a germline PTEN mutation.

Gorlin syndrome is nevoid basal cell carcinoma syndrome. Patients have an increased risk for medulloblastoma.

Von Hippel-Lindau disease is associated with hemangioblastomas in the cerebellum.

Von Recklinghausen disease is another name for neurofibromatosis 1.

13. C

Gliomatosis cerebri is a malignant infiltrating tumor that spreads to multiple lobes of the brain. It may spread bilaterally and/or to the brainstem, cerebellum, and spinal cord.

14. B

The first step is to start Decadron.

Anti-epileptic drugs (AEDs) are not recommended for prevention of the first seizure. If an AED is indicated, enzyme-inducing AEDs should be avoided because they can affect the metabolism of chemotherapy drugs and steroids.

Temozolomide is a treatment for brain tumors, but it is not the first step.

A MEG scan may be helpful later, but does not need to be done first.

15. A

Central neurocytoma resembles an oligodendroglioma but stains positively for synaptophysin and is found in the ventricles.

16. B

Paraganglioma of the filum terminale is an oval or sausage-shaped, WHO grade I neuroendocrine tumor of the filum terminale. On MRI, serpentine vessels may be seen. On histopathology, this tumor mimics an ependymoma with pseudorosettes but stains positive for synaptophysin and chromogranin.

17. A

This patient has posterior fossa syndrome, which is otherwise known as cerebellar mutism. It can occur in patients, especially children, who have undergone posterior fossa surgery.

18. C

Gangliogliomas, hemangioblastomas, pilocytic astrocytomas, and pleomorphic xanthoastrocytomas have the appearance of a cyst with an enhancing mural mass.

Gangliomas are located throughout the CNS (i.e., brain, optic nerve, pituitary, pineal gland, and spinal cord), but the majority are in the temporal lobe. Dysplastic gangliocytoma of cerebellum is called Lhermitte-Duclos disease.

Hemangioblastomas are located in the cerebellum.

Pilocytic astrocytoma the most common type of glioma in children, and most occur in the cerebellum. The most common pediatric supratentorial site is the optic pathway/hypothalamus.

Pleomorphic xanthoastrocytoma is typically in a superficial location over the meninges and cerebrum, mostly supratentorial, and especially in the temporal lobes.

19. A

The most common pineal tumor is the germinoma. Germinomas are radiosensitive and have a good prognosis. Germinomas stain with placental alkaline phosphatase. Alpha-fetoprotein (AFP) is a marker for yolk sac tumors. Human chorionic gonadotropin (HCG) is a marker for choriocarcinoma. Of the germ cell tumors, pure germinomas are most common in the pineal region. Other germ cell tumors (nongerminomas) include choriocarcinomas (which stain with β-HCG), embryonal carcinomas, yolk sac or endodermal sinus tumors (which stain with AFP), teratomas, and mixed germ cell tumors.

20. True

To be diagnosed as pituitary adenocarcinoma, the tumor must have metastasized.

21. D

Dysembryoplastic neuroepithelial tumor is a low-grade tumor that is prone to causing seizures. It is most commonly found in the temporal lobe. There may be molding of overlying bone. Its microscopic features include oligodendroglioma-like cells and neurons that appear to be floating. There may be accompanying cortical dysplasia.

22. C

This patient has a ganglioglioma.

Gangliogliomas, hemangioblastomas, pilocytic astrocytomas, and pleomorphic xanthoastrocytomas have the appearance of a cyst with an enhancing mural mass.

Gangliogliomas, pilocytic astrocytomas, and pleomorphic xanthoastrocytomas have eosinophilic granular bodies.

Craniopharyngiomas typically occur in the sellar region. There may be a cystic component, which may be filled with "machine oil-like" fluid. The histopathology of adamantinomatous craniopharyngioma is characterized by "wet keratin." There are cords of squamous epithelial cells. Calcifications are common.

23. A

L-Asparaginase can cause cerebral venous thrombosis due to antithrombin III deficiency. It can also cause altered mental status.

Busulfan, chlorambucil, and ifosfamide can cause seizures but are less likely to result in a sagittal sinus thrombosis.

Cytarabine can cause a cerebellar syndrome, encephalopathy, and aseptic meningitis (intrathecal).

Bevacizumab can cause stroke, cerebral hemorrhage, and posterior reversible encephalopathy syndrome. Bevacizumab is an antibody that targets vascular endothelial growth factor (VEGF). It has been used in patients with recurrent malignant glioma.

24. D

Primary CNS lymphoma is diffuse, and there can be multiple lesions. The spinal cord, the CSF, or the eye may be involved. Primary CNS lymphoma occurs in immunocompromised individuals. It is associated with human immunodeficiency virus (HIV) and Epstein-Barr virus (EBV) infection. Most commonly, these are diffuse, large B-cell lymphomas. Cells tend to have an angiocentric arrangement. CNS lymphoma is treated with chemotherapy and radiation. These tumors are very responsive to steroids but recur. Biopsy is recommended before steroids are given.

25. D

Hypothalamica hamartomas are associated with behavioral problems, gelastic seizures, and precocious puberty. They are non-neoplastic and do not metastasize.

26. B

If an epidermoid or dermoid cyst leaks, chemical meningitis can occur. Dermoid tumors contain hair follicles and sebaceous glands, are located in the midline, manifest earlier in life, and produce oily secretions. Epidermoid tumors are most common in the cerebellopontine angle cistern, followed by the parasellar and suprasellar regions. They contain keratin and cholesterol crystals.

Neurenteric cysts tend to occur in the spinal canal and are thought to be derived from respiratory/gastrointestinal tract remnants.

Rathke's cleft cysts occur between the anterior and posterior lobes of the pituitary gland and are thought to arise from remnants of the pharyngeal epithelial pouch.

27. A

Colloid cysts arise near the foramen of Monro, where they can have a ball-valve effect. There can be acute or recurrent hydrocephalus. Patients may present with headaches of sudden onset, drop attacks, or sudden death.

28. C

Mutation in isocitrate dehydrogenase 1 (IDH1) and IDH2 predicts a better prognosis in oligodendrogliomas and grade III astrocytomas. Alpha-thalassemia/mental retardation syndrome X-linked (*ATRX*) mutations suggest astrocytic lineage, whereas telomerase reverse transcriptase (TERT) promoter mutations suggest oligodendroglial lineage.

IDH1 mutations are enriched in secondary glioblastoma multiforme (GBM) cases and in younger individuals and are associated with increased patient survival. IDH1 mutations generally occur in the progressive form of glioma, rather than in de novo GBM.

Among the molecular subtypes of GBM, the proneural subtype has the best prognosis. These tumors have overexpression of platelet-derived growth factor receptor-α (PDGFRA) and mutations of the *IDH1* gene.

Classic GBM is associated with phosphatase and tensin homolog (PTEN) deletions and mutations as well as epidermal growth factor receptor (EGFR) amplification and mutations. The mesenchymal subtype of GBM, which is characterized by mutations in *NF1*, has the worst prognosis.

Methylation of the O^6-methylguanine-DNA methyltransferase (MGMT) promoter also affects prognosis in GBM. If MGMT is methylated, then the tumor is more susceptible to alkylating chemotherapy agents such as temozolomide and is associated with better overall survival;

A 1p/19q codeletion has been correlated with both chemosensitivity and improved prognosis in oligodendrogliomas. Patients who have anaplastic oligodendroglioma with 1p/19q loss of heterozygosity have improved survival when treated with both radiation and the chemotherapeutic agents procarbazine, CCNU (lomustine), and vincristine (PCV).[1]

29. A

Of the options listed, a pituitary mass is most likely to cause bitemporal hemianopsia.

30. A

Of the lesions mentioned, pituitary adenoma is the most common pituitary lesion.

Pituitary adenomas typically arise from the anterior pituitary. Microadenomas are smaller than 10 mm in diameter, and macroadenomas are larger than 10 mm.

A pituitary carcinoma may be a metastasis, especially from breast cancer.

Lymphocytic hypophysitis occurs in association with pregnancy or shortly after delivery. It is characterized by infiltration of the pituitary by lymphocytes.

Pituitary apoplexy can also occur during pregnancy.

31. C

The most common type of pituitary adenoma is the prolactinoma.

32. D

Dopamine agonists such as bromocriptine are first-line treatment for prolactinomas, even if the patient has a visual field defect. However, if the lesion does not respond quickly, surgery is considered.

Dopamine inhibits prolactin-secreting pituitary cells. Dopamine agonists decrease prolactin production and decrease the size of the tumor.

33. A

Medulloblastoma and pilocytic astrocytoma are the two most common brain tumors of childhood.

34. D

This patient has opsoclonus-myoclonus, which is a paraneoplastic syndrome seen in patients with neuroblastoma. *N-myc* amplification, late age at onset, diploidy, and reduced catecholamine metabolite production are associated with poor prognosis.

35. A

This patient has atypical teratoid/rhabdoid tumor (AT/RT). AT/RT is a malignant tumor (WHO grade IV) that usually manifests in children younger than 3 years of age but can occur in adults. This tumor has small blue cells, similar to medulloblastoma. Rhabdoid cells present, and the tumor stains positive for vimentin. It is associated with a mutation in *INI1/hSNF5* on chromosome 22.

36. A

This patient has glioblastoma multiforme.

The butterfly pattern is also seen in CNS lymphoma. If CNS lymphoma is suspected, it is recommended that steroids be postponed until after biopsy, if possible.

Anaplastic astrocytoma (AA), which is WHO grade III, differs from glioblastoma (WHO grade IV) in that it does not have necrosis, pseudopalisading, or microvascular proliferation as histologic features. AA exhibits hypercellularity and hyperchromatic, irregular "naked nuclei" within a fibrillary background. Several mitoses are present; there is glial fibrillary acidic protein (GFAP) reactivity; and the proliferation marker MIB-1 is seen in several tumor cells of AA.

37. D

Gangliogliomas, pilocytic astrocytomas, and pleomorphic xanthoastrocytomas have eosinophilic granular bodies; subependymomas do not.

38. C

SEGAs are associated with tuberous sclerosis complex. Everolimus (Afinitor) is being used to treat SEGAs.

Patients with ataxia-telangiectasia are at increased risk for leukemia and lymphoma.

Von Hippel-Lindau disease, which is caused by mutations on chromosome 3, is associated with hemangioblastomas, pheochromocytomas, and renal cell carcinomas. It is caused by mutations in the gene *VHL*, which encodes a protein that inhibits vascular endothelial growth factor.

Neurofibromatosis 1 (NF type 1) is associated with pilocytic astrocytomas, most commonly in the optic pathway. Optic pathway gliomas in patients with NF type 1 often do not progress and typically can be managed conservatively.[2]

39. C

LOH for 1p and 19q predicts sensitivity to chemotherapy with PCV in oligodendrogliomas.

40. True

Areas of necrosis can be seen in low-grade ependymomas. Necrosis does not have the same meaning in ependymomas as in astrocytomas.

41. D

Both pilocytic astrocytoma and hemangioblastoma can appear as cysts with a mural nodule in the cerebellum. In this patient, the histology findings (i.e., Rosenthal fibers, eosinophilic granular bodies, microcysts, and bipolar cell processes) is consistent with pilocytic astrocytoma.

42. True

Carcinomatous meningitis and lymphomatous meningitis can be associated with very low glucose levels.

43. C

Retinoblastoma is a PNET associated with Flexner-Wintersteiner (real) rosettes. The gene is on chromosome 13. It is the most common eye malignancy in children. It typically manifests as leukocoria or strabismus.

Patients with hereditary retinoblastoma are at risk for second neoplasms, such as osteosarcoma and melanoma.

The term *trilateral retinoblastoma* is used if a patient has bilateral retinoblastomas and an intracranial tumor in the suprasellar or pineal region, such as a pineoblastoma.

44. D

Women diagnosed with anti-*N*-Methyl-D-aspartate (anti-NMDA) receptor encephalitis should be evaluated for an ovarian teratoma.

45. A

Anti-Hu and anti-CV2 autoantibodies can cause pseudo-obstruction.

Anti-Hu antibodies are associated with small-cell lung cancer (SCLC). If patients have encephalomyelitis and

SCLC, anti-Hu antibodies should be suspected. Anti-Hu antibodies can also cause brainstem encephalitis, limbic encephalitis, cerebellar ataxia, and sensory neuronopathy.

Anti-amphiphysin antibodies, which are associated with breast cancer, can cause stiff-person syndrome and encephalomyelitis. Anti-glutamic acid decarboxylase (anti-GAD) antibodies are also associated with stiff-person syndrome, but they are typically nonparaneoplastic.

Anti-Ri antibodies cause opsoclonus-myoclonus, brainstem encephalitis, and cerebellar degeneration.

Anti-Yo antibodies occur with gynecologic and breast cancers. They cause cerebellar degeneration.

Cerebellar degeneration is also seen with anti-Tr antibodies, which have been found in patients with Hodgkin lymphoma.

46. B

Antibodies to P/Q-type voltage-gated calcium channels cause Lambert-Eaton myasthenic syndrome.

Anti-α-amino-3-hydroxyl-5-methyl-4-isoxazole-propionate (anti-AMPA) receptor antibodies cause limbic encephalitis.

Antibodies to voltage-gated potassium channels occur in neuromyotonia. They can occur with malignant thymoma.

Antibodies to mGluR1 cause cerebellar degeneration.

Antibodies to LGI1 cause faciobrachial dystonic seizures.

47. a) B and b) C

Antoni A and Antoni B patterns and Verocay bodies are seen in schwannomas. Antoni A refers to the densely packed tissue, Antoni B refers to the loosely packed tissue, and Verocay bodies refers to the pattern of nuclear palisades seen in these tumors.

Schwannomas arising from cranial nerve VIII are the most common tumor in the cerebellopontine angle. They stain with S100, whereas meningiomas arising in this region do not.

The second most common tumor in the cerebellopontine angle is meningioma. There are multiple histologic variants of meningiomas. Some common findings are whorls and psammoma bodies. Calcification or cysts may be present.

Ependymomas can occur in the cerebellopontine angle, but they are not as common. Ependymomas are characterized by perivascular pseudorosettes.

Central neurocytomas are low-grade intraventricular tumors. The cells of the tumor can have perinuclear halos, similar to oligodendrogliomas, but they are synaptophysin positive and GFAP negative.

Bilateral schwannomas of the vestibular nerve are characteristic of NF type 2.

NF type 2 is also associated with astrocytomas, ependymomas, and meningiomas.

Tuberous sclerosis complex is associated with subependymal giant cell astrocytomas.

NF type 1 is associated with optic nerve gliomas, astrocytomas, schwannomas, meningiomas, neurofibromas, and malignant peripheral nerve sheath tumors. Optic nerve gliomas are the most common tumor in NF type 1. Sphenoid wing dysplasia and areas of myelin vacuolization (formerly referred to as "unidentified bright objects") may also be seen on brain MRI in patients with NF type 1.

48. D

Of the medications listed, methotrexate is most likely to cause chronic encephalopathy. It can cause aseptic meningitis and acute, subacute, and chronic encephalopathy. Radiation is a risk factor for methotrexate-induced encephalopathy. Patients may also have a stroke-like syndrome from methotrexate. They may have a hemiparesis that changes from one side to the other.

Cyclosporin, etoposide, ifosfamide, and tamoxifen can cause acute encephalopathy. Methylene blue and thiamine have been used to treat encephalopathy caused by ifosfamide.

49. A

Charcot-Marie-Tooth disease is a risk factor for severe neuropathy from vincristine. Patients should be screened for neuropathy before receiving vincristine.

50. D

Chromosome 22 deletions are common in meningiomas. Mutations in the *NF2* gene (at chromosome 22q12.2) are frequent. The *NF2* gene encodes for the protein merlin. The mutations can be seen in patients without neurofibromatosis.

Mutations in chromosome 22 are also found in ependymomas, neurofibromas, schwannomas, and atypical teratoid/rhabdoid tumors (see Box 17.1).

Box 17.1 TUMORS ASSOCIATED WITH CHROMOSOME 22 DELETIONS

- Atypical teratoid/rhabdoid tumors
- Ependymomas
- Meningiomas
- Neurofibromas
- Schwannomas

Mutations in v-akt murine thymoma viral oncogene homolog 1 (*AKT1*) and in smoothened, frizzled class receptor (*SMO*) have been found in some meningiomas. AKT1 regulates the phosphatidylinositol 3-kinase pathway, and SMO is a component of the hedgehog pathway.[2]

REFERENCES

1. De Groot JF. High-grade gliomas. *Continuum (Minneap Minn)* 2015;21:332–344.
2. Daras M, Kaley TJ. Benign brain tumors and tumors associated with phakomatoses. *Continuum (Minneap Minn)* 2015;21:397–414.

18.

NEURO-OPHTHALMOLOGY

QUESTIONS

1. **What is the term for the region of the retina with the greatest visual acuity?**
   A. Fovea
   B. Macula
   C. Optic disc

2. **Which of the following is the best description of an image on the retina compared to the actual object?**
   A. The image on the retina is inverted compared to the object.
   B. The image on the retina is reversed compared to the object.
   C. The image on the retina is reversed and inverted compared to the object.

3. **When comparing rods and cones, which of the following statements are true for rods, and which are true for cones?**
   1) More numerous
   2) More prevalent at the region of greatest visual acuity
   3) Detect colors
   4) Poor spatial and temporal resolution
   5) More useful in dim lighting
   A. True for rods
   B. True for cones

4. **In the retina, which cells receive impulses directly from the photoreceptors?**
   A. Amacrine cells
   B. Bipolar cells
   C. Ganglion cells
   D. Horizontal cells

5. **The optic nerve is formed from the axons of which type of cells?**
   A. Amacrine cells
   B. Bipolar cells
   C. Ganglion cells
   D. Horizontal cells

6. **Where do most fibers of the optic tract synapse?**
   A. Lateral geniculate body of the thalamus
   B. Midbrain
   C. Optic chiasm

7. **Fill in the blank: The primary visual cortex is known as Brodmann area _____.**
   A. 7
   B. 8
   C. 17
   D. 18

8. **True or False?**
   The pupillary light reflex does not involve the cortex.

9. **Which of the following muscles does *not* affect eyelid position?**
   A. Levator palpebrae superioris
   B. Superior tarsal muscle (Müller's muscle)
   C. Orbicularis oculi
   D. All of the above affect eyelid position.

10. **Which of the following muscles is *not* innervated by the oculomotor nerve?**
    A. Ciliary muscle
    B. Iris sphincter
    C. Müller's muscle
    D. Superior rectus

11. **True or False?**
    A nuclear third nerve palsy can cause bilateral ptosis.

12. **True or False?**
    A nuclear third nerve palsy can cause bilateral gaze abnormalities.

13. **A lesion in which area can cause alternating anisocoria (i.e., the ipsilateral pupil is larger in the light but smaller in the dark)?**
    A. Cavernous sinus
    B. Hypothalamus
    C. Orbit
    D. Brainstem

14. **A lesion in which area can cause bilateral fourth nerve palsies?**
    A. Anterior medullary vellum
    B. Cavernous sinus
    C. Meckel's cave
    D. Orbit

15. **True or False?**
    Injury to the right trochlear nucleus causes a right fourth nerve palsy but can also cause an ipsilateral Horner syndrome if the adjacent sympathetic fibers are involved.

16. **If a patient has an abducens palsy and an ipsilateral postganglionic Horner syndrome, where is the lesion most likely to be?**
    A. Anterior medullary vellum
    B. Cavernous sinus
    C. Meckel's cave
    D. Orbit

17. What is the difference between orbital apex syndrome and cavernous sinus syndrome?
    A. CN 4 is involved in the cavernous sinus syndrome but not in the orbital apex syndrome.
    B. CN 5 (V1) is involved in the cavernous sinus syndrome but not in the orbital apex syndrome.
    C. CN 5 (V2) is spared in orbital apex syndrome, but the optic nerve may be involved.
    D. CN 6 is involved in the cavernous sinus syndrome but not in the orbital apex syndrome.

18. Fill in the blank: The frontal eye field is located in the posterior part of the middle frontal gyrus, which is known as Brodmann area _____.
    A. 7
    B. 8
    C. 17
    D. 18

19. Fill in the blank: The frontal eye fields regulate _____ _____.
    A. Saccadic eye movements
    B. Smooth pursuit
    C. Vertical eye movements

20. Which of the following conditions is *least* likely to affect the eye?
    A. Neurofibromatosis type 1
    B. Tuberous sclerosis complex
    C. Sturge-Weber syndrome
    D. Von Hippel-Lindau disease
    E. Rett syndrome

21. A female patient with a history of infantile spasms is found to have chorioretinal lacunae. Which of the following findings is likely to be present on magnetic resonance imaging (MRI)?
    A. Agenesis of the corpus callosum
    B. Double cortex
    C. Lissencephaly
    D. Periventricular nodular heterotopia

22. Which of the following visual defects is caused by a lesion of the left temporal optic radiations?
    A. Right superior quadrantanopia
    B. Right inferior quadrantanopia
    C. Right homonymous hemianopia with macular sparing
    D. Left inferior quadrantanopia
    E. Right homonymous sectoranopia

23. A 70-year-old woman with diabetes, hypercholesterolemia, and coronary artery disease presents with double vision that improves when she covers one of her eyes. She has no headache, vomiting, or pain. On examination, she cannot abduct the right eye. What is the most likely diagnosis?
    A. Temporal arteritis
    B. Ischemic right abducens palsy
    C. Cavernous sinus thrombosis
    D. Myasthenia gravis

24. A 19-year-old woman presents with decreased vision and pain with eye movement. The symptoms started a few days earlier. She has a left afferent pupil defect, red desaturation, and a central scotoma in the left eye. The funduscopic examination is normal. What is the most likely diagnosis?
    A. Optic neuritis
    B. Idiopathic intracranial hypertension
    C. Multiple sclerosis
    D. Tonic pupil

25. A 50-year-old man presents with decreased vision in the left eye. On examination, he also has decreased color vision in the left eye. He has optic nerve edema on the right. He also has decreased olfaction. What is the most likely diagnosis?
    A. Anterior ischemic optic neuropathy
    B. Leber hereditary optic neuropathy
    C. Olfactory groove meningioma
    D. Optic neuritis

26. A 55-year-old man with hypertension and diabetes presents with sudden, painless vision loss. He does not have a headache or systemic symptoms. He has a field defect affecting central vision and a relative afferent defect. On funduscopic examination, the optic disc is swollen and there are flame-shaped hemorrhages. The erythrocyte sedimentation rate (ESR) and C-reactive protein (CRP) level are normal. What is the most likely diagnosis?
    A. Arteritic anterior ischemic optic neuropathy
    B. Nonarteritic anterior ischemic optic neuropathy
    C. Posterior ischemic optic neuropathy
    D. Tolosa-Hunt syndrome

27. What is the most common cause of optic nerve infarct (anterior ischemic optic neuropathy)?
    A. Carotid occlusive disease
    B. Temporal arteritis
    C. Idiopathic

28. Match the visual field defect with the location of the lesion. (One option will not be used.)
    1) Monocular vision loss
    2) Bitemporal hemianopia
    3) Contralateral inferior quadrantanopia
    A. Optic nerve
    B. Optic chiasm
    C. Parietal lobe
    D. Temporal lobe

29. What is the cause of binasal hemianopia?
    A. A lesion that compresses the chiasm
    B. Calcified internal carotid arteries
    C. Transection of the optic nerve at the chiasm

30. A 24-year-old postpartum woman presents with severe headache and impaired vision. There is a central scotoma in the right eye, and there is a superior temporal

quadrantanopia in the left eye. What is the most likely diagnosis?
- A. Sinus venous thrombosis
- B. Pituitary apoplexy
- C. Brainstem stroke
- D. Stroke in the posterior cerebral artery distribution

31. A patient is nonresponsive and has pinpoint pupils in midposition that do not move with the doll's eye maneuver. Where is the lesion?
- A. Thalamus
- B. Midbrain
- C. Pons
- D. Medulla

32. Which of the following statements is *false*?
- A. Visual loss from cataracts can cause a relative afferent pupillary defect.
- B. Lesions of the optic tract can cause a relative afferent pupillary defect.
- C. Excluding trauma, the presence of anisocoria and a relative afferent pupillary defect indicates that two disease processes are occurring.
- D. Significant retinal disease can cause a relative afferent pupillary defect.
- E. Pretectal lesions can cause a contralateral relative afferent pupillary defect without visual field loss.

33. A 27-year-old woman is involved in a motor vehicle crash. She reports eye and neck pain. On examination, she has ptosis and miosis. What is the most likely diagnosis?
- A. Cavernous sinus thrombosis
- B. Carotid dissection
- C. Frontal lobe contusion
- D. Hypothalamic hematoma

34. Which of the following structures is *not* involved in causing the pupil to constrict with light in the pupillary light reflex?
- A. Ganglion cells of the retina
- B. Pretectal nucleus
- C. Edinger-Westphal nucleus
- D. Ciliospinal center
- E. Ciliary ganglion

35. A 20-year-old woman presents with double vision. When she looks to the left, neither eye moves. She is not able to adduct the right eye but is able to abduct it. She cannot adduct the left eye. What is her diagnosis?

- A. Internuclear ophthalmoplegia
- B. One-and-a-half syndrome
- C. Left cranial nerve VI palsy
- D. Right cranial nerve III palsy

36. True or False?
The vestibulo-ocular reflex is preserved with supranuclear lesions.

37. A 40-year-old woman presents with double vision. On examination, she has ptosis on the right, her right eye is deviated downward and outward, and her right pupil is dilated. Which diagnosis is most likely?
- A. Cavernous sinus thrombosis
- B. Increased intracranial pressure
- C. Posterior communicating artery aneurysm
- D. Vasculopathy

38. A woman presents with impaired upgaze, impaired convergence, and abnormal pupillary responses. Where is the lesion?
- A. Midbrain
- B. Pons
- C. Medulla
- D. Flocculonodular lobe of the cerebellum

39. A patient has unusual eye movements. His eyes beat to one side, slow, stop, and then beat to the other side. This repeats every 2 minutes. Where is the lesion?
- A. Midbrain
- B. Pons
- C. Medulla
- D. Flocculonodular lobe of the cerebellum

40. A 16-year-old patient complains of headaches at the back of his head. He has downbeat nystagmus. Which diagnosis is most likely?
- A. Multiple sclerosis
- B. Arnold-Chiari malformation
- C. Retinoblastoma
- D. Pituitary tumor

41. Sudden blindness may result from occlusion of which branch of the ophthalmic artery?
- A. Central retinal artery
- B. Supraorbital artery
- C. Frontal artery
- D. Lacrimal artery

NEURO-OPHTHALMOLOGY

ANSWERS

1. A

The fovea is the area of the retina with the greatest visual acuity. Cones are closely packed in the fovea, and color discrimination is most precise here. No ganglion cells are present in the fovea.

The macula also has high visual acuity. It surrounds the fovea.

The optic disc is where the axons from the ganglion cells leave the retina to become the optic nerve. There are no photoreceptors over this area. The lack of photoreceptors over the optic disc creates a blind spot.

2. C

The image on the retina is reversed and inverted compared to the object.

3.

1) A
2) B
3) B
4) A
5) A

Rods have poor spatial and temporal resolution but are more numerous and more useful in dim lighting. Rods contain rhodopsin.

Cones are more prevalent at the region of greatest visual acuity (the fovea) and detect color.

4. B

Bipolar cells receive impulses directly from the photoreceptors.

Visual information entering the eye first reaches the layer containing rods and cones, which are photoreceptor cells. Pigments in these photoreceptor cells transform energy from light into electrical signals, which are transmitted to the bipolar cells. This information is then carried to ganglion cells.

Photoreceptors and bipolar cells are unusual compared to other neurons because they do not use action potentials. Neurotransmitters are released in a graded manner that depends on the membrane potential.

5. C

The optic nerve is formed from the axons of ganglion cells.

Amacrine cells and horizontal cells are interneurons that increase visual contrast through their interactions with other cells.

6. A

Most fibers of the optic tract synapse in the lateral geniculate body. Layers 2, 3, and 5 of the lateral geniculate body receive uncrossed fibers; layers 1, 4, and 6 receive crossed fibers.

Fibers from the optic tract also travel to the superior colliculus and the pretectal nuclei in the midbrain. The superior colliculus is involved with saccades, and the pretectal nuclei are involved in pupillary responses. Information travels from the superior colliculus and pretectal nuclei to the pulvinar and then to the temporoparieto-occipital association cortex.

Fibers from the optic tract also travel to the suprachiasmatic nucleus, which regulates circadian rhythms.

7. C

Information regarding the form, color, and motion of visual stimuli is carried from the lateral geniculate nucleus to the visual cortex through the optic radiations. The primary visual cortex, which is Brodmann area 17, is located in the calcarine fissure of the occipital lobe. Layer 4 of the visual cortex is relatively thick due to the amount of input.

The calcarine cortex consists of the cuneus and the lingual gyrus. The cuneus, which is superior to the lingual gyrus, receives information from the upper quadrants of the retina. The lingual gyrus receives information from the lower retina.

Brodmann areas 18 and 19 are visual association cortex. They are responsible for color perception and object recognition.

Further visual processing is performed in the parieto-occipital association cortex and the occipitotemporal association cortex. Information regarding motion and spatial relationships travels from the primary visual cortex to the parietal lobe in the "where" pathway, also called the dorsal pathway. Information regarding shape and color travels to the temporal lobe from the primary visual cortex in the "what" pathway, also known as the ventral pathway.

8. True

Patients with cortical blindness have preserved pupil light reflexes. They can also have normal visual evoked potentials (see Fig. 18.1).

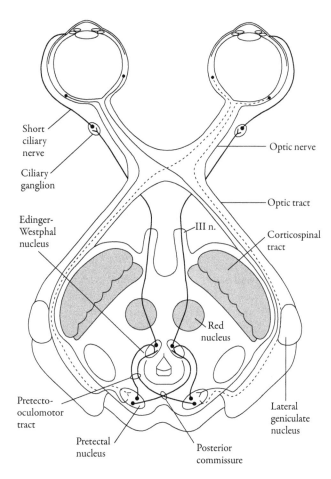

Figure 18.1 Light reflex pathway. (From Sundaram V, Barsam A, Alwitry A, Khaw P. *Training in Ophthalmology*, Fig. 9.1. New York, Oxford University Press, 2009.)

Short ciliary nerve

Ciliary ganglion

Edinger-Westphal nucleus

III n.

Optic nerve

Optic tract

Corticospinal tract

Red nucleus

Pretecto-oculomotor tract

Pretectal nucleus

Posterior commissure

Lateral geniculate nucleus

9. D

The levator palpebrae superioris elevates the upper eyelid. It is innervated by cranial nerve III (CN 3).

The superior tarsal muscle is also responsible for elevating the eyelid. It is innervated by sympathetic nerves.

The orbicularis oculi is responsible for eyelid closure and is innervated by CN 7.

10. C

Müller's muscle is innervated by sympathetic nerves.

The superior rectus, iris sphincter, and ciliary muscle are innervated by CN 3.

11. True

Due to the central caudal nucleus, a nuclear third nerve palsy can cause bilateral ptosis. The central caudal nucleus is one of the subnuclei of the oculomotor nucleus. It innervates both levator palpebrae superior muscles.

12. True

The superior rectus is innervated by the contralateral CN 3 nucleus.

Fibers from one superior rectus nucleus decussate and cross through the contralateral superior rectus nucleus

before proceeding to the muscle. Therefore, a nuclear third nerve palsy can cause bilateral superior rectus weakness.

13. A

A cavernous sinus lesion can cause both a Horner syndrome and CN 3 palsy, which can result in alternating anisocoria.

Horner syndrome typically causes anisocoria that is worse in the dark. Anisocoria is worse in the light with third nerve palsies and with tonic pupils.

14. A

A lesion in the anterior medullary vellum, where the trochlear nerves decussate, can cause bilateral CN 4 palsies. For example, head trauma can cause injury to the anterior medullary vellum. Patients with bilateral trochlear nerve palsies have a characteristic "chin down" position.

15. False

Injury to the right trochlear nucleus causes a *left* fourth nerve palsy because the nerve decussates. There may also be a Horner syndrome on the right if the adjacent sympathetic fibers are involved in the lesion.

Horner syndrome with a contralateral fourth nerve palsy suggests a lesion of the fourth nerve nucleus or its fascicle prior to decussation in the anterior medullary vellum.

16. B

A lesion in the cavernous sinus can cause an abducens palsy with an ipsilateral postganglionic Horner syndrome.

The anterior medullary vellum is where the trochlear nerves decussate.

The trigeminal ganglion is located in Meckel's cave.

17. C

The orbital apex syndrome, cavernous sinus syndrome, and superior orbital fissure syndrome can all involve CN 3, CN 4, the V1 division of CN 5, and CN 6. Involvement of CN 2 helps to differentiate the orbital apex syndrome from the superior orbital fissure syndrome: CN 2 is involved in the former but spared in latter. Involvement of the V2 division of CN 5 suggests cavernous sinus syndrome. Cavernous sinus syndrome may also involve the carotid artery and oculosympathetic fibers. Division V3 can be involved if there is spread to Meckel's cave.

18. B

The frontal eye fields are in the middle frontal gyrus in Brodmann area 8.

19. A

Voluntary saccades are controlled by the contralateral frontal lobe. There are projections from the frontal lobe to the superior colliculus and to the brainstem saccade centers. There is also a parietocollicular pathway that produces reflexive saccades.

Burst neurons in the paramedian pontine reticular formation (PPRF) initiate horizontal saccades. The nucleus prepositus hypoglossi and the medial vestibular nucleus act as horizontal gaze neural integrators.

The rostral interstitial nucleus of the medial longitudinal fasciculus (riMLF) and interstitial nucleus of Cajal are responsible for vertical saccades.

Smooth pursuit requires an intact ipsilateral occipital lobe.

20. E

Rett syndrome is least likely to involve the eye.

Ataxia-telangiectasia is associated with bilateral bulbar conjunctival telangiectasias but also with abnormal eye movements. Initially, patients have ocular motor apraxia. Then, smooth pursuit is impaired. Later, patients develop complete supranuclear ophthalmoplegia.

Klippel-Trenaunay-Weber, which is a disorder of soft tissue and bony hypertrophy and cutaneous vascular abnormalities, is associated with multiple eye findings: orbital varix, heterochromia iridis, varicosities of the retina, and choroidal angioma.

Neurofibromatosis type 1 is associated with Lisch nodules. Also, patients can have an optic pathway glioma.

Sturge-Weber syndrome is associated with glaucoma, typically ipsilateral to the facial angioma. Patients can also have choroidal hemangiomas, heterochromia iridis, and angiomas of the conjunctiva and sclera.

Tuberous sclerosis complex is associated with retinal astrocytic hamartomas.

Von Hippel-Lindau disease is associated with retinal hemangioblastomas, which are also known as retinal angiomas.

Wyburn-Mason syndrome, also known as retinocephalic vascular malformation, is associated with ocular arteriovenous malformations (AVMs) such as AVM of the retina, in the orbit, or involving the optic nerve, as well as intracranial AVM.

21. A

This is Aicardi syndrome, which is X-linked dominant. Patients with Aicardi syndrome have the triad of infantile spasms, agenesis of the corpus callosum, and chorioretinal lacunae.

22. A

A lesion of the left temporal optic radiations causes a right superior quadrantanopia.

A lesion of the left parietal optic radiations causes a right inferior quadrantanopia.

A right homonymous hemianopia with macular sparing occurs with left occipital lobe lesions.

A right homonymous sectoranopia occurs with lesions of the left lateral geniculate nucleus.

23. B

This patient has an ischemic abducens palsy, which can occur with microvascular disease. The lack of headache

makes temporal arteritis less likely. Other cranial nerves would probably be involved if the patient had a cavernous sinus thrombosis.

24. A

This is retrobulbar optic neuritis. Optic neuritis can be associated with papillitis, in which case the disc is swollen.

She does not have papilledema, so idiopathic intracranial hypertension is unlikely.

There is not enough information to diagnose the patient as having multiple sclerosis.

A patient with a tonic pupil, or Adie's tonic pupil, has anisocoria that is worse in the light. The pupil reacts slowly to sustained bright light. It reacts with accommodation but then redilates slowly. The fact that the pupil reacts better with accommodation than with light is referred to as light-near dissociation. A tonic pupil would *not* have an afferent pupil defect or red desaturation (see Box 18.1).

Box 18.1 CAUSES OF LIGHT-NEAR DISSOCIATION

- Adie's tonic pupil
- Argyll Robertson pupil
- Diabetes
- Optic neuropathy
- Parinaud syndrome
- Retinopathy (severe)

Light-near dissociation is caused by degeneration of the ciliary ganglion and postganglionic parasympathetic fibers. The postganglionic parasympathetics travel from the ciliary ganglion through the short ciliary nerves. These nerves innervate the ciliary muscle, which is responsible for accommodation, and the iris sphincter, which is responsible for pupil constriction.

A tonic pupil can be accompanied by decreased reflexes. This is known as Holmes-Adie syndrome.

25. C

This patient has Foster Kennedy syndrome, which is caused by an olfactory groove meningioma. Patients with Foster Kennedy syndrome have decreased visual acuity and color vision and have optic atrophy in the ipsilateral eye due to compression of the optic nerve by the tumor. There is papilledema in the contralateral eye due to increased intracranial pressure. These patients may have anosmia as well.

Leber hereditary optic neuropathy is a mitochondrial disorder that usually manifests in childhood or young adulthood. Patients may present with sudden vision loss. A cecocentral scotoma (affecting central vision and extending to the blind spot) is characteristic. Initially, the symptoms are unilateral, but severe bilateral vision loss eventually occurs.

26. B

The patient's history and examination findings are consistent with nonarteritic anterior ischemic optic neuropathy (NAION).

The presence of optic disc edema excludes posterior ischemic optic neuropathy, in which ischemia is retrobulbar.

Arteritic anterior ischemic optic neuropathy (AAION) is associated with giant cell arteritis (GCA).

GCA can cause fever, headache, jaw claudication, scalp tenderness, malaise, anorexia, weight loss, and polymyalgia rheumatica. The temporal artery may be pulseless. Laboratory studies show elevated inflammatory markers such as CRP and ESR. The patient may have thrombocytosis or anemia. Temporal artery biopsy is diagnostic. Treatment is with steroids. Prompt recognition and treatment are required to prevent permanent vision loss. If GCA is suspected, steroids should be initiated before a temporal artery biopsy is obtained.

A pale optic disc with edema is more likely to be AAION. Disc edema with flame-shaped hemorrhages is more characteristic of NAION. In addition, this patient does not have a headache, systemic symptoms, or elevated inflammatory markers, so AAION is less likely.

27. C

Most cases of anterior ischemic optic neuropathy are idiopathic.

28.

1) A. Monocular vision loss occurs with optic nerve lesions.
2) B. A lesion at the optic chiasm, such as a pituitary tumor, can cause bitemporal hemianopia.

3) C. A lesion affecting the optic radiations traveling through the parietal lobe causes a contralateral inferior quadrantanopia.

29. B

Calcified internal carotid arteries can cause binasal hemianopia (see Fig. 18.2).

30. B

This patient has pituitary apoplexy. The visual field defect (junctional scotoma) is consistent with chiasmal compression. Junctional scotoma has been attributed to Wilbrand's knee: At the chiasm, inferonasal fibers decussate and make a forward loop, traveling anteriorly with the contralateral optic nerve before joining the optic tract. (However, this concept is now under scrutiny.)

Chiasmal compression can also cause bitemporal hemianopia.

Pituitary apoplexy can cause Addisonian crisis.

31. C

A lesion in the pons causes pinpoint pupils that are in midposition.

32. A

Cataracts do not usually cause a relative afferent pupillary defect (RAPD).

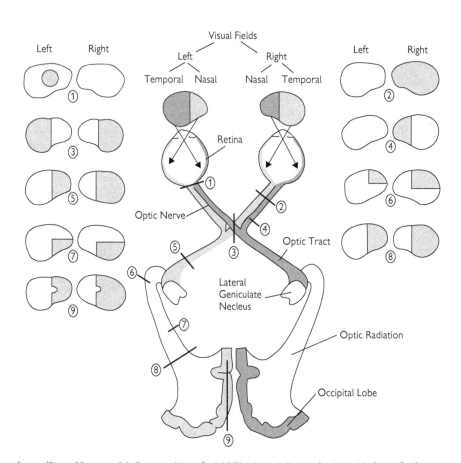

Figure 18.2 The optic pathway. (From Harrison M. *Revision Notes for MCEM Part A*, Fig. A.6.3. New York, Oxford University Press, 2011.)

RAPD/Marcus-Gunn pupil is tested with the swinging flashlight test: The affected pupil dilates when the light is directed to it, instead of constricting, because less light is perceived (see Box 18.2).

Box 18.2 CAUSES OF A RELATIVE AFFERENT
PUPILLARY DEFECT (RAPD)

- Optic nerve disease
- Significant retinal disease
- Optic tract (when there are more crossed than uncrossed fibers)
- Pretectal lesions (RAPD is contralateral)

---

33. B

Carotid dissection, which can occur after trauma, can manifest as a painful Horner syndrome.

34. D

The ciliospinal center, which is located in the intermediolateral (IML) cell column at the C8-T2 level of the spinal cord, is part of the oculosympathetic pathway and dilates the pupil. The ciliospinal reflex causes pupillary dilation when the skin of the neck is pinched.

35. B

This patient has one-and-a-half syndrome.

In the one-and-a-half syndrome, neither eye moves to the side of the lesion (in this case the left side). The only horizontal movement is abduction of the contralateral eye (in this case the right eye). The patient has a conjugate horizontal gaze palsy to the left and an internuclear ophthalmoplegia on right gaze (i.e., impaired adduction when looking to the right). Convergence is normal. This syndrome is caused by a lesion of the medial longitudinal fasciculus (MLF) plus the ipsilateral paramedian pontine reticular formation (PPRF) or the ipsilateral CN 6 nucleus.

A lesion of the MLF alone causes internuclear ophthalmoplegia (INO). The MLF connects the abducens nucleus with the contralateral oculomotor nucleus. With a lesion of the right MLF, the right eye does not adduct with lateral gaze to the left. The left eye abducts and often has nystagmus. Convergence is relatively preserved. Bilateral INO can occur in multiple sclerosis.

36. True

The vestibulo-ocular reflex is preserved with supranuclear lesions.

37. C

This patient has a CN 3 palsy with pupillary involvement, which is most likely caused by a posterior communicating artery aneurysm.

If the pupil were spared, a vasculopathy would be more likely in an older patient.

A cavernous sinus thrombosis would likely cause other cranial nerve palsies as well.

Increased intracranial pressure is more likely to cause an isolated CN 6 palsy than a CN 3 palsy.

38. A

This patient has Parinaud syndrome, which is caused by a midbrain lesion. It is characterized by impaired upgaze, impaired convergence, and light-near dissociation of the pupils.

39. D

This patient has periodic alternating nystagmus, which is associated with lesions of the flocculonodular lobe of the cerebellum.

40. B

Downbeat nystagmus is seen in patients with lesions at the cervicomedullary junction and can be seen in patients with Arnold-Chiari I malformation.

41. A

Sudden blindness may result from occlusion of the central retinal artery.

The ophthalmic artery is a branch of the internal carotid artery. The central retinal artery is a branch of the ophthalmic artery. The central retinal artery has four branches, each of which supplies blood to a quadrant of the retina.

19.

NEURO-OTOLOGY

QUESTIONS

1. Which structure carries auditory information from the superior olivary complex to the inferior colliculus?
   A. Cochlear nuclei
   B. Lateral lemniscus
   C. Medial lemniscus
   D. Medial geniculate nucleus

2. Which of the following structures is important in sound localization in the horizontal plane?
   A. Inferior olivary nucleus
   B. Semicircular canals
   C. Superior olivary nucleus
   D. Utricle and saccule

3. Which structure transfers information between the left and right auditory cortices?
   A. Anterior commissure
   B. Posterior commissure
   C. Corpus callosum
   D. Hippocampal commissure

4. **True or False?**
   A unilateral lesion at the midpons or higher does *not* cause deafness.

5. A 40-year-old man presents with recurrent episodes of vertigo. The episodes last 30 minutes and are associated with tinnitus and a feeling of fullness in his right ear. He has fallen abruptly after a feeling of being pushed to the ground. His neurologic examination is normal between episodes except for decreased hearing in the right ear. His brain MRI is normal. Which procedure needs to be performed?
   A. Audiometry
   B. Electroencephalography
   C. Epley maneuver
   D. Sinus computed tomography (CT)

6. A 55-year-old man presents with vertigo when he sits up in the morning every morning for the past 2 weeks. He feels better when he lies down. The events last about 30 seconds. He has no hearing loss. His neurological examination is normal. The Dix-Hallpike maneuver is negative. Which treatment should be offered?
   A. Canalith repositioning procedure
   B. Meclizine
   C. Prednisone
   D. Scopolamine

NEURO-OTOLOGY

ANSWERS

1. B

Information from the cochlear nuclei travels to either the ipsilateral or the contralateral superior olive. The crossing fibers are found in the trapezoid body in the pons.

The lateral lemniscus carries auditory information from the superior olivary complex to the inferior colliculus.

Brainstem auditory evoked potential pathway (BAEP) consists of seven peaks: Cranial nerve 8 (Wave I) → Cochlear nuclei in the medulla (Wave II) → Superior olivary complex in the pons (Wave III) → Lateral lemniscus in the pons (Wave IV) → Inferior colliculus in the midbrain (Wave V) →Medial geniculate nucleus in the thalamus (Wave VI) → Auditory radiations (Wave VII)

The BAEP pathway can be remembered by the mnemonic NCSLIMA (see Box 19.1).

The stapedius nerve, which is innervated by the facial

Box 19.1 **PEAKS OF THE BRAINSTEM AUDITORY EVOKED POTENTIAL: NCSLIMA**

- Nerve (cochlear)
- Cochlear nuclei
- Superior olive
- Lateral lemniscus
- Inferior colliculus
- Medial geniculate
- Auditory cortex

---

nerve, dampens sound.

2. C

The superior olivary nucleus is involved in sound localization in the horizontal plane.

The semicircular canals, utricle, and saccule are part of the vestibular system. The semicircular canals detect angular acceleration. The utricle and saccule are involved in detection of linear acceleration.

3. C

The corpus callosum transfers information between the left and right auditory cortices.

4. True

A unilateral lesion at the midpons or higher does not cause hearing loss. Bilateral injury to primary auditory cortex can cause a variety of symptoms depending on the lesions. For instance, bilateral injury can cause cortical deafness, pure word deafness, or auditory agnosia. Even with cortical deafness, the audiogram may be normal.

5. A

This patient has Ménière disease. Audiometry should be performed.

Patients with Ménière disease have episodes of vertigo lasting for at least 20 minutes. They can fall abruptly as if pushed to the ground. In addition, patients with Ménière disease have tinnitus or a sensation of fullness in the ear, and low-frequency hearing loss occurs. (With aging, high-frequency hearing loss usually occurs.) Ménière disease is associated with endolymphatic hydrops. Electrocochleography can help to confirm the diagnosis; there is a characteristic pattern with hydrops. Salt restriction is recommended for patients with Ménière disease.

There is an association between Ménière disease and migraine. Vestibular migraine may be difficult to differentiate from early Ménière disease, and some patients have both. Significant hearing loss does not occur in vestibular migraine. Vestibular migraine is a common cause of recurrent spontaneous vertigo. The patient with vestibular migraine has both vestibular symptoms and headaches with migrainous features.

6. A

This patient has benign paroxysmal positional vertigo (BPPV). The typical patient has episodes of vertigo with nystagmus that occur in certain positions. A negative Dix-Hallpike maneuver does not rule out BPPV.

BPPV is the most frequent cause of episodic vertigo in adults. It results from the presence of calcium carbonate (otoconia) debris in the semicircular canal, typically the posterior canal. Common causes of otoconia release include head trauma, infection, ischemia of the inner ear, and vigorous exercise. Also, otoconia may fall into the posterior semicircular canal when the head is extended back below horizontal for a few minutes. The treatment is a canalith repositioning procedure, such as the Epley maneuver.

20.

NEUROPATHOLOGY

QUESTIONS

1. **In a normal brain, it is most common to find neurons in the white matter in which area?**
   A. Frontal lobe
   B. Parietal lobe
   C. Temporal lobe
   D. Occipital lobe

2. **Normal ependymal cells stain strongly with which of the following?**
   A. Glial fibrillary acidic protein (GFAP)
   B. Luxol fast blue
   C. Synaptophysin
   D. Vimentin

3. **Which of the following statements is _false_?**
   A. Astrocytes are unable to proliferate.
   B. Astrocytes, oligodendrocytes, and ependymal cells are of ectodermal origin.
   C. Astrocytes have intermediate filaments that contain glial fibrillary acidic protein (GFAP).
   D. Astrocytes can be found in the white matter.

4. **True or False?**
   Microglia in the central nervous system are derived from monocytes.

5. **Fill in the blank: On sections stained with hematoxylin and eosin, red neurons are seen in the setting of ___**
   _____.
   A. Hypoxia/ischemia
   B. A virus
   C. A storage disease

6. **Which of the following cells are most susceptible to hypoxic-ischemic injury?**
   A. Astrocytes
   B. Hippocampal pyramidal cells of Sommer's sector (CA1)
   C. Neurons of cortical layers III, V, and VI
   D. Oligodendrocytes

7. **Which of the following features is characteristic of apoptosis?**
   A. Activation of intracellular proteases
   B. Rupture of the cell membrane
   C. Inflammation
   D. Random DNA degradation

8. **Which type of astrocytes can be found in hyperammonemia but are especially associated with Wilson disease?**

   A. Alzheimer type I astrocytes
   B. Alzheimer type II astrocytes
   C. Bergmann glia
   D. Creutzfeldt astrocytes

9. **Which type of astrocytes are associated with demyelination?**
   A. Alzheimer type I astrocytes
   B. Alzheimer type II astrocytes
   C. Bergmann glia
   D. Creutzfeldt astrocytes

10. **What is tau?**
    A. A microfilament
    B. An intermediate filament
    C. An aggregate of tubulin
    D. A microtubule-associated protein

11. **Which of the following is _not_ a synucleinopathy?**
    A. Multiple system atrophy
    B. Lewy body dementia
    C. Parkinson disease
    D. Chronic traumatic encephalopathy

12. **Which of the following is most likely to be found in the intradural extramedullary space?**
    A. Astrocytoma
    B. Ependymoma
    C. Oligodendroglioma
    D. Schwannoma

13. **Which of the following is _not_ characteristic of Alzheimer disease?**
    A. Neurofibrillary tangles
    B. Senile plaques
    C. Granulovacuolar degeneration
    D. Hirano bodies
    E. Lewy bodies

14. **Which of the following is the major component of neurofibrillary tangles?**
    A. Hyperphosphorylated tau protein
    B. Neurofilament protein
    C. Ubiquitin
    D. Amyloid

15. **The severity of Alzheimer dementia is _least_ likely to correlate with which of the following?**
    A. Quantity of diffuse plaques
    B. Distribution of neurofibrillary tangles
    C. Quantity of neuritic plaques
    D. Location of β-amyloid plaques

16. A low Braak stage indicates that neurofibrillary tangles are limited to which of the following areas?
    A. Transentorhinal cortex and CA1 region of the hippocampus
    B. Subiculum and amygdala
    C. Basal nucleus of Meynert and substantia nigra
    D. Thalamus and hypothalamus

17. Which of the following diseases is most likely to be associated with myoclonus, alien limb phenomenon, cortical sensory loss, neuronal degeneration in the precentral and postcentral gyrus, and swollen neurons?
    A. Alzheimer disease
    B. Corticobasal degeneration
    C. Diffuse Lewy body disease
    D. Progressive supranuclear palsy
    E. Amyotrophic lateral sclerosis (ALS)

18. Which of the following conditions is associated with early falls, square-wave jerks, slowing of vertical saccades, retrocollis, and a "Mickey mouse midbrain"?
    A. Progressive supranuclear palsy
    B. Corticobasal degeneration
    C. Multiple system tauopathy with dementia
    D. Dementia with Lewy bodies

19. Which of the following conditions is associated with visual hallucinations, REM sleep disorder, neuroleptic sensitivity, loss of neurons in the substantia nigra and basal nucleus of Meynert, granulovacuolar degeneration in the hippocampus, neurofibrillary tangles, and senile plaques?
    A. Alzheimer disease
    B. Corticobasal degeneration
    C. Dementia with Lewy bodies
    D. Parkinson disease

20. Which of the following conditions causes rigidity, gait disturbance, and globose neurofibrillary tangles?
    A. Corticobasal degeneration
    B. Dementia with Lewy bodies
    C. Frontotemporal dementia
    D. Progressive supranuclear palsy

21. Which disease is characterized by alpha-synuclein immunopositive glial intracytoplasmic inclusions found in oligodendrocytes?
    A. Corticobasal degeneration
    B. Multiple system atrophy (MSA)

C. Frontotemporal dementia
D. Progressive multifocal leukoencephalopathy

22. In which of the following conditions do patients have atrophy of the frontotemporal regions, depigmentation of the substantia nigra, and loss of anterior roots?
    A. ALS-Parkinsonism-dementia of Guam
    B. Cortical basal degeneration
    C. Multiple system atrophy
    D. Progressive supranuclear palsy

23. Rosenthal fibers are very prominent in which of the following diseases, some forms of which are caused by mutations in the glial fibrillary acidic protein (GFAP) gene?
    A. Alexander disease
    B. Canavan disease
    C. Krabbe disease
    D. Niemann-Pick disease type C

24. Which of the following is most likely to cause hemorrhagic lesions in the putamen?
    A. Carbon monoxide poisoning
    B. Kernicterus
    C. Methanol poisoning
    D. Nitrous oxide poisoning

25. A 20-year-old man is bitten by a bat. Three weeks later, he develops fever, headache, confusion, and hydrophobia. He later dies. Which of the following is most likely to be found in the brain?
    A. Cowdry A bodies
    B. Cowdry B bodies
    C. Lafora bodies
    D. Negri bodies

26. Which cell population is affected earliest in Huntington disease?
    A. Interneurons in the cortex
    B. Interneurons in the striatum
    C. Medium spiny neurons in the striatum
    D. Pyramidal cells

27. What is the term for the eosinophilic spheric structures that store oxytocin and vasopressin in the neurohypophysis?
    A. Bunina bodies
    B. Herring bodies
    C. Hirano bodies
    D. Marinesco bodies

NEUROPATHOLOGY

ANSWERS

1. C

In a normal brain, some neurons can be found in the white matter. This is most commonly seen in the temporal lobe.

2. D

Normal ependymal cells stain strongly with vimentin, which is an intermediate filament expressed in a number of cell types. Ependymal cells line the ventricles. The side of the cell adjacent to the ventricle has cilia and microvilli. Desmosomes connect the cells and create a barrier between the brain and the cerebral spinal fluid (CSF). The central canal of the spinal cord is also lined with ependymal cells.

Most normal ependymal cells do not stain for GFAP. However, ependymomas may stain positive for GFAP, which can cause confusion with astrocytic neoplasms.

Luxol fast blue stains myelin.

Synaptophysin is a neuronal marker.

3. A

Astrocytes are the most numerous type of glial cell. In general, protoplasmic astrocytes are found in the cortex, and fibrillary astrocytes are found in the white matter.

Astrocytes provide structural support to neurons and contribute to the blood-brain barrier. In response to injury, astrocytes proliferate and swell.

4. True

Microglia are derived from the monocyte/macrophage lineage; they are of mesodermal origin, not neuroepithelial origin. They phagocytose debris and are important in the inflammatory response.

5. A

Neurons affected by hypoxia/ischemia appear red on hematoxylin and eosin staining.

6. B

Neurons are the cells most sensitive to hypoxic-ischemic injury.

The most sensitive neurons are hippocampal pyramidal cells of Sommer's sector (CA1) and Purkinje cells in the cerebellar cortex, followed by neurons of cortical layers III, V, and VI.

7. A

Apoptosis is associated with activation of intracellular proteases.

Rupture of the cell membrane, inflammation, and random DNA degradation occur with necrosis.

Necrosis and apoptosis are both forms of cell death. Necrosis is a disorganized, unintentional, inflammatory process. Apoptosis is an organized, intentional form of cell death.

In necrosis, water flows into the cell. This leads to swelling of the cytoplasm, nucleus, and mitochondria. The cell membrane ruptures, and the cell contents leak into surrounding tissue.

Apoptosis is programmed cell death which ultimately leads to release of cytochrome *c* from mitochondria, activation of a caspase cascade, and fragmentation of DNA at specific locations.

8. A

Both Alzheimer type I and Alzheimer type II astrocytes are found in hyperammonemia, but the former are more common in Wilson disease.

9. D

Creutzfeldt astrocytes are associated with demyelination.

Bergmann glia act as guides for migrating granular cell neurons during cerebellar development.

10. D

Tau is a microtubule-associated protein. The gene for tau is on chromosome 17.

11. D

Chronic traumatic encephalopathy (CTE) is a tauopathy. CTE is a neurodegenerative disease that occurs in some patients who have experienced repetitive traumatic brain injury.

Parkinson disease, Lewy body dementia, and multiple system atrophy are synucleinopathies.

12. D

Of the tumors listed, schwannoma is most likely to occur in the intradural extramedullary space. Neurofibromas and meningiomas also are found in that space.

Astrocytomas, ependymomas, and oligodendrogliomas are intramedullary neoplasms.

Metastases and bone cancers tend to be extradural.

13. E

Lewy bodies are intraneuronal cytoplasmic inclusions found in patients with Parkinson disease or diffuse Lewy body disease.

Neurofibrillary tangles, senile plaques, granulovacuolar degeneration, and Hirano bodies are found in patients with Alzheimer disease.

14. A

Neurofibrillary tangles are composed of hyperphosphorylated tau protein.

Neuritic plaques are composed of amyloid and dystrophic neurites. Neuritic plaques contain Aβ peptide, which is a derivative of amyloid precursor protein (APP). The dystrophic neurites contain phosphorylated tau.

15. A

Diffuse plaques contain Aβ peptide, similar to the neuritic plaques in Alzheimer disease, but diffuse plaques are found in elderly patients who have no cognitive impairment.

Multiple pathologic classification systems are used to assess the brains of patients with suspected Alzheimer disease (see Table 20.1).

Table 20.1 PATHOLOGIC CLASSIFICATION OF ALZHEIMER DISEASE

CLASSIFICATION SYSTEM	LESIONS USED FOR CLASSIFICATION
CERAD	Neuritic plaques
Braak and Braak	Neurofibrillary tangles
Thal	β-amyloid plaques

Neuritic plaques correlate better with cognitive impairment than diffuse plaques do. The Consortium to Establish a Registry for Alzheimer's Disease (CERAD) classification is based on the extent of neuritic plaques.

Neurofibrillary tangles tend to occur in specific locations in Alzheimer disease. The Braak and Braak classification is used to assess the distribution of neurofibrillary tangles.

The Thal score is determined by the location of β-amyloid plaques. The lowest score corresponds to the presence of β-amyloid plaques solely in the neocortex.

16. A

The Braak and Braak score is a pathologic classification scheme for Alzheimer disease that is based on the distribution of neurofibrillary tangles. The lowest score in this classification indicates that neurofibrillary tangles are limited to the transentorhinal cortex and CA1 region of the hippocampus.

17. B

Corticobasal degeneration causes asymmetric atrophy of the parasagittal perirolandic cortices. There is neuronal loss and astrocytosis in the primary motor and sensory cortices, substantia nigra, and basal ganglia. There are neuronal and glial lesions containing tau. Astrocytic plaques are found in the cortex. There are tau-positive coiled bodies within oligodendrocytes. Also, swollen, achromatic neurons are seen.

18. A

Progressive supranuclear palsy (PSP) causes selective atrophy of the midbrain tegmentum with relative preservation of the cerebral peduncles and tectum; this can result in the appearance of Mickey mouse midbrain on axial magnetic resonance imaging (MRI).

Early oculomotor abnormalities in patients with PSP include slowed vertical saccadic movements, hypometric saccades, decreased blinking, and square-wave jerks. Later, supranuclear vertical gaze palsy occurs. Typically, downgaze is affected first. Also, patients have lid retraction, rare blinking, and eyelid apraxia. Late oculomotor findings include supranuclear horizontal gaze palsy.

19. C

Diffuse Lewy body disease causes diffuse cortical atrophy. The substantia nigra and locus coeruleus become pale. Lewy bodies are found in the cortex and brainstem. These are immunoreactive for alpha-synuclein, ubiquitin, and neurofilament. Neuritic plaques and neurofibrillary tangles may be seen, as in patients with Alzheimer disease.

20. D

Progressive supranuclear palsy (PSP) causes atrophy of the midbrain tegmentum. Sometimes the pons is affected as well. Neurofibrillary tangles and neuropil threads are found in the brainstem and basal ganglia. Globose neurofibrillary tangles are characteristic of PSP. Tuft-shaped astrocytes are also characteristic.

21. B

In patients with MSA, glial intracytoplasmic inclusions that stain for alpha-synuclein are found in oligodendrocytes.

Corticobasal degeneration (CBD) is characterized by swollen, achromatic neurons; astrocytic plaques in the cortex; and tau-positive coiled bodies in oligodendrocytes.

Frontotemporal dementia (formerly known as Pick disease) causes atrophy of the frontal and temporal lobes. There may be relative sparing of the posterior superior temporal gyrus. Pick bodies are found in the mesial temporal lobe, especially in the dentate granule cells. These are argyrophilic intracytoplasmic inclusions composed of polymerized tau. Pick cells are neurons with neurofilament in the cytoplasm.

Atypical astrocytes with bizarre, pleomorphic nuclei are found in progressive multifocal leukoencephalopathy

(PML). Also in PML, oligodendrocytes have ground-glass intranuclear inclusions due to JC virus.

22. A

Patients with amyotrophic lateral sclerosis (ALS)-Parkinsonism-dementia of Guam have atrophy of the frontotemporal regions, depigmentation of the substantia nigra, and loss of anterior roots.

23. A

Rosenthal fibers are prominent in Alexander disease. They are also found in tumors such as pilocytic astrocytomas. They occur normally in the pineal gland.

24. C

Methanol poisoning causes hemorrhagic lesions in the putamen.

Carbon monoxide poisoning causes bilateral lesions of the globus pallidus.

Kernicterus is associated with changes in the globus pallidus, subthalamus, and Ammon's horn.

Nitrous oxide causes a myeloneuropathy that resembles vitamin B12 deficiency.

25. D

This patient has rabies, which is characterized by Negri bodies. Negri bodies are eosinophilic cytoplasmic inclusions that are found most often in pyramidal cells of the hippocampus and Purkinje cells.

Cowdry A bodies are eosinophilic intranuclear inclusions found in patients with certain infections, such as cytomegalovirus (CMV), herpes, and subacute sclerosing panencephalitis (SSPE).

Cowdry B bodies are eosinophilic intranuclear inclusions found in patients with acute poliomyelitis.

Lafora bodies are intracytoplasmic inclusions found in patients with Lafora disease, a progressive myoclonic epilepsy.

26. C

GABA-ergic medium spiny neurons in the striatum are affected early in Huntington disease.

Pyramidal cells are involved to a lesser extent, and interneurons are relatively spared.

27. B

Herring bodies store oxytocin and vasopressin.

Bunina bodies are intracytoplasmic inclusions found in patients with amyotrophic lateral sclerosis (ALS).

Hirano bodies are found in patients with Alzheimer disease.

Marinesco bodies are eosinophilic intranuclear inclusions that are found in the substantia nigra and locus coeruleus with age.

21.

NEUROPHARMACOLOGY

QUESTIONS

1. What is the term for the effect that a medication has on the body?
   A. Pharmacodynamics
   B. Pharmacogenomics
   C. Pharmacokinetics
   D. Potency

2. Which of the following can affect absorption?
   A. Antacids
   B. Gastric motility
   C. Proton pump inhibitors
   D. All of the above

3. Fill in the blank: The amount of drug in the body divided by the concentration of the drug in the blood is the _____.
   A. Absorption
   B. Potency
   C. Therapeutic index
   D. Volume of distribution

4. Which of the following is the most important factor in determining a medication's concentration in the blood?
   A. Clearance
   B. Half-life
   C. Potency
   D. Therapeutic index
   E. Volume of distribution

5. True or False?
   The effectiveness of a medication does *not* depend on its potency.

6. Which of the following can affect a medication's half-life?
   A. Volume of distribution
   B. Protein binding
   C. Lipid solubility
   D. Illness
   E. All of the above

7. Which term best describes the situation in which a specific amount of drug is eliminated per unit time, regardless of the blood concentration?
   A. Zero-order kinetics
   B. First-order kinetics

C. Bioavailability
D. Bioequivalence

8. Fill in the blank: The loading dose of a medication is calculated by multiplying the target concentration by the _____.
   A. Clearance
   B. Rate of elimination
   C. Volume of distribution

9. Which of the following medications does *not* undergo biotransformation?
   A. Gabapentin
   B. Phenytoin
   C. Diazepam
   D. Clopidogrel

10. For which of the following drugs is the transport mechanism for absorption from the intestine saturable at therapeutic doses?
    A. Carbamazepine
    B. Gabapentin
    C. Phenytoin
    D. Valproic acid

11. Which of the following cytochrome P450 (CYP) enzymes is strongly inhibited by grapefruit juice?
    A. CYP2C9
    B. CYP2C19
    C. CYP2D6
    D. CYP3A4

12. Which cytochrome P450 enzyme is primarily responsible for metabolizing carbamazepine?
    A. CYP2C19
    B. CYP2D6
    C. CYP3A4

13. For patients of Asian background, a standard dose of diazepam may be toxic because of decreased metabolism by which enzyme?
    A. CYP2C9
    B. CYP2C19
    C. CYP2D6
    D. CYP3A4

14. Patients with reduced function of which enzyme have a reduced response to clopidogrel?
    A. CYP2C19
    B. CYP2D6

C. CYP2E1

D. CYP3A4

15. Which of the following is *least* likely to affect carbamazepine metabolism?
    A. HLA-B*1502 genotype
    B. Erythromycin
    C. Cyclosporin
    D. Fluoxetine
    E. Lamotrigine

16. Which enzyme helps to metabolize warfarin and phenytoin and is inhibited by fluconazole and amiodarone?
    A. CYP1A2
    B. CYP2C9
    C. CYP2C19
    D. CYP2D6

17. Genotype testing to assess metabolism is *least* necessary for which of the following medications?
    A. Warfarin
    B. Azathioprine
    C. Tetrabenazine
    D. Vigabatrin

18. Which of the following enzymes is responsible for metabolism of codeine (i.e., poor metabolizers have no analgesia from codeine, whereas ultrametabolizers develop opioid intoxication with typical doses of codeine)?
    A. CYP1A2
    B. CYP2C9
    C. CYP2C19
    D. CYP2D6

19. Which of the following medications is metabolized by UDP-glucuronosyltransferases (UGTs)?
    A. Clobazam
    B. Clonazepam
    C. Lamotrigine
    D. Phenytoin

20. A patient who is taking valproic acid develops hyperammonemia. Which of the following would be the most effective treatment?
    A. Carnitine
    B. Citric acid/potassium citrate
    C. Lactulose
    D. Sodium benzoate

21. A 7-year-old patient with spastic quadriplegia is implanted with a baclofen pump. What is the mechanism of action for baclofen?
    A. It is a GABA-A receptor agonist.
    B. It is a GABA-B receptor agonist.
    C. It is a GABA-B receptor antagonist.
    D. It is a glycine receptor agonist.

22. Phenelzine, selegiline, tranylcypromine, and isocarboxacid can all contribute to serotonin syndrome. What is the mechanism?
    A. Increased serotonin release
    B. Decreased serotonin metabolism

C. Inhibition of serotonin reuptake

D. They are direct serotonin receptor agonists.

23. Fill in the blank: Patients who are taking a monoamine oxidase (MAO) inhibitor should avoid _____.
    A. Arginine
    B. Serine
    C. Taurine
    D. Tyramine

24. Which of the following medications is *least* likely to cause serotonin syndrome?
    A. Dapsone
    B. Doxepin
    C. Lithium
    D. Ritonavir
    E. Tramadol

25. Which of the following medications would be most helpful in treating serotonin syndrome?
    A. Amantadine
    B. Bromocriptine
    C. Cyproheptadine
    D. Dextromethorphan
    E. Tryptophan

26. Which of the following has antiserotonergic properties?
    A. Bromocriptine
    B. Buspirone
    C. Chlorpromazine
    D. Lysergic acid diethylamide (LSD)
    E. Meperidine

27. Which of the following features is more characteristic of anticholinergic syndrome than of serotonin syndrome?
    A. Absent bowel sounds
    B. Mydriasis
    C. Tachycardia
    D. Tremor
    E. Agitation

28. Which of the following medications is a selective norepinephrine reuptake inhibitor?
    A. Atomoxetine
    B. Guanfacine
    C. Dextroamphetamine
    D. Bupropion

29. A patient presents with an overdose of benzodiazepines. Which of the following is the most effective treatment?
    A. Flumazenil
    B. Fomepizole
    C. Naloxone
    D. Pralidoxime
    E. Physostigmine

30. Fill in the blank: Tolcapone and entacapone inhibit _____.
    A. Acetylcholinesterase
    B. Catechol-*O*-methyltransferase (COMT)

C. Monoamine oxidase A (MAO-A)
D. Monoamine oxidase B (MAO-B)

31. Which of the following is a muscarinic receptor agonist?
    A. Atropine
    B. Pilocarpine
    C. Scopolamine
    D. Tacrine

32. Which of the following medications is *least* likely to cause seizures?
    A. Buspirone
    B. Isoniazid
    C. Lithium
    D. Propoxyphene
    E. Theophylline

33. Which of the following medications is *least* likely to cause cardiac rhythm changes?
    A. Clobazam
    B. Ezogabine
    C. Lacosamide
    D. Rufinamide

34. Which of the following medications is *least* likely to affect cardiac rhythm?
    A. Amantadine
    B. Citalopram
    C. Gabapentin
    D. Galantamine
    E. Tetrabenazine

35. Which of the following medications is *least* likely to cause peripheral edema?
    A. Amantadine
    B. Amitriptyline
    C. Gabapentin
    D. Lacosamide
    E. Pramipexole

36. Which of the following medications is most likely to cause Lhermitte's sign, ototoxicity, and nephrotoxicity?
    A. Busulfan
    B. Cisplatin
    C. Cytarabine
    D. Ifosfamide
    E. ʟ-Asparaginase

NEUROPHARMACOLOGY

ANSWERS

1. A

The term *pharmacodynamics* refers to the effects of a drug on the body, including its mechanism of action.

Pharmacokinetics refers to the effect of the body on the drug. This includes absorption, metabolism, distribution, and elimination.

Pharmacogenomics is the study of the relationship between an individual's genetic background and his or her response to medication.

Potency is the dose or concentration of a medication that is needed to produce 50% of its maximal effect.

2. D

The term *absorption* refers to the quantity of medication that enters the body. It is affected by the rate and degree of transfer into the blood. Multiple factors affect absorption. These include drug concentration, drug formulation, surface area available for absorption, blood flow, gastric motility, pH, drug solubility, and drug binding.

3. D

The amount of drug in the body divided by the concentration of the drug in the blood is the volume of distribution. Drugs that stay in the vascular system have a smaller volume of distribution. The volume of distribution is greater if the drug is lipophilic. Multiple factors affect volume of distribution (Box 21.1).

Box 21.1 FACTORS THAT AFFECT VOLUME OF DISTRIBUTION

- Age
- Gender
- Pregnancy
- Organ failure
- Protein binding
- Tissue binding
- Edema or other fluid collections
- Drug acidity

4. A

Clearance is the major factor affecting drug concentration in the blood. Clearance is defined as the removal of a drug from the body. Clearance of a drug is equal to its rate of elimination divided by the concentration. The dose of the medication, blood flow to the organs, and liver and kidney function affect clearance. Excretion and metabolism are methods by which elimination occurs. Elimination can occur through the liver, kidneys, lungs, and other organs. Excretion is the removal of a drug through body waste.

The therapeutic index is the ratio of the median effective dose to the median toxic dose.

5. True

The effectiveness of a medication does not depend on its potency but rather on its maximal efficacy. Maximal efficacy is the maximal response that can be produced by a drug.

6. E

Half-life is the time required for the amount of drug in the body to be reduced by half. Half-life depends on the volume of distribution and the clearance of the drug. Therefore, factors that affect volume of distribution or clearance can affect the half-life.

7. A

In first-order kinetics, the rate of elimination is proportionate to the concentration. The metabolism is linear: A constant fraction of the drug is metabolized in a given amount of time. Most drugs exhibit first-order kinetics.

In zero-order kinetics, the rate of elimination is constant. This is nonlinear metabolism: The amount of drug eliminated in a given amount of time does not depend on the concentration of the drug.

Phenytoin demonstrates first-order kinetics at lower concentrations. However, at higher concentrations, saturation of hepatic enzymes occurs, and there is a change to zero-order kinetics. Therefore, the clearance of phenytoin depends on its concentration. Aspirin and ethanol also have capacity-limited elimination and demonstrate zero-order kinetics.

Bioavailability refers to the fraction of drug that is absorbed (i.e., not affected by first-pass elimination). Intravenous dosing results in the highest bioavailability.

Bioequivalence refers to the condition in which two drugs with the same active ingredient have similar bioavailability and physiologic effect.

8. C

A loading dose of a medication is the product of the target concentration and the volume of distribution.

9. A

Biotransformation is the conversion of a drug into a water-soluble compound for the purpose of excretion. Phase I and phase II reactions make the compound more polar. Phase I reactions include hydrolysis, oxidation, and reduction. Conjugation occurs in phase II reactions. Not all medications undergo biotransformation. Gabapentin and pregabalin, both of which bind to calcium channel α2δ subunits, do not undergo biotransformation. They are not metabolized.

10. B

Gabapentin has saturable absorption at therapeutic doses, which results in nonlinear pharmacokinetics. Gabapentin, which has a structure resembling an amino acid, is transported by a low-capacity L-amino acid transporter in the small intestine. At higher doses, the bioavailability of gabapentin decreases as a result of saturation of this transporter. Therefore, the bioavailability of gabapentin is dose dependent. The bioavailability of gabapentin is also affected by antacids.

Gabapentin has unique pharmacokinetics. It has saturable absorption at therapeutic doses, it is not bound to plasma proteins, and it is not metabolized. It is excreted unchanged in the urine.

Phenytoin and carbamazepine have poor absorption from the gastrointestinal tract, especially in young children.

At therapeutic doses, protein binding of valproic acid is saturable.

11. D

CYP3A4 is inhibited by grapefruit juice.

12. C

Carbamazepine is primarily metabolized by CYP3A4. Carbamazepine induces its own metabolism, resulting in nonlinear pharmacokinetics. It also induces metabolism of oral contraceptives (OCPs), increasing the risk for pregnancy.

Other medications that induce the metabolism of OCPs include felbamate, phenobarbital, phenytoin, primidone, and rufinamide. Higher doses of topiramate and oxcarbazepine are also associated with lower OCP levels. Gabapentin, lacosamide, lamotrigine, levetiracetam, pregabalin, valproic acid, vigabatrin, and zonisamide do not lower OCP levels. Folate is recommended for menstruating females who are taking any anti-epileptic medication.

Vitamin D levels are also a concern in patients taking anti-epileptic medication, especially in those taking enzyme inducers, such as carbamazepine.

13. B

Patients of Asian background may have reduced activity of CYP2C19, which is responsible for metabolism of diazepam.

14. A

Patients with reduced function of CYP2C19 have a reduced response to clopidogrel. There is also a variant that causes an increased response, resulting in an increased risk for bleeding.

15. E

Lamotrigine is least likely to effect carbamazepine metabolism.

Asians with the HLA-B*1502 genotype are more likely to develop Stevens-Johnson syndrome from carbamazepine. Patients can be screened for this genotype before being prescribed carbamazepine.

Erythromycin, cyclosporine, and fluoxetine are inhibitors of CYP3A4, which metabolizes carbamazepine.

16. B

CYP2C9 is involved in the metabolism of warfarin and phenytoin. CYP2C19 also plays an important role in metabolism of phenytoin.

17. D

Vigabatrin is not metabolized.

Azathioprine is methylated by thiopurine methyltransferase (TPMT). Some patients have reduced or absent TPMT, which results in increased myelotoxicity. Genotyping helps to identify these patients.

Tetrabenazine is metabolized by CYP2D6. The activity of this enzyme varies by genotype.

Metabolism of warfarin is also affected by genotype. For example, certain variants of CYP2C9 and vitamin K epoxide reductase complex, subunit 1 (VKORC1) are associated with slow warfarin metabolism.

18. D

CYP2D6 metabolizes multiple medications, including codeine, amitriptyline, atomoxetine, dextromethorphan, tetrabenazine, and haloperidol. Inhibitors of CYP2D6 include fluoxetine, paroxetine, and quinidine.

19. C

Uridine 5′-diphospho-glucuronosyltransferases (UDP-glucoronosyltransferases, or UGTs) perform glucuronidation, which is a type of phase II reaction. Lamotrigine is one of the medications metabolized by UGTs. Valproic acid inhibits glucuronidation of lamotrigine, leading to an increase in its half-life.

20. A

Carnitine is used in the treatment of hyperammonemia due to valproic acid. Valproic acid use can deplete carnitine, which is important in its metabolism. Carnitine is a cofactor in the β-oxidation of fatty acids.

Risk factors for hyperammonemia due to valproic acid include hepatic dysfunction, carnitine deficiency, urea cycle disorders, infancy, polypharmacy, and poor nutritional status. Also, the combination of topiramate and valproic acid can produce hyperammonemia, which may be associated with encephalopathy.

Valproic acid is contraindicated in patients with inborn errors of metabolism. For instance, it is contraindicated in urea cycle disorders (e.g., ornithine transcarbamylase deficiency); carnitine deficiency; and mitochondrial diseases. Mitochondrial β-oxidation is one of the pathways by which valproic acid is metabolized. There is an increased risk for liver failure and death in patients with mutations in the mitochondrial DNA polymerase γ (POLG) gene.

21. B

Baclofen is a GABA-B receptor agonist. Side effects of baclofen include hypotonia, drowsiness, nausea, headache, and dizziness.

Intrathecal baclofen overdose can cause somnolence, cephalad progression of hypotonia, seizures, hypotension, and respiratory depression. Coma can occur.

Signs of withdrawal from intrathecal baclofen include pruritus, paresthesias, muscle rigidity, fever, seizures, altered mental status, and diaphoresis. Rhabdomyolysis and multiple organ failure can occur.

22. B

Phenelzine, selegiline, tranylcypromine, and isocarboxacid are monoamine oxidase (MAO) inhibitors, which decrease serotonin metabolism. Serotonin is metabolized by MAO to 5-hydroxyindole acetaldehyde, which is then metabolized by aldehyde dehydrogenase to 5-hydroxyindoleacetic acid (5-HIAA).

Linezolid, which is an MAO-A inhibitor, also increases serotonin levels due to reduced metabolism.

23. D

Patients who are taking an MAO inhibitor should avoid tyramine. MOA enzymes in the intestine and liver digest tyramine. If tyramine metabolism is inhibited by an MAO inhibitor, tyramine accumulates in adrenergic nerves. This results in release of norepinephrine and epinephrine, which can cause a hypertensive crisis. Tyramine can be found in alcoholic beverages, cured meats, and "aged" foods, such as cheese. Patients taking nonselective MOA inhibitors and MAO-A inhibitors are at higher risk than those taking MAO-B inhibitors. However, at higher doses, MAO-B inhibitors, such as selegiline, can inhibit both MAO-A and MAO-B.

Sympathomimetic medications should also be avoided to prevent hypertensive crisis.

The combination of an MAO inhibitor and a serotonin reuptake inhibitor can result in serotonin syndrome.

24. A

Dapsone is the least likely to cause serotonin syndrome. It can cause methemoglobinemia.

Doxepin, lithium, ritonavir (which is used to treat human immunodeficiency virus infection), and tramadol can increase serotonin levels. Triptans and dopamine agonists can as well.

25. C

Tryptophan increases serotonin synthesis and should be avoided in serotonin syndrome. Amantadine, bromocriptine, and dextromethorphan also can worsen serotonin syndrome.

Serotonin syndrome is treated with removal of the contributing agent or agents and supportive care including intravenous fluids and treatment of fever. Benzodiazepines have been used to treat serotonin syndrome. Also, cyproheptadine, which is a nonspecific serotonin receptor blocker, has been used.

26. C

Chlorpromazine has antiserotonergic properties. The others are serotonergic. Bromocriptine increases serotonin activity. Buspirone and LSD are serotonin receptor agonists. Meperidine prevents serotonin reuptake.

27. A

Patients with anticholinergic syndrome have dry skin, normal deep tendon reflexes, and absent bowel sounds. Diarrhea, hyperreflexia, and diaphoresis are seen in serotonin syndrome.

Neuroleptic malignant syndrome (NMS) and serotonin syndrome have similar symptoms, but NMS has a slower progression of symptoms and is characterized by decreased movement rather than hyperkinetic activity. Pupillary dilation and diarrhea are more suggestive of serotonin syndrome than of NMS.

Clonus and myoclonus are also suggestive of serotonin syndrome rather than NMS or anticholinergic syndrome.

28. A

Atomoxetine is a selective norepinephrine reuptake inhibitor.

Like clonidine, guanfacine is an α_2-agonist. It has been used to treat attention deficit hyperactivity disorder (ADHD) because of its action in the prefrontal cortex.

Amphetamine and dextroamphetamine increase release of monoamines (norepinephrine, serotonin, and dopamine), interfere with monoamine reuptake, and inhibit monoamine oxidase (MAO).

Bupropion is a norepinephrine and dopamine reuptake inhibitor.

29. A

Flumazenil, which is a benzodiazepine antagonist, is used in benzodiazepine overdose. However, it can cause seizures due to benzodiazepine withdrawal.

Fomepizole is used to treat methanol or ethylene glycol poisoning.

Naloxone is an opioid antagonist. It can cause withdrawal in patients with opioid dependence.

Pralidoxime is used in organophosphate poisoning. It regenerates active acetylcholinesterase that had been involved in an organophosphorus-cholinesterase complex.

Physostigmine is a cholinesterase inhibitor that is used to treat anticholinergic poisoning. It should not be used if there is prolongation of the PR, QRS, or QTc interval.

30. B

Tolcapone and entacapone inhibit COMT, which converts dihydroxyphenylacetic acid to homovanillic acid.

31. B

Pilocarpine is a muscarinic receptor agonist. It is used to treat dry mouth in patients with Sjögren syndrome and in those who have received chemotherapy. It is also used to treat glaucoma.

Atropine and scopolamine are antagonists to the muscarinic receptor; they block the effect of acetylcholine. Atropine counteracts vagal tone to the heart, causing tachycardia at higher doses. It results in dry mouth, decreased sweating, decreased secretions in the respiratory tract, dilated pupils, and decreased gastrointestinal motility. At higher doses, it can cause hallucinations and restlessness.

Tacrine and donepezil are anticholinesterase agents.

32. A

Buspirone is least likely to cause seizures. Bupropion can cause seizures at therapeutic doses. Isoniazid, lithium, propoxyphene, and theophylline also lower the seizure threshold.

33. A

Clobazam is least likely to cause changes in cardiac rhythm.

Lacosamide can prolong the PR interval and rarely causes atrioventricular (AV) block.

Ezogabine prolongs the QT interval.

Rufinamide shortens the QT interval.

34. C

Patients with long QT syndrome are advised not to take amantadine, citalopram, galantamine, or tetrabenazine. Galantamine can also cause bradycardia and AV block.

Gabapentin is least likely to cause cardiac rhythm changes.

35. D

Lacosamide is least likely to cause peripheral edema.

Amantadine, amitriptyline, gabapentin, pregabalin, and pramipexole can cause peripheral edema.

36. B

Cisplatin can cause Lhermitte's sign, ototoxicity, and nephrotoxicity.

Busulfan can cause electroencephalogram (EEG) abnormalities and generalized seizures.

Cytarabine causes cerebellar dysfunction.

Ifosfamide can cause encephalopathy, which can be treated with methylene blue.

L-Asparaginase can cause venous sinus thrombosis.

22.

NEUROPHYSIOLOGY

1. Fill in the blank: At rest, the axonal membrane of a nerve is _____ when the inside is compared to the outside.
   A. Negatively polarized
   B. Positively polarized
   C. Neutral

2. Fill in the blank: The resting membrane potential of the axonal membrane is closest to the equilibrium potential for _____.
   A. Calcium
   B. Chloride
   C. Potassium
   D. Sodium

3. Fill in the blank: The concentration of _____ is greater inside the axonal membrane of the nerve than outside it.
   A. Chloride
   B. Potassium
   C. Sodium

4. What is the mechanism of action of 4-aminopyridine, which has been used in patients with multiple sclerosis?
   A. Calcium channel blocker
   B. Chloride channel blocker
   C. Potassium channel blocker
   D. Sodium channel blocker

5. What is the function of myelin?
   A. It reduces the capacitance of the nerve.
   B. It increases the capacitance of the nerve.
   C. It decreases transmembrane resistance.

6. How does depolarization occur in myelinated nerves?
   A. It occurs transversely across the diameter of the nerve underneath the myelin sheath.
   B. It occurs longitudinally along the nerve underneath the myelin.
   C. It occurs at gaps in the myelin.

7. Which of the following nerve types conducts the fastest?
   A. A large myelinated nerve
   B. A small myelinated nerve
   C. A large unmyelinated nerve
   D. A small unmyelinated nerve

8. Which of the following is required at the presynaptic neuron for an action potential to result in release of neurotransmitters into the synaptic cleft?

A. Calcium influx
B. Zinc efflux
C. Potassium influx
D. Acetylcholine binding

9. Fill in the blank: At the neuromuscular junction, when acetylcholine binds to the postsynaptic acetylcholine receptor, there is _____, which results in depolarization.
   A. An influx of sodium
   B. An influx of potassium
   C. An influx of chloride
   D. An efflux of calcium

10. Fill in the blank: In the monosynaptic stretch reflex, _____ excites _____, which synapse on the anterior horn cells that innervate the muscle that was stretched, causing muscle contraction.
    A. Stretch of a muscle spindle excites group Ia sensory afferent axons
    B. Stretch of a nuclear chain excites group II afferent fibers
    C. Stretch of Golgi tendon organs excites C fibers
    D. Stretch of Pacinian corpuscles excites Aδ fibers

11. A 30-year-old woman is scheduled for electromyography (EMG) and nerve conduction studies (NCS). Her extremities are found to be cold. Which of the following could result from the cold temperature?
    A. Slowed conduction velocities
    B. Prolonged distal latencies
    C. Increased duration of the motor unit action potential (MUAP)
    D. All of the above

12. True or False?
    Unmyelinated (C) fibers are *not* tested with standard nerve conduction studies.

13. Which nerve conduction studies (NCS) record the largest nerve fibers?
    A. Motor NCS
    B. Sensory NCS
    C. Mixed NCS

14. A child is diagnosed with Guillain-Barré syndrome/acute inflammatory demyelinating polyradiculopathy (AIDP). Which of the following is *not* expected on EMG/NCS?
    A. Early involvement of the sural nerve sensory action potential
    B. Prolonged F waves
    C. Slowed conduction velocities
    D. Prolonged distal latencies

15. A patient presents with acute leg weakness and decreased deep tendon reflexes. Conduction velocities are slow, and a demyelinating polyneuropathy is suspected. Which of the following differentiates acquired demyelinating polyneuropathy from hereditary demyelinating neuropathies?
    A. Prolonged distal latencies
    B. Prolonged F waves
    C. Slow conduction velocities
    D. Conduction block

16. Which of the following statements is *false*?
    A. Excluding technical factors, low-amplitude sensory nerve action potentials (SNAPs) are indicative of a peripheral nerve disorder.
    B. SNAPs are normal in a patient who has a radiculopathy.
    C. The nerve conduction velocity is determined by the fastest conducting fibers.
    D. Abnormal motor conduction studies localize to the peripheral nerve.

17. Which of the following findings is most consistent with myopathy?
    A. Large, polyphasic motor unit action potentials
    B. Pseudoconduction block
    C. Small, short-duration motor unit potentials
    D. Satellite potentials

18. Testing of which muscles helps to determine whether an ulnar nerve lesion is located proximal to the elbow or at the wrist?
    A. Abductor digiti minimi and flexor pollicis brevis
    B. Adductor pollicis and flexor digiti minimi
    C. Flexor carpi ulnaris and flexor digitorum profundus
    D. Flexor pollicis brevis and flexor digiti minimi

19. If there appears to be conduction block of the ulnar nerve at the elbow and no other abnormalities are found on EMG/NCS, which of the following needs to be considered?
    A. Martin-Gruber anastomosis
    B. Charcot-Marie Tooth
    C. An accessory ulnar nerve
    D. B12 deficiency

20. A Martin-Gruber anastomosis occurs when there is a branch from the _____ nerve to the ____ _____ nerve in the forearm.
    A. Median nerve to the posterior interosseous nerve
    B. Median nerve to the ulnar nerve
    C. Radial nerve to the ulnar nerve
    D. Ulnar nerve to the radial nerve

21. Which of the following statements aids in differentiating an L5 radiculopathy from a peroneal neuropathy?
    A. EMG of the gluteus medius and tensor fascia lata are abnormal in an L5 radiculopathy.
    B. EMG of the iliopsoas is abnormal in an L5 radiculopathy.
    C. EMG of the gastrocnemius is abnormal in an L5 radiculopathy.
    D. EMG of the tibialis anterior is abnormal in a peroneal neuropathy.

22. When do very slow nerve conduction velocities (<35 m/s in the arms, <30 m/s in the legs) *not* indicate a demyelinating lesion?
    A. In regenerating nerve fibers after complete transection
    B. In hereditary peripheral nerve diseases
    C. In the hyperacute period of an axonal lesion

23. True or False?
    Routine motor nerve conduction studies are usually normal in postsynaptic disorders of the neuromuscular junction (NMJ).

24. True or False?
    A positive edrophonium test is specific for myasthenia gravis.

25. What is the most sensitive test for myasthenia gravis?
    A. Rapid repetitive nerve stimulation
    B. Slow repetitive nerve stimulation
    C. Single-fiber EMG

26. An intravenous drug user presents with vomiting and abdominal pain. He has diplopia and blurred vision. On examination, he has impaired accommodation. He develops ophthalmoplegia, areflexia, and a flaccid quadriparesis. The weakness progresses rapidly in a descending pattern. What is the EMG most likely to show?
    A. Large, polyphasic motor unit action potentials
    B. Complex repetitive discharges
    C. An incremental response with rapid repetitive nerve stimulation
    D. Absence of insertional activity

27. Which of the following is most likely to be associated with a "dive bomber" sound on EMG?
    A. Duchenne muscular dystrophy
    B. Oculopharyngeal muscular dystrophy
    C. Facioscapulohumeral muscular dystrophy
    D. Myotonic dystrophy

28. Which of the following types of discharges can be found in hyperkalemic periodic paralysis, myotubular myopathy, and polymyositis?
    A. Complex repetitive discharges
    B. Myokymic discharges
    C. Myotonic discharges
    D. Neuromyotonic discharges

29. In which metabolic disease are myotonic discharges most likely to occur?
    A. Acid maltase deficiency
    B. Metachromatic leukodystrophy
    C. Krabbe disease
    D. Adrenoleukodystrophy

30. Which of the following can be observed in patients with brainstem neoplasms, multiple sclerosis, or a history of radiation therapy?
    A. Contractures
    B. Cramp potentials
    C. Myokymic discharges
    D. Neuromyotonic discharges

31. Which of the following are caused by spontaneous discharge of muscle fibers in near-synchrony and with uniform frequency? (They can be seen in anterior horn cell diseases, in muscular dystrophies, and in certain normal muscles.)
    A. Complex repetitive discharges
    B. Myokymic discharges
    C. Myotonic discharges
    D. Neuromyotonic discharges

32. A patient receiving steroids for dermatomyositis presents with worsening weakness. Which of the following statements differentiates steroid myopathy from polymyositis or dermatomyositis?
    A. Myotonic discharges are seen in steroid myopathy.
    B. Positive sharp waves are seen in steroid myopathy.
    C. Steroid myopathy causes proximal weakness.
    D. There is a lack of spontaneous activity on EMG in patients with steroid myopathy.

33. How much of the cortex must be activated to generate activity on scalp electroencephalography (EEG)?
    A. 3 cm^2
    B. 6 cm^2
    C. 15 cm^2
    D. 20 cm^2

34. Asynchronous sleep spindles are seen in a 1-year-old child. What is the most likely explanation?
    A. Agenesis of the corpus callosum
    B. Infantile spasms
    C. Ohtahara syndrome
    D. This finding is normal in this age group.

35. A patient is thought to have lambda waves on her EEG. What can be done to verify this?
    A. Ask her to close her eyes; the lambda waves should disappear when she does so.
    B. Ask her to move her hands.
    C. Wake her up from sleep.
    D. Repeat hyperventilation.

36. A patient undergoes removal of a small right frontal tumor (lesionectomy). An EEG performed 3 months later shows sharp, higher-amplitude activity over the right frontal area without epileptiform discharges. What is this activity called?
    A. Bancaud phenomenon
    B. Breach rhythm
    C. Small sharp spikes
    D. Wicket spikes

37. Which of the following is most closely associated with seizures?
    A. Frontal intermittent rhythmic delta activity (FIRDA)
    B. Subclinical rhythmic electrographic discharges of adults (SREDA)
    C. Temporal intermittent rhythmic delta activity (TIRDA)
    D. 14- and 6-Hz positive bursts

38. True or False?
    Interictal discharges are more prominent in rapid eye movement (REM) sleep than in non-REM sleep.

39. In which animal model of epilepsy was levetiracetam shown to work?
    A. Maximal electroshock
    B. Pentylenetetrazol
    C. Kindling

40. Which of the following findings is *least* consistent with sporadic Creutzfeldt-Jakob disease?
    A. Periodic sharp wave complexes occurring every 15 seconds
    B. Increased signal in the basal ganglia on MRI
    C. Increased signal in the cortical ribbon on MRI
    D. Increased 14-3-3, tau, and neuron-specific enolase in the cerebrospinal fluid

41. On EEG, patients with which of the following conditions may have prolonged slowing with hyperventilation?
    A. Hypocalcemia
    B. Hypoglycemia
    C. Hyponatremia
    D. Hypomagnesemia

42. A 15-year-old girl presents for an EEG after her first generalized tonic-clonic seizure. During photic stimulation, she has myoclonic jerks followed by another generalized tonic-clonic seizure. What is the term for this response to photic stimulation?
    A. Photoconvulsive response
    B. Photomyogenic response/photomyoclonic response
    C. Photoparoxysmal response

43. A photoparoxysmal response is seen in which of the following conditions?
    A. Dentatorubral-pallidoluysian atrophy (DRPLA)
    B. Lafora body disease
    C. Neuronal ceroid lipofuscinosis
    D. Unverricht-Lundborg disease
    E. All of the above

44. A 20-year-old woman describes her seizure as beginning with a rising feeling in her stomach. Her family says that she then stares, smacks her lips, and performs odd movements with her left hand. Her right hand is in an unusual posture. Where is the seizure most likely beginning?
    A. Left occipital lobe
    B. Left temporal lobe
    C. Right frontal lobe
    D. Right parietal lobe

45. A baby at 27 weeks corrected gestational age would most likely have which EEG finding?
    A. Tracé discontinu
    B. Tracé alternant

C. Activité moyenne
D. Continuous slow-wave sleep during quiet sleep

46. **Delta brushes are seen in premature infants. In which condition are extreme delta brushes seen?**
    A. Angelman syndrome
    B. Anti-NMDA receptor encephalitis
    C. Baclofen overdose
    D. Rett syndrome

47. **Periodic epileptiform discharges are *least* likely to be seen in which of the following conditions?**
    A. Subacute sclerosing panencephalitis (SSPE)
    B. Stroke
    C. Herpes encephalitis
    D. West Nile encephalitis

48. **True or False?**
    With near-field potentials, the amplitude recorded is higher the closer the recording electrode is to the source.

49. **What is indicated by unilateral prolongation of P100 on a visual evoked potential?**
    A. A prechiasmatic lesion of the optic pathway
    B. Glaucoma
    C. An occipital lesion
    D. A lesion in the lateral geniculate nucleus

50. **Somatosensory evoked potentials evaluate which pathway?**
    A. Corticospinal tract
    B. Posterior column-medial lemniscal pathway
    C. Spinocerebellar tract
    D. Spinothalamic tract

51. **Which structure produces wave I on brainstem auditory evoked potentials?**
    A. Cochlear nucleus
    B. Cranial nerve VIII (CN 8)
    C. Lateral lemniscus
    D. Medial geniculate nucleus

NEUROPHYSIOLOGY

ANSWERS

1. A

At rest, the axonal membrane of a nerve is negatively polarized when the inside is compared to the outside.

2. C

The resting membrane potential is closest to the equilibrium potential for potassium.

3. B

The resting membrane potential of the nerve is results from the presence of a semipermeable membrane and the sodium-potassium (Na^+/K^+) pump. The concentrations of potassium and large anions are greater inside the axonal membrane of the nerve than outside it. The Na^+/K^+ pump causes sodium to move outside and potassium to move inside. Depolarization results in influx of sodium and opening of potassium channels. When depolarization occurs, sodium is driven into the cell by the concentration and electrical gradients.

The concentrations of chloride and sodium are greater outside the axonal membrane.

4. C

The compound 4-aminopyridine is an antagonist to voltage-gated potassium channels (the delayed rectifier potassium channel). It increases the chance that the axon will depolarize.

5. A

Myelin reduces the capacitance of the nerve and increases the transmembrane resistance.

6. C

In myelinated nerves, depolarization occurs by saltatory conduction. Depolarization occurs at the nodes of Ranvier, gaps where the nerve is not myelinated. The highest density of sodium channels is at the nodes of Ranvier.

7. A

Conduction velocity of a nerve depends on its diameter and whether it is myelinated. Large nerves have less electrical resistance than small nerves and conduct faster. Myelinated nerves conduct faster than unmyelinated nerves. Less nerve membrane is depolarized in myelinated nerves because of saltatory conduction. The action potential travels from node to node rather than continuously along the nerve. More current is needed for saltatory conduction.

8. A

At the synapse, exocytosis of a synaptic vesicle depends on calcium influx. Synaptotagmin acts as a calcium sensor on the vesicle.

The term *quanta* refers to the number of neurotransmitter molecules within a single vesicle. Spontaneous release of a single quanta of acetylcholine produces a miniature endplate potential (MEPP).

The term *quantal content* refers to the number of synaptic vesicles released by the action potential. It is determined by the number of synaptic vesicles available at the presynaptic terminal multiplied by the probability of quantal release.

9. A

Two acetylcholine molecules must bind to each subunit of the acetylcholine receptor to open the channel. When the channel opens, there is an influx of sodium. This results in depolarization and an endplate potential (EPP). The size of the EPP depends on the amount of acetylcholine that binds to the receptor. If the EPP is above the muscle membrane's threshold, a muscle fiber action potential is generated.

10. A

In the monosynaptic stretch reflex, stretch of a muscle spindle excites group Ia sensory afferent axons. These synapse on the anterior horn cells that innervate the muscle that was stretched, causing muscle contraction.

11. D

Cold temperature results in slowed conduction velocities and prolonged distal latencies. Also, amplitude and duration of potentials are increased on nerve conduction studies. Sensory nerve action potentials (SNAPs) are more affected than compound muscle action potentials (CMAPs). In addition, motor unit action potentials (MUAPs) are increased in duration and amplitude and have more phases on EMG.

12. True

Small myelinated (Aδ, β) and unmyelinated (C) fibers are *not* tested with standard nerve conduction studies. Unmyelinated fibers carry pain, temperature, and autonomic information.

13. C

The largest and fastest nerve fibers are the Ia fibers. Ia fibers mediate the afferent limb of the muscle stretch reflex. Ia fibers are assessed in mixed nerve studies but not in pure motor or pure sensory NCS, so mixed nerve studies are faster than routine NCS. These fibers also have the greatest amount of myelin. They are affected early by demyelinating lesions. Therefore, mixed nerve studies are typically more sensitive to demyelination than routine NCS. For example, a palmar mixed nerve study may detect carpal tunnel syndrome before routine NCS.

14. A

The sural sensory response tends to be spared in Guillain-Barré syndrome (GBS)/AIDP, even when other sensory responses are affected.

Initially, routine motor NCS may be normal. Typically, the earliest finding in GBS is delayed or absent F waves and H responses. Later, prolonged distal latencies, conduction block, and temporal dispersion are seen.

Low-amplitude CMAPs predict a poor prognosis in GBS. These can occur with distal conduction block or axonal loss.

The axonal variants of GBS are acute motor axonal neuropathy (AMAN) and acute motor sensory polyneuropathy (AMSAN). These tend to progress more rapidly than typical GBS. Patients with AMAN or AMSAN may require ventilation and may have dysautonomia. AMAN is often associated with *Campylobacter jejuni* infection. Porphyria is also an acute axonal polyneuropathy and should be included in the differential diagnosis of AMAN and AMSAN.

15. D

Conduction block, temporal dispersion, and abnormal phase cancellation occur in acquired demyelinating polyneuropathy because of the variable degrees of demyelination. They do *not* occur in hereditary demyelinating neuropathies; patients with these conditions have uniform conduction slowing. Hereditary demyelinating neuropathies and acquired demyelinating polyneuropathy are both associated with prolonged distal latencies, prolonged F waves, prolonged H waves, and slow conduction velocities.

16. D

An abnormal motor NCS does not necessarily localize to the peripheral nerve. It can be abnormal with anterior horn cell, nerve root, neuromuscular junction, or muscle lesions. In contrast, low-amplitude SNAPs do indicate a peripheral nerve disorder.

A patient may have sensory loss with normal SNAPs if the lesion is proximal to the dorsal root ganglia, if there is a proximal demyelination lesion, or if there is a hyperacute axonal loss lesion.

In patients with brain lesions, spinal cord lesions, or radiculopathies, the SNAPs are normal because the lesion is proximal to the dorsal root ganglia. Since SNAPs are normal in radiculopathy and abnormal in plexopathy, they are helpful in differentiating the two conditions. Patients with a radiculopathy may have sensory loss with normal SNAPs. However, EMG studies may show neuropathic changes in the paraspinal muscles in a patient with radiculopathy.

17. C

Small, short-duration motor unit action potentials are consistent with myopathy. In acute myopathy, short-duration, small-amplitude polyphasic motor unit action potentials (MUAPs) are seen. Recruitment is normal or early. (Recruitment refers to the addition of more MUAPs with increased firing rates.) The MUAPs in chronic myopathies may be difficult to differentiate from those of chronic neuropathy on EMG. However, in chronic myopathy, recruitment is normal or early. Sensory NCS are normal in myopathy. Motor NCS may be normal in a proximal myopathy because the NCS usually study distal muscles.

Large, polyphasic MUAPs are consistent with reinnervation. For example, they are seen in motor neuron diseases and in chronic axonal injury.

Immediately after a lesion causing axonal loss, NCS will be normal if stimulation and recording are performed distal to the lesion. Acutely, the only finding on EMG is decreased recruitment in the weak muscles. With chronic axonal injury, decreased recruitment and large, polyphasic MUAPs are seen.

In central nervous system (CNS) disorders, MUAPs and recruitment are normal; however, there is decreased activation. The ability to increase firing frequency (activation) is a central process.

Satellite potentials can be seen in myopathy and in neuropathy. For example, they are seen in early reinnervation. A satellite potential is a small action potential that consistently follows a main action potential; satellite potentials they are time locked.

Pseudoconduction block can occur in the setting of nerve transection or nerve infarction, as seen in vasculitic neuropathy. Pseudoconduction block is seen in acute axonal loss if stimulation is performed both distal and proximal to the lesion. With distal stimulation, the amplitude is normal; with proximal stimulation, the amplitude is reduced. This gives the appearance of a conduction block. However, when the study is repeated later (after Wallerian degeneration), low amplitudes are seen with both proximal and distal stimulation.

18. C

If both the flexor carpi ulnaris and flexor digitorum profundus are abnormal with axonal loss, the lesion is proximal to the elbow.

The ulnar nerve innervates multiple muscles in the hand (i.e., abductor digiti minimi, opponens digiti minimi, flexor digiti minimi, third and fourth lumbricals, first dorsal and first palmar interossei, adductor pollicis, and flexor pollicis brevis). It also innervates the flexor carpi ulnaris and the flexor digitorum profundus III and IV in the forearm.

19. A

If there appears to be conduction block of the ulnar nerve at the elbow and no other abnormalities are found, a Martin-Gruber anastomosis should be considered.

20. B

A Martin-Gruber anastomosis is a connection between the median and ulnar nerves. In patients with this condition, the median nerve innervates muscles typically innervated by the ulnar nerve: the first dorsal interosseous, abductor digiti minimi, and adductor pollicis. Some authorities would also include the deep head of the flexor pollicis brevis.

Anomalous innervation can also occur in the lower extremity. There may be an accessory peroneal nerve innervating the extensor digitorum brevis (EDB). The accessory peroneal nerve is a branch of the superficial peroneal nerve. Typically, the deep peroneal nerve innervates the EDB. The deep peroneal nerve is a branch of the common peroneal nerve.

21. A

There are multiple lesions that can cause foot drop. In the peripheral nervous system, these include lesions of the deep peroneal nerve, common peroneal nerve, sciatic nerve, lumbosacral plexus, and L5 nerve root. EMG of the tibialis anterior can be abnormal with any of these lesions. Weakness of ankle inversion in addition to foot drop indicates that the lesion also affects the tibial nerve. Involvement of the tibial and peroneal nerves indicates that the lesion involves the sciatic nerve, lumbosacral plexus, or L5 nerve root. If the gluteus medius and the tensor fascia lata are involved, the patient has a lumbar plexopathy or an L5 radiculopathy. Abnormalities in the paraspinal muscles indicate that the patient has an L5 radiculopathy rather than a lumbar plexopathy.

EMG of the iliopsoas and gastrocnemius muscles should be normal in an L5 radiculopathy (see Table 22.1).

EMG of the tibialis anterior does not help to differentiate a peroneal neuropathy from an L5 radiculopathy. It may be abnormal with either lesion.

Table 22.1   INNERVATION OF SELECTED LOWER EXTREMITY MUSCLES

MUSCLE	INNERVATION (SPINAL ROOTS)
Iliopsoas	L1, L2, L3
Gluteus medius and tensor fascia lata	L4, L5, S1
Gastrocnemius	S1, S2

22. A

Typically, very slow nerve conduction velocities indicate a demyelinating lesion. An exception occurs in the setting of nerve injury. After complete nerve transection, regenerating nerve fibers can have very slow nerve conduction velocities.

23. True

NMJ disorders can be mistaken for myopathy. Sensory conduction studies are normal. Distal latencies, conduction velocities, and late responses are normal on motor studies. Also, CMAP amplitudes are typically normal in postsynaptic disorders such as myasthenia gravis (MG). However, CMAP amplitudes are decreased in presynaptic NMJ disorders such as Lambert-Eaton syndrome (LEMS) and botulism. In botulism and LEMS, the number of quanta released is reduced.

Repetitive nerve stimulation helps to differentiate an NMJ disorder from a myopathy. Both MG and LEMS show a decrement with 3-Hz stimulation. However, LEMS shows a significant increment with rapid repetitive nerve stimulation or brief intense exercise. Clinically, LEMS is associated with reduced deep tendon reflexes and autonomic dysfunction, which are not typical of MG.

24. False

A positive edrophonium test is *not* specific for myasthenia gravis. Amyotrophic lateral sclerosis, Lambert-Eaton syndrome, and brainstem lesions can also result in a positive edrophonium test.

25. C

Single-fiber EMG (SF-EMG) is very sensitive for myasthenia gravis (MG) but is not specific. SF-EMG of weak muscles demonstrates increased jitter in patients with MG. However, increased jitter can be seen many other conditions, including myopathic diseases, neuropathic diseases, and other NMJ disorders.

26. C

This patient has wound botulism. The rapid progression, decreased reflexes, and autonomic dysfunction help to clinically differentiate it from myasthenia gravis.

Botulinum toxin causes reduced CMAPs. Latencies and conduction velocities are normal. Sensory nerve conduction studies are normal. Slow repetitive nerve stimulation can cause a decrement. Rapid repetitive nerve stimulation can cause an incremental response. Lack of an increment does *not* rule out botulism.

In most NMJ disorders, there is no abnormal spontaneous activity. Botulism is the exception. Fibrillation potentials and positive sharp waves, which are signs of denervation, are seen.

Botulism is in the differential diagnosis of AIDP.

27. D

Myotonic discharges, as seen in myotonic dystrophy, cause a dive bomber sound on EMG. The discharges wax and wane in amplitude and frequency.

28. C

Myotonic discharges can be seen in hyperkalemic periodic paralysis, polymyositis, myotubular myopathy, myotonic dystrophy, myotonia congenita, and paramyotonia congenita.

29. A

Myotonic discharges are seen in the paraspinal muscles of patients with acid maltase deficiency.

30. C

Myokymic discharges are spontaneous, rhythmic discharges arising from a motor unit. Rippling of the muscle may be seen clinically. These discharges can be seen in cases of radiation-induced nerve damage. They can help to differentiate radiation plexitis from neoplastic invasion of the brachial plexus. Facial myokymia can be seen in multiple sclerosis and in brainstem neoplasms.

Contractures are electrically silent on EMG. They can be seen in metabolic diseases, such as glycolytic enzyme defects.

Cramp potentials are rapid discharges of motor axons.

31. A

Complex repetitive discharges result from the spontaneous discharge of muscle fibers in near-synchrony and with uniform frequency (see Table 22.2). A single muscle fiber depolarizes, and there is direct spread from it to another muscle membrane (ephaptic spread). Complex repetitive discharges can be seen in anterior horn cell diseases, in muscular dystrophies, and in certain normal muscles.

Neuromyotonic discharges are seen in Isaac syndrome. In this condition, muscles do not relax; patients have continuous muscle fiber activity. The patient experiences stiffness and muscle cramps. Myokymia can be seen. Patients have delayed muscle relaxation. However, in contrast to patients with myotonia, percussion does not cause muscle contraction. Patients may have hyperhidrosis. Some patients have a malignancy, such as thymoma or small cell lung cancer. Some patients with Isaac syndrome have Morvan syndrome, which is characterized by hallucinations, insomnia, and autonomic dysfunction. Some patients with Morvan syndrome have potassium channel antibodies, and some have thymoma.

Table 22.2 EMG SPONTANEOUS WAVEFORM SOURCE GENERATORS

GENERATOR	TYPES OF WAVEFORMS
Motor neuron/axon	Cramp, fasciculation, myokymia, neuromyotonia, tetany
Neuromuscular junction	Endplate noise
Terminal axon	Endplate spike
Multiple muscle fibers	Complex repetitive discharges
Single muscle fiber	Fibrillation, myotonia, positive wave

32. D

Proximal weakness occurs in steroid myopathy, polymyositis, and dermatomyositis. The lack of spontaneous activity on EMG in patients with steroid myopathy helps to differentiate it from dermatomyositis and polymyositis. Insertional activity is normal in steroid myopathy. There are no positive sharp waves or fibrillations. Steroid myopathy tends to affect type II fibers. EMG tends to assess type I fibers.

Fibrillations and positive waves are seen in inflammatory myopathies such as polymyositis and dermatomyositis. There are small, short-duration, polyphasic motor units in patients with polymyositis and dermatomyositis.

Just as dermatomyositis and its treatment can each cause myopathy, both human immunodeficiency virus (HIV) and zidovudine (AZT) can cause myopathy. Zidovudine myopathy is associated with ragged red fibers due to mitochondrial injury. These help to differentiate it from HIV myopathy.

33. B

To generate activity on a scalp EEG, 6 cm² of cerebral cortex must be activated. The EEG is generated from postsynaptic potentials of cortical neurons.

Focal epileptiform activity results from a paroxysmal depolarization shift at the cellular level.

Irregular focal slow activity is caused by a focal subcortical lesion or dysfunction.

A cortical lesion can cause focal voltage attenuation.

34. D

Asynchronous sleep spindles are normal until age 2 years. Sleep spindles appear at 2 month, but may be asynchronous until 2 years of age because of insufficient myelination.

35. A

Lambda waves occur during wakefulness. They are positive discharges seen over the occipital region. They occur with scanning and should disappear with eye fixation or closure.

Mu rhythm is seen over the central regions. It is 7- to 11-Hz arch-shaped activity that resolves with movement of the contralateral hand.

36. B

After surgery, a breach rhythm can be seen. This activity is more sharp and higher in amplitude because of the skull defect.

Bancaud phenomenon is the term used for unilateral lack of attenuation of the alpha rhythm with eye opening.

Small sharp spikes are a pseudoepileptiform pattern seen in adolescents and adults in sleep.

Wicket spikes are also normal waveforms seen in adults, but they can be mistaken for epileptiform temporal spikes.

37. C

TIRDA is most closely associated with increased risk for seizures.

FIRDA can be seen in adults with diffuse encephalopathy.

In children, occipital intermittent rhythmic delta activity (OIRDA) may be seen instead of FIRDA. OIRDA can also be found in patients with childhood absence epilepsy.

SREDA is a normal variant seen in adults older than 50 years of age.

The pattern of 14- and 6-Hz positive bursts is a pseudoepileptiform pattern. These bursts can occur in normal adolescents in drowsiness and sleep. They have also been described in Reye syndrome.

38. False

Interictal discharges are *less* prominent in REM than in non-REM sleep.

39. C

Levetiracetam was shown to be effective in the kindling model of epilepsy.

40. A

Periodic sharp wave complexes are seen in sporadic Creutzfeldt-Jakob disease (CJD) but not in variant CJD. The frequency of discharges in CJD is every 0.5 to 1 second.

41. B

Hyperventilation is an activation procedure performed during an EEG. Children often have symmetric slowing of the background with hyperventilation. Occasionally, this may be associated with staring. If no epileptiform activity is present, then this finding can be considered normal. Hyperventilation may cause absence seizures in at-risk individuals.

Hypoglycemia may result in prolonged slowing with hyperventilation.

Rebuildup can occur in patients with moyamoya, who should *not* be hyperventilated; impressive slowing is seen a few minutes after hyperventilation has been completed. Hyperventilation can cause decreased carbon dioxide and alkalosis. It may result in vasospasm and decreased cerebral perfusion. Hyperventilation is *contraindicated* in patients with cerebrovascular disease and intracranial hemorrhage. It is also contraindicated in sickle cell disease and trait, congenital heart disease, cystic fibrosis, and active asthma.

Occasionally, tetany can be induced by hyperventilation in patients with hypocalcemia.

42. A

The term *photoparoxysmal response refers to* epileptiform activity (without clinical correlate) resulting from photic stimulation. It is classically seen in genetic generalized epilepsies, especially juvenile myoclonic epilepsy. Patients with Dravet syndrome may also have a photoparoxysmal response.

A photoconvulsive response is a clinical seizure resulting from photic stimulation.

A photomyogenic (or photomyoclonic) response occurs when the frontalis muscle contracts in response to photic stimulation; the contractions are time locked with the flashes of light. Risk factors are alcohol withdrawal and barbiturate withdrawal.

43. E

A photoparoxysmal response may be seen in any of the conditions listed. In addition, patients with progressive myoclonic epilepsy may have a photoparoxysmal response. Patients with neuronal ceroid lipofuscinosis tend to have a photoparoxysmal response at low frequencies.

44. B

This description is consistent with a left temporal lobe seizure. Patients with temporal lobe epilepsy often describe a rising epigastric sensation at the beginning of the seizure. Ipsilateral automatisms and contralateral dystonic posturing are also typical.

45. A

Tracé discontinu is the EEG pattern seen in the most premature infants. It is characterized by periods of higher-voltage activity separated by periods of low-voltage activity measuring less than 25 microvolts. By 36 weeks, it is seen only during quiet sleep. By term, tracé alternant replaces tracé discontinu in quiet sleep. Tracé alternant resembles tracé discontinu (i.e., higher-amplitude activity separated by periods of lower-amplitude activity), but the lower-voltage activity is greater than 25 microvolts.

46. B

Anti-*N*-Methyl-D-aspartate (NMDA) receptor encephalitis is an autoimmune encephalitis that causes fever, behavioral changes, movement disorders, seizures, and autonomic dysfunction. It is diagnosed by the finding of antibodies to the NMDA glutamate receptor in serum or CSF. (The antibodies are usually to the NR1 subunit.) EEG may show an extreme delta brush pattern. Positron-emission tomography (PET) may show frontal and temporal hypermetabolism with occipital hypometabolism. Brain magnetic resonance imaging (MRI) may be normal. Some women with anti-NMDA receptor encephalitis have an ovarian teratoma or develop one later.

Baclofen is a GABA-B receptor agonist. Baclofen overdose can cause multiple EEG abnormalities including triphasic waves, generalized periodic discharges, and a burst-suppression pattern.

Angelman syndrome causes rhythmic delta activity over the frontal regions.

In Rett syndrome, spikes may be seen over the central head region.

47. D

Periodic lateralizing epileptiform discharges (PLEDs) are seen in patients with stroke or herpes encephalitis. Stroke

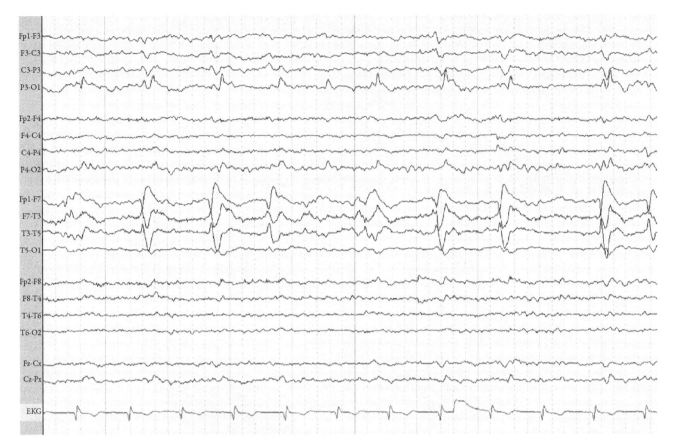

Figure 22.1 Example of PLEDS. (From Misulis KE. Atlas of EEG, Seizure Semiology, and Management, Fig. 4-73. New York, Oxford University Press, 2013.)

is the most common cause, but PLEDs are a classic finding in herpes encephalitis.

Sporadic Creutzfeldt-Jakob disease (CJD) and SSPE cause generalized periodic epileptiform discharges. The frequency of discharges in CJD is every 0.5 to 1 second. The frequency of discharges in SSPE is every 4 to 15 seconds.

Anoxia can cause generalized periodic epileptiform discharges (GPEDs) or bilateral independent periodic lateralizing epileptiform discharges (BiPLEDs).

West Nile encephalitis does not typically cause periodic discharges (see Figs. 22.1 and 22.2).

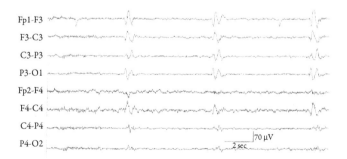

Figure 22.2 SSPE with periodic discharges. (From Misulis KE. Atlas of EEG, Seizure Semiology, and Management, Fig. 4-80. New York, Oxford University Press, 2013.)

48. True

With near-field potentials, the amplitude recorded is higher the closer the recording electrode is to the source. A far-field potential is seen simultaneously at all recording electrodes even though one of them is closer to the source.

49. A

Unilateral prolongation of P100 on visual evoked potential testing indicates a prechiasmatic lesion of the optic pathway. Optic neuritis is one example.

Visual evoked potentials are affected by anesthesia and are not usually tested intraoperatively.

50. B

Somatosensory evoked potentials (SSEPs) evaluate the posterior column-medial lemniscal pathway. Intraoperative SSEPs monitor the integrity of this pathway.

Intraoperative SSEPs can also identify sensorimotor cortex. With the use of median nerve SSEPs, the location of the central sulcus can be determined by the phase reversal of N20.

Giant SSEPs are seen in patients with cortical myoclonus, such as patients with progressive myoclonic epilepsies.

51. B

Brainstem auditory evoked potentials (BAEPs) are useful for monitoring peripheral and central auditory pathways intraoperatively. In the operating room, sudden loss of the BAEP can occur with ischemia involving the internal auditory nerve.

Wave I on the BAEP corresponds to the peripheral portion of CN 8.

If wave I is absent but the other waves are normal, the patient has peripheral hearing loss.

Brain death may result in loss of all waveforms or loss of all waveforms after wave I.

A vestibular schwannoma can cause a prolonged latency between waves I and III.

Demyelinating disease may result in increased latency between waves III and V. (Wave III corresponds to the superior olivary complex in the pons, and wave V corresponds to the inferior colliculus in the midbrain.) Wave V may be absent in patients with multiple sclerosis.

The BAEP pathway can be remembered by the mnemonic NCSLIMA: Cranial nerve 8 (Wave I) → **C**ochlear nuclei in the medulla (Wave II) → **S**uperior olivary complex in the pons (Wave III) → **L**ateral lemniscus in the pons (Wave IV) → **I**nferior colliculus in the midbrain (Wave V) → **M**edial geniculate nucleus in the thalamus (Wave VI) → **A**uditory radiations (Wave VII).

23.

NEUROTOXICOLOGY

QUESTIONS

1. A mother brings her 3-year-old child for evaluation because of change in personality and lethargy. The physical examination is remarkable for a line around the gum margins. Laboratory studies show a microcytic anemia. Radiographic studies show opaque bands at the metaphysis of the lower femur and upper tibia. Which of the following is most likely responsible?
   A. Arsenic poisoning
   B. Cadmium exposure
   C. Lead toxicity
   D. Mercury poisoning

2. Which of the following is the most likely presentation of lead toxicity in adults?
   A. Insomnia
   B. Paresthesias
   C. Tremor
   D. Wrist drop

3. A 50-year-old woman presents with lower extremity paresthesias. On examination, she has alopecia and palmar and plantar keratosis. There are white lines across her nails. She has decreased ankle reflexes and decreased pinprick, vibration, and proprioception in her feet. Exposure to which of the following best explains her symptoms?
   A. Arsenic
   B. Bismuth
   C. Magnesium
   D. Mercury

4. Which of the following substances causes erethism?
   A. Arsenic
   B. Cyanide
   C. Mercury
   D. Thallium

5. Fill in the blank: Alopecia can occur with _____ _____ toxicity.
   A. Copper
   B. Lead
   C. Nickel
   D. Thallium

6. What is the mechanism of action of botulinum toxin?
   A. It decreases acetylcholine release.
   B. It blocks the acetylcholine receptor.
   C. It inhibits acetylcholinesterase.

D. It antagonizes the glycine receptor.
   E. It acts as an agonist at the glutamate receptor.

7. A 6-year-old presents with vomiting, altered mental status, miosis, bradycardia, and wheezing after visiting a farm. On examination, he is weak and has fasciculations. What is the mechanism of action of the agent to which he was exposed?
   A. It inactivates acetylcholinesterase.
   B. It prevents release of acetylcholine.
   C. It blocks the acetylcholine receptor.
   D. It antagonizes the glycine receptor.
   E. It acts as an agonist at the glutamate receptor.

8. Which of the following is found in reef fish, opens the sodium channel, and causes paresthesias and paradoxical sensory disturbances?
   A. Ciguatoxin
   B. Tetrodotoxin
   C. Saxitoxin
   D. Latrotoxin

9. Which marine toxin is a glutamate receptor agonist and causes amnestic shellfish poisoning?
   A. Brevetoxin
   B. Domoic acid
   C. Tetrodotoxin
   D. Mu conotoxin

10. A 23-year-old man is bitten by a black widow spider. What is the mechanism of action of its venom?
    A. It acts as an agonist at the glutamate receptor.
    B. It antagonizes the glycine receptor.
    C. It blocks the acetylcholine receptor.
    D. It increases the release of neurotransmitters.
    E. It inhibits acetylcholinesterase.

11. Exposure to which of the following is *least* likely to affect the basal ganglia?
    A. Carbon monoxide
    B. Copper
    C. Manganese
    D. Nickel

12. A 20-year-old ingests *N*-methyl-4-phenyl-1,2,3,6-tetrahydropyridine (MPTP). What symptoms are expected?
    A. Parkinsonian symptoms
    B. Schizophrenia symptoms
    C. Miosis and sedation
    D. Superhuman strength

13. Which of the following chemicals causes retinal ganglion cell degeneration and necrosis of the putamina?
    A. Ethylene glycol
    B. Hexane
    C. Methanol
    D. Trichloroethylene

14. A 20-year-old man presents with unsteady gait and tingling in his legs. He has decreased vibration and position sensation in a stocking-glove distribution. Ankle reflexes are decreased, but patellar reflexes are hyperreactive. Which of the following is the most likely cause?
    A. Nitrous oxide abuse
    B. Strychnine poisoning
    C. Tetanus
    D. Toluene abuse

15. A 3-year-old presents with bradycardia, somnolence, and miosis. Which of the following is the most likely cause?
    A. Clonidine toxicity
    B. Diphenhydramine overdose

C. MDMA (3,4-methylenedioxy-methamphetamine)
D. Salicylate poisoning

16. Excessive zinc ingestion can cause a myelopathy due to which of the following?
    A. Copper deficiency
    B. Magnesium deficiency
    C. Vitamin B12 deficiency
    D. Vitamin E deficiency

17. Which of the following is a treatment for cyanide poisoning?
    A. Acetylcysteine
    B. Fomepizole
    C. Hydroxocobalamin hydrochloride
    D. Methylene blue
    E. Penicillamine

18. Which of the following is *least* likely to cause hyperthermia?
    A. Baclofen withdrawal
    B. Gamma-hydroxybutyrate ingestion
    C. Salicylate toxicity
    D. Serotonin syndrome

NEUROTOXICOLOGY

ANSWERS

1. C

This patient has been exposed to lead. Lead toxicity causes lead lines along the gums and in the long bones. It can cause microcytic anemia, and basophilic stippling of red blood cells may be seen. Lead toxicity can also cause proximal renal tubular dysfunction. Lead encephalopathy caused by inorganic lead (found in paint) is treated with chelation.

Cadmium causes flu-like symptoms.

2. D

The most common presentation of lead toxicity in adults is wrist drop. Lead causes an asymmetric motor neuropathy involving the wrist and finger extensors.

3. A

This patient has chronic arsenic toxicity. It manifests as a sensorimotor peripheral neuropathy. Other characteristic features are Mees lines (white lines across the nails due to growth disruption), hyperkeratosis of the palms and soles, and alopecia.

Acute arsenic poisoning may manifest with an ascending peripheral neuropathy resembling Guillain-Barré syndrome. Gastrointestinal symptoms are severe. Patients have vomiting and "rice water" diarrhea. The patients' breath may have a garlic odor. Chelating agents such as dimercaprol and succimer are used to treat arsenic poisoning.

Bismuth can cause acute renal failure. Chronic exposure can cause a myoclonic encephalopathy similar to Creutzfeldt-Jakob disease. Blue-black gum discoloration is also characteristic of chronic bismuth poisoning.

4. C

Exposure to mercury can occur during the production of chemicals, paints, paper, plastics, and fungicides. Mercury can be found in multiple forms.

Inorganic mercury includes elemental mercury vapor and mercury salts. Inhaled mercury vapor primarily affects the brain. Mercury salts tend to affect the gastrointestinal tract and the kidneys. Acute poisoning with inorganic mercury causes delirium. It is associated with respiratory distress, profuse vomiting, metallic breath/taste, bloody diarrhea, and renal failure. Chronic exposure to inorganic mercury causes personality changes, polyneuropathy, and tremor. Gingivitis and renal dysfunction also occur. The personality changes seen with inorganic mercury poisoning are referred to as *erethism*. Initially, shyness and withdrawal are seen. Later, irritability occurs. The term "mad as a hatter" is derived from the personality changes seen in manufacturers of felt hats, who were exposed to mercuric salts. Acrodynia ("pink disease") occurs with chronic inorganic mercury poisoning in children. It is characterized by a painful neuropathy (painful erythematous digits) with autonomic symptoms.

Organic mercury includes those compounds in which mercury is bonded to a structure with carbon atoms. Exposure to organic mercury causes cognitive problems, ataxia, constricted visual fields, polyneuropathy, and circumoral and acral paresthesias. Methylmercury, which is a type of organic mercury, is found in certain fish. Minamata disease is caused by methylmercury poisoning; the classic outbreak occurred in humans who consumed fish and shellfish that were contaminated with methylmercury, which had been dumped by a chemical plant into Minamata Bay in Japan.

5. D

Alopecia can occur with thallium toxicity. Thallium is found in rodenticides and insecticides. It competes with potassium ion transport in the Na^+/K^+ adenosine triphosphatase (ATPase) system.

Acutely, thallium can cause altered mental status, vomiting, optic neuropathy, autonomic dysfunction (including hypertension), and a painful ascending neuropathy. With chronic exposure, alopecia and Mees lines are seen. Arsenic can also cause alopecia and Mees lines.

Thallium poisoning is in the differential diagnosis of Guillain-Barré syndrome. Alopecia helps to differentiate thallium poisoning. Reflexes are relatively preserved in thallium poisoning, but there may be cranial nerve involvement. Patients with thallium poisoning also have painful joints.

6. A

Botulinum toxin is produced by the bacteria, *Clostridium botulinum*. The toxin causes decreased acetylcholine release, which results in muscle relaxation.

7. A

This patient has organophosphate poisoning. Organophosphates inactivate acetylcholinesterase, resulting in decreased hydrolysis of acetylcholine.

Cholinergic poisoning, such as from organophosphates, causes altered mental status, miosis, lacrimation, rhinorrhea, salivation, diaphoresis, bradycardia, bronchospasm, vomiting, diarrhea, urination, muscle fasciculations, and weakness.

Atropine is an antagonist at muscarinic receptors; it helps prevent increased secretions, bronchoconstriction, and bradycardia in patients with organophosphate poisoning. However, it is not effective against the neuromuscular effects that result from moderate to severe intoxication. Pralidoxime (2-PAM), which is a cholinesterase reactivator, treats weakness due to organophosphate poisoning.

8. A

The most common food poisoning illness caused by seafood is ciguatera. Multiple toxins have been found in ciguatera. The most common is ciguatoxin. Ciguatoxin is produced by dinoflagellates found in reef fish such barracuda, grouper, and snapper. It opens sodium channels, causing depolarization. Vomiting and diarrhea appear within 8 hours after ingestion. Paradoxical sensory disturbances are characteristic (e.g., hot feels cold and vice versa). Fatigue, weakness, and areflexia may be present.

Saxitoxin is a sodium channel blocker. It causes paralytic shellfish poisoning.

Latrotoxin is found in the black widow spider.

9. B

Domoic acid, which is an ingestible marine toxin that affects the central nervous system, is produced by a diatom found in shellfish. It is a glutamate receptor agonist that has an affinity for the hippocampus. It can cause headache, acute encephalopathy, permanent memory loss, seizures, and coma. It also produces gastrointestinal symptoms.

Tetrodotoxin is a fatal toxin found in pufferfish. The sodium channels that are responsible for initiation of axonal action potentials are sensitive to tetrodotoxin. Tetrodotoxin, saxitoxin, and mu conotoxin all bind to the sodium voltage-gated ion channels and block sodium influx.

Brevetoxin, which is produced by red tide dinoflagellates in shellfish, opens slow sodium channels along sensory axons. Similar to ciguatoxin, it can cause reversal of hot and cold temperature sensation. It also causes paresthesias and ataxia.

10. D

The black widow spider releases latrotoxin. α-Latrotoxin stimulates neuronal calcium channels, causing release of synaptic vesicles. It causes presynaptic facilitation of neurotransmitter release (e.g. acetylcholine, GABA, glutamate). Symptoms include muscle and chest pain, dysarthria, hyperhidrosis, and anxiety.

11. D

Carbon monoxide causes bilateral globus pallidus necrosis. Carbon monoxide poisoning can be treated with hyperbaric oxygen.

In Wilson disease, copper accumulates in multiple tissues, including the brain. Patients may have chorea, dystonia, tremor, or parkinsonian symptoms. Magnetic resonance imaging (MRI) shows increased T2 signal in the basal ganglia and thalamus. The "face of the giant panda" sign may be seen in the midbrain on axial T2-weighted images.

Manganese can cause parkinsonism. Increased T1 signal is seen in the striatum bilaterally, especially the globus pallidus.

Nickel can cause cerebral edema acutely.

12. A

MPTP, an analog of meperidine, causes loss of melanin-containing dopaminergic neurons in the substantia nigra, which results in Parkinsonian symptoms.

13. C

Methanol ingestion can cause hemorrhagic necrosis of the putamina. It also can cause retinal edema, degeneration of ganglion cells, and blindness.

Methanol can be found in antifreeze, solvents, and adulterated alcoholic beverages. It causes discoordination, headache, vomiting, and impaired vision. It also produces a metabolic acidosis with a large anion gap and an elevated osmolar gap.

Methanol is metabolized by alcohol dehydrogenase to formaldehyde. Then formaldehyde is converted to formic acid by aldehyde dehydrogenase. Formic acid is a neurotoxin. Fomepizole, which inhibits alcohol dehydrogenase, has been used as an antidote to methanol poisoning. Ethanol, which competes with the metabolism of methanol, has also been used to treat methanol toxicity. Bicarbonate may be required to treat the metabolic acidosis.

Ethylene glycol is in antifreeze. Ingestion of ethylene glycol causes organic acidosis, coma, and renal failure.

Thallium and trichloroethylene can cause cranial neuropathies. Toxicity from trichloroethylene can cause trigeminal neuropathy.

Hexane causes a peripheral neuropathy. Axonal swellings are characteristic. Automotive technicians may be exposed to hexane. Glue sniffing and gasoline sniffing may also result in hexane toxicity.

14. A

This patient's examination findings are consistent with nitrous oxide abuse, which can produce a myelopathy resembling that caused by vitamin B12 deficiency. A proposed mechanism is that nitrous oxide inhibits methionine synthase, which converts homocysteine to methionine. B12 is a cofactor in this reaction.

Strychnine is found in rat poisoning. It can cause painful muscle spasms, seizures, and rhabdomyolysis. Tetanospasmin, which causes tetanus, and latrotoxin from the black widow spider can also cause severe muscle spasms. Although opisthotonus and risus sardonicus are classic signs of tetanus, they can also occur with strychnine poisoning. Benzodiazepines are helpful in the treatment of muscle spasms caused by strychnine, tetanospasmin, or latrotoxin.

Toluene is found in certain glues and paints. Acutely, it can cause headache, unsteadiness, hallucinations, tremors, seizures, and coma. It can also cause vomiting, respiratory depression, renal tubular acidosis, and chemical pneumonitis. Chronically, it can cause leukoencephalopathy. It can cause tremor, ataxia, cerebellar atrophy, and an abnormal brainstem auditory evoked response (BAER).

15. A

Clonidine can cause sedation, bradycardia, respiratory depression, and miosis. It resembles opiate toxicity but is only partially responsive to naloxone. Opiates cause sedation, miosis, and respiratory depression. They can cause flash pulmonary edema. Other causes of miosis are barbiturates, cholinergics, organophosphates, phenothiazines, and ethanol. Phencyclidine (PCP) can cause miosis or mydriasis. Nystagmus may be present in patients with PCP intoxication as well.

MDMA, which is known as Ecstasy, is a derivative of methamphetamine. It also has some structural similarities to the hallucinogen mescaline, which is found in peyote.

MDMA causes a sympathomimetic syndrome, similar to that caused by amphetamines, methamphetamine, cocaine, crack, epinephrine, ephedra (in dietary supplements), ephedrine, pseudoephedrine, and monoamine oxidase inhibitors. It causes agitation, pressured speech, mydriasis, tachycardia, hypertension, hyperthermia, hyperreflexia, rhabdomyolysis, and tremor. Beta-blockers should be avoided to prevent unopposed alpha-induced vasoconstriction.

MDMA acts primarily at the serotonin transporter (SERT). In addition to increasing serotonin levels, it increases dopamine and norepinephrine levels. Since MDMA affects serotonin, it can contribute to serotonin syndrome.

Serotonin syndrome causes agitation, mydriasis, hyperthermia, tachycardia, diaphoresis, vomiting, diarrhea, shivering, hyperreflexia, clonus (including ocular), and myoclonus. Many medications can contribute to serotonin syndrome, including selective serotonin reuptake inhibitors (SSRIs), serotonin-norepinephrine reuptake inhibitors (SNRIs), tricyclic antidepressants (TCAs), monoamine oxidase inhibitors (MAOIs), stimulants, lithium, tramadol, dextromethorphan, meperidine, fentanyl, triptans, linezolid, St. John's wort, and tryptophan. Cyproheptadine is used in the treatment of serotonin syndrome.

Neuroleptic malignant syndrome (NMS) and serotonin syndrome have similarities. Both cause fever, altered mental status, and autonomic dysfunction. Therefore, antipsychotics should be avoided in suspected serotonin syndrome, in case the patient actually has NMS. NMS tends to have longer onset than serotonin syndrome. Bradykinesia is more consistent with NMS, whereas hyperreflexia, clonus, myoclonus, and shivering are more consistent with serotonin syndrome (see Table 23.1).

Table 23.1 NEUROTOXICOLOGY SYNDROMES

SYNDROME	DISTINGUISHING FEATURES
Anticholinergic syndrome	Dry, flushed skin and absent bowel sounds
Sympathetic syndrome	Diaphoresis and normal bowel sounds
Serotonin syndrome	Hyperreflexia, clonus, myoclonus, and shivering
Neuroleptic malignant syndrome	Rigidity, bradykinesia

In addition to hyperthermia, mental status changes, and autonomic instability, NMS causes rigidity and leukocytosis. Rhabdomyolysis can occur, resulting in elevated creatine phosphokinase (CPK) levels. Liver function enzyme levels are high, and iron is low. NMS that is caused by an antipsychotic usually occurs within the first 2 weeks of treatment. It can also occur when a patient who is taking a dopaminergic medication abruptly discontinues it.

NMS is treated with supportive care. Fluid resuscitation is important to protect kidney function, and alkalinization of the urine may be necessary. Benzodiazepines, dopamine agonists, and dantrolene have been used for treatment.

In addition to NMS, antipsychotics can cause dystonic reactions, extrapyramidal side effects, anticholinergic side effects, and orthostatic hypotension. Some have serotonergic effects as well.

Anticholinergic medications, such as diphenhydramine and tricyclic antidepressants, also cause confusion, tachycardia, and hyperthermia, but bowel sounds are absent in anticholinergic poisoning and present in sympathomimetic poisoning. In addition, anticholinergic poisoning causes dry, flushed skin; whereas sympathomimetics cause diaphoresis. Diphenhydramine can also cause seizures.

16. A

Excessive zinc ingestion can result in copper deficiency, which can lead to myelopathy. Zinc is found in cold medicines and dental adhesives.

Copper deficiency can also occur with malabsorption, for instance after bariatric surgery.

Myelopathy due to copper deficiency resembles subacute combined degeneration due to vitamin B12 deficiency. Patients have decreased vibration and joint position sensation, paresthesias, sensory ataxia, spasticity, brisk deep tendon reflexes, and extensor plantar responses.

17. C

Hydroxocobalamin hydrochloride is used to treat cyanide toxicity. In addition to intentional poisoning or exposure during manufacturing, cyanide toxicity can occur with smoke inhalation. Cyanide interacts with cytochrome oxidase. It causes cardiovascular collapse and coma. Classically, cyanide has been associated with a "bitter almond" odor, but this may not be present. Patients have evidence of hypoxia but may not be cyanotic until later. The skin initially may be flushed. Lactic acidosis is also a clue.

Acetylcysteine is used to treat acetaminophen poisoning.

Fomepizole is used to treat methanol and ethylene glycol poisoning. Ethanol is also used to treat these conditions.

Methylene blue is the treatment for methemoglobinemia. Multiple medications can cause methemoglobinemia. One is benzocaine, which is found in some forms of Orajel.

Penicillamine is used to treat lead, mercury, and copper poisoning.

18. B

Anticholinergic syndrome, baclofen withdrawal, salicylate toxicity, serotonin syndrome, and neuroleptic malignant syndrome can cause hyperthermia.

Gamma-hydroxybutyrate (GHB) is used to treat narcolepsy. It reduces daytime sleepiness and cataplexy. It can also cause amnesia, leading to its abuse. GHB withdrawal can cause hyperthermia. GHB intoxication can cause hypothermia. GHB intoxication also causes central nervous system and respiratory depression, myoclonic jerks and seizure-like activity, vomiting, and bradycardia. Patients may recover suddenly several hours after ingestion.

Salicylate poisoning first results in hyperventilation and respiratory alkalosis. This is followed by metabolic acidosis with an increased anion gap. Patients can have hyperthermia, vomiting, seizures, coma, and cardiovascular collapse.

24.

PAIN AND HEADACHE

QUESTIONS

1. A 70-year-old woman presents with chronic severe headache, weight loss, anemia, and aching shoulders. Which test should be performed first?
   A. Erythrocyte sedimentation rate (ESR)
   B. Thyroid-stimulating hormone
   C. Liver function tests
   D. Reticulocyte count

2. A 14-year-old presents with worsening headaches. He denies photophobia and phonophobia but endorses vomiting. The headaches are most severe when he awakens. They worsen when he bends over to put on his shoes in the morning. The physical examination, including funduscopy, is normal. Which of the following should be done first?
   A. Prescribe ondansetron and obtain a headache diary
   B. MRI of the brain
   C. Trial of sumatriptan
   D. Initiate topiramate

3. A 20-year-old woman presents with weekly headaches for the past 4 months. She has a feeling of pressure on both sides of her head. The pain is mild to moderate and lasts an hour. She is able to continue her activities but loses her appetite. She has some photophobia. The funduscopic examination is normal. What is the most likely diagnosis?
   A. Cluster headache
   B. Migraine headache
   C. Tension-type headache
   D. Pseudotumor cerebri

4. A mother brings in her 7-year-old son because she thinks he has migraines. He also tends to get motion sickness. Which of the following suggests a diagnosis other than migraine?
   A. He has bilateral pain.
   B. He does not complain of photophobia.
   C. He has occipital pain.
   D. He tends to get motion sickness.

5. Which of the following is more typical of migraine without aura than of migraine with aura?
   A. Cortical spreading depression
   B. A relationship to the menstrual cycle
   C. Increased risk for ischemic stroke
   D. Visual changes

6. A 9-year-old boy presents with a 3-month history of headaches. He has severe pain at his right temple, nausea, and photophobia. The headaches start before lunch, can last all day, and do not respond to acetaminophen, which he takes when he gets home from school. The headaches are occurring at least twice a week. Which of the following is recommended?
   A. Start a preventive medication.
   B. Prescribe acetaminophen with codeine for severe headaches.
   C. Prescribe butalbital for severe headaches.
   D. Prescribe prednisone.

7. An 8-year-old patient presents with episodes of unsteadiness, double vision, and dysarthria. These are typically followed by headache. Computed tomography (CT) of the head and the results of laboratory studies are normal. Which of the following is the most likely cause?
   A. Abdominal migraine
   B. Benign paroxysmal vertigo
   C. Exploding head syndrome
   D. Migraine with brainstem aura

8. What is the mechanism of action of sumatriptan?
   A. It is a 5-HT1A receptor antagonist.
   B. It is a 5-HT1D receptor agonist.
   C. It is a 5-HT 2A/2C receptor antagonist.
   D. It is a 5-HT3 agonist.

9. A 30-year-old patient with a previous diagnosis of migraines presents with a complaint of daily headaches for the past 3 months. Unlike her migraines, these headaches are not associated with photophobia or vomiting. She says the headaches are constant, so she must take ibuprofen at least twice daily. Her examination findings are normal. Which of the following topics needs to be discussed with this patient?
   A. The benefits of naproxen over ibuprofen
   B. The benefits of alternating ibuprofen and acetaminophen
   C. The benefits of indomethacin over ibuprofen
   D. Medication-overuse headache

10. A 24-year-old woman with a history of migraine with aura presents with a 4-day history of headache. She said it started like her usual headache, with an aura of squiggly lines, and then was followed by throbbing pain, nausea, vomiting, and photophobia. However, it did not respond to sumatriptan as her headaches usually do. Her last dose of sumatriptan was 2 hours before

arrival in the emergency department. Which of the following medications should be avoided *at this time*?

   A. Intravenous magnesium
   B. Metoclopramide
   C. Dihydroergotamine
   D. Ketorolac

11. Which of the following conditions may be followed by migraine variants and eventually by migraine with aura when the patient is older. (Some cases of this condition have been linked to mutations in *CACNA1A*.)

   A. Benign paroxysmal torticollis of infancy
   B. Episodic ataxia 1
   C. Paroxysmal kinesigenic dyskinesia
   D. Paroxysmal tonic upgaze of infancy

12. A 30-year-old man presents to the emergency department with severe, stabbing pain above his right eye. He reports that this has happened several times before. Alcohol seems to be a trigger. He has headaches several days in a row, and then they recur about 2 months later. Often they wake him from sleep. On examination, he has ptosis, conjunctival injection, and rhinorrhea ipsilateral to his pain. He appears restless, and he reports that his pain is worse when he lies down. Which of the following is the best treatment option?

   A. Indomethacin
   B. Oxygen via a nonrebreather
   C. Prednisone
   D. Caffeine

13. A 32-year-old woman presents with episodes of brief, intense pain involving her right cheek and jaw. Applying makeup can trigger an attack. After the pain occurs, there is a period of time during which she can apply makeup without pain. What is her diagnosis?

   A. Hemicrania continua
   B. Short-lasting unilateral neuralgiform headache attacks with cranial autonomic features (SUNA)
   C. Short-lasting unilateral neuralgiform headache attacks with conjunctival injection and tearing (SUNCT)
   D. Trigeminal neuralgia

14. A 45-year-old man presents with recurrent headache when he coughs. He has sudden, bilateral head pain when he coughs, lasting for a few seconds. He does not have any other types of headaches. What is the most effective treatment?

   A. Antitussives
   B. Indomethacin
   C. Naproxen
   D. Verapamil

15. A 26-year-old man presents with a headache that worsens when he stands. He also complains of nausea and photophobia. On examination, he is afebrile and his blood pressure is normal. He does have mild neck stiffness. MRI shows diffuse pachymeningeal enhancement. What is the diagnosis?

   A. Intracranial hypotension
   B. Subarachnoid hemorrhage
   C. Viral meningitis
   D. Migraine

16. A 20-year-old woman presents with constant, diffuse headaches; blurry vision; and pulsatile tinnitus. She says she is trying to be healthy but hates to exercise, so she takes four One-a-Day vitamins per day. She is taking no other medications. The findings from CT and MRI ordered by her primary care physician were normal. Which of the following diagnoses should be suspected?

   A. Intracranial hypertension
   B. Migraine
   C. Tension headache
   D. Refractive error

17. Which of the following conditions is characterized by acute onset of a daily headache in which the pain becomes continuous and unremitting within 24 hours of onset and lasts for longer than 3 months.

   A. Colloid cyst of the third ventricle
   B. New daily persistent headache
   C. Thunderclap headache
   D. Reversible cerebral vasoconstriction syndrome

18. Match each term with its definition.

   1) Allodynia
   2) Hyperalgesia
   3) Hyperpathia
   4) Dysesthesia
   5) Causalgia

   A. Delayed, increased pain from a noxious stimulus
   B. Pain from a non-noxious stimulus
   C. Pain from a noxious stimulus that is significantly greater than expected
   D. Unpleasant sensation (spontaneous or provoked)
   E. A burning pain occurring after peripheral nerve injury

19. Neuropathic pain is more common in neuropathies involving which of the following?

   A. Aα and Aβ nerve fibers
   B. Aβ and Aδ nerve fibers
   C. Aα and C nerve fibers
   D. C and Aδ nerve fibers

20. Which of the following is the gold standard for diagnosis of small-fiber neuropathy?

   A. Electromyography (EMG)
   B. Nerve conduction studies (NCS)
   C. Skin biopsy
   D. Sural nerve biopsy

21. Which of the following is part of the spinothalamic system?

   A. Bare nerve endings
   B. Golgi tendon organs
   C. Meissner's corpuscles
   D. Pacinian corpuscles

22. Which of the following neuropeptides/neurotransmitters is most specific to pain pathways involving C fibers?
    A. Adenosine
    B. Substance P
    C. Neuropeptide Y
    D. Neurotensin

23. A 36-year-old woman reports frequent episodes of brief stabbing pain in the distribution of the maxillary division of the trigeminal nerve (V2). Which of the following statements is *false*?
    A. Features that help to distinguish symptomatic trigeminal neuralgia from classic trigeminal neuralgia include sensory deficits and bilateral involvement.
    B. If symptomatic trigeminal neuralgia is suspected, MRI or trigeminal reflex testing is reasonable.
    C. Carbamazepine and oxcarbazepine are first-line treatments for classic trigeminal neuralgia (no established etiology).
    D. Topical ophthalmic anesthesia is helpful in treating classic trigeminal neuralgia.

24. A 50-year-old woman with a history of herpes zoster presents with persistent pain despite resolution of the rash 4 months ago. Which of the following treatments is *least* likely to be helpful?
    A. Gabapentin
    B. Lidocaine patch
    C. Nortriptyline
    D. Indomethacin

25. A 20-year-old woman with a recent radius fracture presents with pain, weakness, and swelling in her right hand. She reports a persistent burning pain involving the whole hand and says that the pain is unbearable when she moves the hand. Her entire hand is swollen. She also reports that the hand sweats less than her normal hand and is more hairy than it used to be. Which of the following is the most likely diagnosis?
    A. Complex regional pain syndrome
    B. Poor casting
    C. Dejerine-Roussy syndrome
    D. Radicular pain

26. Mutations in which of the following channels can cause increased pain sensitivity? (Other mutations in this channel can cause congenital inability to experience pain.)
    A. Chloride
    B. Potassium
    C. Sodium
    D. Magnesium

27. According to the American Academy of Neurology guideline regarding treatment of painful diabetic neuropathy, which medication has the strongest evidence?
    A. Amitriptyline
    B. Capsaicin
    C. Gabapentin
    D. Pregabalin

28. Which of the following medications does *not* act on the $\alpha_2\delta$ subunit of N-type calcium channels?
    A. Capsaicin
    B. Gabapentin
    C. Pregabalin
    D. Topical lidocaine

PAIN AND HEADACHE

ANSWERS

1. A

This scenario is concerning for giant cell arteritis (GCA), which is also known as temporal arteritis.

GCA can cause headache with fever, weight loss, malaise, anorexia, jaw claudication, and scalp tenderness. Polymyalgia rheumatica may be present. Inflammatory markers, such as ESR and C-reactive protein, are elevated. The patient may also have thrombocytosis or anemia. On biopsy, granulomatous inflammation is seen in the temporal artery, which may be pulseless. Prednisone is the treatment. Steroids should be initiated immediately if GCA is suspected in order to prevent vision loss.

2. B

This patient's symptoms are concerning for increased intracranial pressure. The funduscopic examination is not always abnormal in a patient with a tumor (e.g., a posterior fossa mass). Worsening headaches, especially if they occur in the morning and are accompanied by vomiting, may indicate increased intracranial pressure. It is also concerning if headache occurs with cough, the Valsalva maneuver, or bending over, all of which increase intracranial pressure. Seizures, focal findings, papilledema, systemic symptoms, and sudden onset also raise concern for an intracranial process.

3. C

This patient has tension-type headache. The pain in tension-type headaches is usually bilateral in location, mild or moderate in intensity, nonpulsating, and not aggravated by activity. It can last 30 minutes to 7 days. Patients with tension-type headache can have photophobia or phonophobia but not both. Nausea or vomiting also excludes the diagnosis.[1]

4. C

In adults who have migraine without aura, the pain is usually unilateral, frontotemporal, pulsating, moderate or severe, and aggravated by physical activity. It usually lasts 4 to 72 hours if untreated. The pain is accompanied by nausea and/or vomiting or photophobia and phonophobia. In children, migraines can be bilateral and can last 2 to 72 hours. Children may not complain of photophobia or phonophobia, but they can be surmised from behavior suggestive of these symptoms. A history of motion sickness is not uncommon in patients with migraine.[1]

Pain over the occipital region is not common in migraine, and other causes need to be considered.

5. B

Migraine *without* aura often has a menstrual relationship. American Academy of Neurology (AAN) headache guidelines state that frovatriptan should be offered for short-term prevention of menstrual-associated migraine.[2]

Nitric oxide, 5-hydroxytryptamine (5-HT), and calcitonin gene-related peptide (CGRP) are thought to be involved in migraine without aura. Cortical spreading depression (spreading hypoperfusion) is more typical of migraine *with* aura. The trigeminovascular system is involved in migraine pain.

A visual aura is the most common type of aura.

Migraine with aura is associated with an increased risk for stroke. AAN primary stroke prevention guidelines state that smoking cessation should be strongly recommended to women who have migraine headaches with aura, and alternatives to oral contraceptives, particularly those with estrogen, may be considered. Also, it is reasonable to try to reduce headache frequency.[3]

6. A

This patient's headaches are characteristic of migraine headaches. Other features characteristic of migraine without aura are pulsating pain quality, aggravation by physical activity, and phonophobia. To meet criteria, the patient should have at least five attacks with the appropriate features.[1] Given this patient's headache frequency, a preventive medication is recommended.

In adults, evidence strongly supports the use of valproic acid, topiramate, propranolol, metoprolol, and timolol for migraine prevention. Topiramate carries a risk for angle-closure glaucoma. Both topiramate and valproic acid place women of child-bearing age at risk for neural tube defects in their children. Folate should be prescribed if either of these drugs is used. Children born to women taking topiramate are at risk for cleft lip and cleft palate. Valproic acid can cause lower intelligence quotient in children born to women taking the medication. The combination of topiramate and valproic acid can cause hyperammonemia. Beta-blockers should be avoided in patients with asthma and diabetes. There is moderate evidence that amitriptyline and venlafaxine are effective in migraine prevention. Lamotrigine is not effective for prevention of migraine.

There is strong evidence that *Petasites* (butterbur) is effective for migraine prevention, but it can cause hepatitis.

The patient's abortive agent could be changed as well. Taking an abortive agent earlier rather than later is more likely to be effective. Ibuprofen has been shown to be effective in migraine. Rizatriptan has been approved for patients age 6 years or older. In adults with prolonged migraines, taking a medication with a longer half-life, such as frovatriptan, may be helpful.

Acetaminophen with codeine and butalbital-containing medications tend to cause medication overuse headaches.

Prednisone has been used for rare, prolonged attacks. It should not be used routinely as an abortive agent.[2,4]

7. D

This patient has migraine with brainstem aura, which was formerly called basilar migraine. For a diagnosis of migraine with brainstem aura to be made, the aura must include two brainstem symptoms such as dysarthria, vertigo, tinnitus, hypacusis, diplopia, ataxia, or decreased level of consciousness. Neither weakness nor retinal symptoms should be present. Typically, the headache follows the aura within 1 hour.

Abdominal migraine is a childhood precursor of migraine. The child has intermittent episodes of abdominal pain without gastrointestinal pathology. At least two of the following symptoms are present with the pain: anorexia, nausea, vomiting, or pallor. Headache does not occur with the episodes.

Exploding head syndrome is a parasomnia. It is not painful. The patient hears a loud noise in his or her head when falling asleep or waking.

Benign paroxysmal vertigo is a precursor of migraine seen in childhood. Intermittent episodes of unsteadiness or vertigo are seen. Other symptoms include nystagmus, vomiting, pallor, and fearfulness. The events last minutes to hours. The patient is normal between events. Other causes of ataxia should be excluded, including posterior fossa tumors, seizures, and vestibular disorders. Audiometry and electroencephalography (EEG) should be performed.[1]

8. B

Sumatriptan is a 5-HT1D receptor agonist.

Most subtypes of 5-hydroxytryptamin (5-HT) or serotonin receptors are G protein coupled. The 5-HT3 receptor is a ligand-gated ion channel. Ondansetron is a 5-HT3 antagonist.

9. D

Medication-overuse headache is defined as headache that occurs at least 15 days per month in a patient with a history of headache and overuse of medication for longer than 3 months.

Combination medications are prone to causing medication-overuse headache, especially if they contain butalbital. Clonazepam or phenobarbital can be used to treat butalbital withdrawal.

10. C

This patient has status migrainosus. She should not be given dihydroergotamine (DHE) at this time because DHE should not be given within 24 hours of a triptan. Both triptans and DHE are vasoconstrictors and should be avoided in patients with uncontrolled hypertension, a history of stroke or myocardial infarction, peripheral vascular disease, or hemiplegic or prolonged (>1 hour) aura. She should be given intravenous fluids. Dopamine receptor antagonists may be helpful in status migrainosus, especially for those patients with vomiting. Akathisia and dystonia are risks of dopamine receptor antagonists. Pretreatment with diphenhydramine or benztropine may help prevent extrapyramidal side effects. Ketorolac is an option, but it can cause gastritis. Greater occipital nerve blockade has been used for status migrainosus. Intravenous magnesium has also been used but can cause hypotension. Corticosteroids may reduce the risk of headache recurrence but are associated with gastritis and, rarely, avascular necrosis. Intravenous valproic acid is an option if there is no contraindication such as liver disease. However, it can cause hyperammonemia in patients taking topiramate. Opioids should be avoided.[5]

11. A

Patients with benign paroxysmal torticollis of infancy may develop migraine variants or migraine with aura when older. This condition has been linked to mutations in *CACNA1A*. The same gene is also linked to familial hemiplegic migraine type 1, spinocerebellar ataxia type 6, and episodic ataxia type 2.

Children with benign paroxysmal torticollis have recurrent episodes of head tilt with pallor, irritability, malaise, vomiting, or ataxia. The child is normal between events.

Cyclic vomiting is also a childhood precursor of migraine.

12. B

This patient has cluster headaches. Oxygen should be administered via a nonrebreather. Cluster headaches are more common in men, and there is an increased risk for cluster headaches in first-degree relatives of patients with cluster headaches. Cluster headache is the most common type of trigeminal autonomic cephalgia (TAC). Cluster headaches are less frequent than the other TACs but last longer.

Cluster headaches are associated with severe orbital, supraorbital, and/or temporal pain with ipsilateral autonomic symptoms such as conjunctival injection, lacrimation, congestion and/or rhinorrhea, eyelid edema, facial diaphoresis, facial flushing, fullness in the ear, miosis, or ptosis. The patient often has a sense of restlessness. The pain lasts from 15 minutes to 3 hours if untreated. Besides oxygen, other options for acute treatment are sumatriptan, zolmitriptan, and dihydroergotamine (DHE). Verapamil can be used to prevent cluster headaches. An electrocardiogram (ECG) should be checked before verapamil is started.

Hypnic headaches are another type of painful headaches that wake the patient from sleep. In contrast to cluster headaches, the pain in hypnic headache is bilateral, there are no autonomic symptoms, and the patient is not restless or agitated. Caffeine can be helpful for hypnic headaches.

Paroxysmal hemicrania shares some features with cluster headache. Both are TACs. Compared with cluster headache, paroxysmal hemicrania is less likely to occur at night, less likely to be triggered by alcohol, and more likely to be triggered by neck movement or pressure on the C2 root. Paroxysmal hemicrania also responds better to indomethacin. It does not respond to oxygen.[6]

13. D

This patient has trigeminal neuralgia. Trigeminal neuralgia usually causes pain in the distribution of the maxillary or mandibular division of the trigeminal nerve, but it can involve the ophthalmic division. In the other conditions listed, pain is usually maximal at the orbit or the temple. All of the conditions listed can cause stabbing pain. Sometimes the pain in trigeminal neuralgia is electric or shock-like.

Trigeminal neuralgia, SUNA, and SUNCT can all be triggered by touching the trigger zone or chewing. However, only trigeminal neuralgia is associated with a refractory period after the pain occurs, during which the pain will not occur with the usual triggers. Severe pain can result in facial contraction in trigeminal neuralgia. The attacks in patients with SUNCT and SUNA are more frequent, are longer in duration, and are associated with more prominent autonomic features than those in patients with trigeminal neuralgia.

SUNA, SUNCT, paroxysmal hemicrania, and cluster headaches cause brief, recurrent unilateral headaches with autonomic symptoms that are ipsilateral to the pain. They are classified as TACs. SUNA and SUNCT attacks occur the most frequently (up to 100 times per day) and have the shortest duration (1 to 10 minutes). Hemicrania continua is also a TAC, but it is a continuous headache with intermittent exacerbations. Autonomic symptoms are present during the exacerbations of hemicrania continua. Patients with hemicrania continua may have a foreign body sensation in the eye ipsilateral to the pain.

TACs can occur with lesions around the pituitary gland, so MRI with special attention to the pituitary gland is recommended in these patients.

Paroxysmal hemicrania and hemicrania continua respond to indomethacin. It is recommended that a proton pump inhibitor or similar medication be used for gastrointestinal protection in patients taking indomethacin. SUNA/SUNCT responds to lamotrigine (see Table 24.1).[6]

Table 24.1 SELECTED TREATMENTS FOR TRIGEMINAL AUTONOMIC CEPHALGIAS

DIAGNOSIS	TREATMENT
Cluster headache	Oxygen by nonrebreather, sumatriptan
Hemicrania continua	Indomethacin
Paroxysmal hemicrania	Indomethacin
SUNA/SUNCT	Lamotrigine

SUNA = Short-lasting unilateral neuralgiform headache attacks with cranial autonomic features; SUNCT = short-lasting unilateral neuralgiform headache attacks with conjunctival injection and tearing.

14. B

This patient has primary cough headache, which responds to indomethacin.

Arnold-Chiari I malformation, which is a common cause of cough headache, needs to be ruled out. Also, cerebrovascular disease and cerebral aneurysms can cause cough headache.

15. A

Orthostatic headache is characteristic of intracranial hypotension. Diffuse pachymeningeal enhancement is seen on MRI. Connective tissue disorders such as Marfan syndrome and Ehlers-Danlos syndrome increase the risk for intracranial hypotension.

16. A

This patient most likely has intracranial hypertension. A funduscopic examination would most likely show papilledema, and lumbar puncture would likely show an elevated opening pressure. In this case, intracranial hypertension may be caused by vitamin A toxicity due to excessive vitamin intake. There are many other possible etiologies. Sinus venous thrombosis is a common cause of intracranial hypertension.

17. B

This patient's symptoms define new daily persistent headache. It can have features of migraines or of tension-type headaches.

A thunderclap headache is a severe headache of abrupt onset that quickly reaches maximum intensity (in <1 minute). To meet criteria for thunderclap headache, the headache should last at least 5 minutes. Intracranial pathology should be ruled out. Subarachnoid hemorrhage is the most common cause of this type of headache pain. Other causes include intracerebral hemorrhage, cerebral venous thrombosis, unruptured vascular malformation, arterial dissection, reversible cerebral vasoconstriction syndrome, pituitary apoplexy, meningitis, cerebrospinal fluid (CSF) hypotension, sinusitis (especially with barotrauma), and colloid cyst of the third ventricle.

In addition to causing thunderclap headache, a colloid cyst of the third ventricle can obstruct the foramen of Monro and cause syncope, hydrocephalus, and sudden death.

Reversible cerebral vasoconstriction syndrome (RCVS) can cause recurrent thunderclap headache. It tends to affect middle-aged women. RCVS is associated with multiple areas of vasoconstriction involving multiple arteries, resulting in a string-of-beads appearance. Initial imaging may be normal, so imaging may need to be repeated. In RCVS, arteries improve significantly within 12 weeks. RCVS can be associated with nonaneurysmal subarachnoid hemorrhage. Stroke can occur with RCVS. Triggers for thunderclap headache in RCVS are the Valsalva maneuver, intercourse, exertion, and emotion. Recurrent thunderclap headaches during intercourse are highly suspicious for RCVS.

18.

1) B
2) C
3) A
4) D
5) E

Nociceptive pain is the term for pain caused by direct activation of pain fibers as a result of tissue injury (see Table 24.2).

Table 24.2 DEFINITIONS OF PAIN TERMS

TERM	DEFINITION
Allodynia	Pain from a non-noxious stimulus
Causalgia	A burning pain occurring after peripheral nerve injury
Dysesthesia	Unpleasant sensation (spontaneous or provoked)
Hyperalgesia	Pain from a noxious stimulus that is significantly greater than expected
Hyperpathia	Delayed, increased pain from a noxious stimulus

Neuropathic pain results from lesions in the nervous system. Allodynia, hyperalgesia, hyperpathia, dysesthesia, and paresthesias characterize neuropathic pain. Neuropathic pain tends to be chronic and to increase with time. There is sensitization of nociceptors in patients with neuropathic pain: Nociceptors respond to subthreshold stimuli or have increased response to a typical stimulus. Inflammation contributes to sensitization.

19. D

Neuropathic pain is more common in neuropathies involving C and Aδ nerve fibers, which are small fibers. Small-fiber neuropathies tend to be painful and length dependent, causing a stocking-glove distribution, but there are exceptions. Although neuropathic pain is more common in small-fiber peripheral neuropathies, it can also occur in large-fiber peripheral neuropathies.

20. C

C and Aδ nerve fibers, which are small fibers, are not assessed with EMG or NCS. Therefore, EMG and NCS are not able to diagnose a small-fiber neuropathy. EMG and NCS assess Aα and Aβ nerve fibers.

The gold standard for diagnosis of small-fiber neuropathy is skin biopsy. The intraepidermal nerve fiber density is assessed.

21. A

Golgi tendon organs, Meissner's corpuscles, muscle spindles, and Pacinian corpuscles are part of the dorsal column system.

Bare nerve endings are part of the spinothalamic system, which carries pain and temperature information. There are three types of these free endings: mechanoreceptors, thermoreceptors, and polymodal nociceptors. Information from these receptors is transmitted by Aδ and C fibers to the dorsal horn of the spinal cord. (Information from cranial pain afferents travels to the spinal trigeminal nucleus.) Aδ fibers are small and thinly myelinated. They transmit pain and temperature information, typically sharp pain. C fibers are small, unmyelinated nerves that are responsible for slow pain and temperature. They transmit dull pain.

Small-diameter sensory fibers, such as Aδ and C fibers, enter the spinal cord in the tract of Lissauer.

22. B

Aδ fibers terminate in lamina I (the marginal zone), lamina II (the substantia gelatinosa), and lamina V in the spinal cord. Aδ fibers transmit pain using glutamate, aspartate, and adenosine triphosphate (ATP).

C fibers use substance P and terminate in lamina II. Neurons in lamina II release enkephalins, endorphins, and dynorphins, which inhibit pain transmission.

Axons of second-order neurons responsible for pain sensation decussate in the anterior spinal commissure of the cord and become the spinothalamic tract. The spinothalamic tract projects to the ventral posterolateral thalamus and then to the primary somatosensory cortex.

23. D

Patients with trigeminal neuralgia of no known etiology and those who may possibly have vascular compression are considered to have classic trigeminal neuralgia. There should be no neurologic deficit. Patients with an identifiable cause (other than possible vascular compression) have symptomatic trigeminal neuralgia. For example, patients with trigeminal neuralgia caused by multiple sclerosis, a tumor, or an abnormality of the skull base have symptomatic trigeminal neuralgia. These patients are more likely to have sensory deficits, bilateral involvement, and abnormal trigeminal reflexes.

First-line agents used to treat trigeminal neuralgia are carbamazepine and oxcarbazepine. Topical ophthalmic anesthesia is not recommended.

Surgery may be considered for patients with trigeminal neuralgia who do not benefit from medical therapy. Microvascular decompression can be performed in patients with trigeminal neuralgia due to vascular compression.[7]

24. D

Postherpetic neuralgia is continuation of the pain of herpes zoster for longer than 3 months after the rash resolves. Treatments that have been proven to be helpful include opioids, tricyclic antidepressants, gabapentin, pregabalin, and lidocaine patches. Acupuncture, indomethacin, lorazepam, and dextromethorphan have not been proven to be helpful.

The AAN guideline that addresses postherpetic neuralgia states that antiviral agents given within 72 hours after the onset of herpes zoster symptoms can reduce the severity and duration of the acute illness and may prevent postherpetic neuralgia. Amitriptyline may also be helpful in this regard.[8]

25. A

This patient has complex regional pain syndrome (CRPS). CRPS is characterized by autonomic changes, sensory abnormalities, motor abnormalities, and trophic changes. CRPS is divided into two types. Type I (reflex sympathetic dystrophy) occurs most often after minor injury to a limb and is less commonly caused by central nervous system abnormalities. Type II (causalgia) occurs after injury to a peripheral nerve that results in focal deficits.

Psychological treatment and physical and occupational therapy are recommended for CRPS. Medications used to treat CRPS include opioids; anti-epileptic medications such as gabapentin, pregabalin, and carbamazepine; antidepressants; calcium-regulating medications; and corticosteroids. In some cases, sympatholytic procedures are performed.

Dejerine-Roussy syndrome is a thalamic syndrome characterized by pain on the contralateral side of the body with anesthesia to pinprick.

Radicular pain is dermatomal. An extramedullary tumor can cause radicular pain.

26. C

Mutations in the sodium channel can cause increased pain sensitivity. For instance, mutations in *SCN9A* cause paroxysmal extreme pain disorder and primary erythermalgia. (Primary erythermalgia causes episodes of painful, red extremities.) Other mutations in *SCN9A* cause congenital insensitivity to pain. Similarly, some mutations in *SCN11* cause intense pain, and others cause insensitivity

to pain. Familial hemiplegic migraine (FHM) type 3 is caused by sodium channel mutations in *SCN1A*. (FHM type 1 is caused by a calcium channel defect, and FHM type 2 is caused by mutations in Na$^+$,K$^+$-ATPase pumps.)

27. D

Pregabalin has the strongest evidence for treating painful diabetic neuropathy. There is less evidence for amitriptyline, capsaicin, duloxetine, gabapentin, valproic acid, and opioids, although these agents can be considered. Oxcarbazepine, mexiletine, clonidine, and lamotrigine are not recommended.[9]

28. A

Capsaicin is an agonist at a vanilloid receptor (TPRV1). It causes release of substance P and calcitonin G related peptide.

Gabapentin, pregabalin, and topical lidocaine act on the $\alpha2\delta$ subunit of N-type calcium channels. Topical lidocaine is useful if allodynia is a problem.

REFERENCES

1. Headache Classification Committee of the International Headache Society (IHS). *The International Classification of Headache Disorders*, 3rd edition (beta version). *Cephalgia* 2013;33:629–808.
2. Silberstein SD, Holland S, Freitag F, et al. Evidence-based guideline update: Pharmacologic treatment for episodic migraine prevention in adults. Report of the Quality Standards Subcommittee of the American Academy of Neurology and the American Headache Society. *Neurology* 2012;78:1337–1345.
3. Meschia JF, Bushnell C, Boden-Albala B, et al. Guidelines for the primary prevention of stroke. A statement for healthcare professionals from the American Heart Association/American Stroke Association. *Stroke* 2014;45:3754–3832.
4. Holland S, Silberstein SD, Freitag F, et al. Evidence-based guideline update: NSAIDs and other complementary treatments for episodic migraine prevention in adults. Report of the Quality Standards Subcommittee of the American Academy of Neurology and the American Headache Society. *Neurology* 2012;78:1346–1353.
5. Rozen T. Emergency and inpatient management. *Continuum (Minneap Minn)* 2015;21:1004–1017.
6. Newman L. Trigeminal autonomic cephalgias. *Continuum (Minneap Minn)* 2015;21:1041–1057.
7. Gronseth G, Cruccu G, Alksne J, et al. Practice parameter: The diagnostic evaluation and treatment of trigeminal neuralgia (an evidence-based review). Report of the Quality Standards Subcommittee of the American Academy of Neurology and the European Federation of Neurological Societies. *Neurology* 2008;71:1183–1190.
8. Dubinsky RM, Kabbani H, El-Chami Z, et al. Practice parameter: Treatment of postherpetic neuralgia. An evidence-based report of the Quality Standards Subcommittee of the American Academy of Neurology. *Neurology* 2004;63:959–965.
9. Bril V, England J, Franklin GM, et al. Evidence-based guideline: Treatment of painful diabetic neuropathy. Report of the American Academy of Neurology, the American Association of Neuromuscular and Electrodiagnostic Medicine, and the American Academy of Physical Medicine and Rehabilitation. *Neurology* 2011;76:1758–1765.

25.

PEDIATRIC NEUROLOGY

QUESTIONS

1. A neonate with microcephaly and hepatosplenomegaly develops seizures. Computed tomography (CT) shows calcifications surrounding the ventricles. Which of the following organisms is most likely responsible?
   A. Cytomegalovirus
   B. Rubella
   C. Syphilis
   D. Toxoplasmosis

2. Which type of brachial plexus injury is most common at birth?
   A. Erb palsy
   B. Middle trunk plexopathy
   C. Klumpke palsy
   D. Complete brachial plexus palsy

3. A newborn is noted to have facial asymmetry. When she cries, her lower lip is pulled to the lower right. The nasolabial folds are symmetric, and the patient closes both eyes well. What additional test should be performed?
   A. Echocardiogram (ECHO)
   B. Eye examination
   C. Hearing screen
   D. Head ultrasound

4. A 3-day-old develops vomiting and diarrhea. On examination, he has hypotonia, cataracts, jaundice, and hepatosplenomegaly. Which of the following diagnoses is most likely?
   A. Adrenomyeloneuropathy
   B. Arginosuccinase deficiency
   C. Classic galactosemia (type 1)
   D. X-linked adrenoleukodystrophy

5. A baby in the newborn nursery with a history of poor fetal movements has poor respiratory effort and is hypotonic. His mother has male-pattern baldness, ptosis, and a persistent grip. Which of the following is the preferred confirmatory test?
   A. Acetylcholine receptor antibodies
   B. DNA methylation
   C. Molecular genetic testing of the gene *DMPK*
   D. Electromyography

6. A mother brings her infant son to the emergency department because she has noticed that he has brief jerks in his sleep. When she wakes him, they resolve.

She has seen the episodes only when the infant is asleep. The patient had a typical event during routine electroencephalography (EEG), and no EEG correlate was seen. The EEG was read as normal. Which of the following is the most likely diagnosis?
   A. Myoclonic seizures
   B. Benign sleep myoclonus
   C. Benign rolandic epilepsy
   D. Tics

7. Which of the following statements is *false*?
   A. The majority of newborns with stroke have focal deficits at birth.
   B. Placental vasculopathy can cause perinatal acute ischemic stroke.
   C. Most neonatal strokes involve the left middle cerebral artery territory.
   D. In most cases, antithrombotic therapy is not indicated for perinatal stroke.

8. An infant with a cranial bruit over the posterior cranium and bounding carotid pulses develops congestive heart failure. What is the most likely cause?
   A. An arteriovenous malformation
   B. Cardiomyopathy
   C. Hypertension
   D. Carotid stenosis

9. Which of the following conditions is *least* likely to be associated with cardiac defects?
   A. DiGeorge syndrome
   B. Menkes disease
   C. Noonan syndrome
   D. Turner syndrome

10. A 2-week-old with a history of poor feeding develops seizures. On examination, the patient has hypertelorism and a high forehead. He is hypotonic and has poor visual fixation. A bone survey shows calcifications of the patellae. Ultrasound studies show renal cysts. Which of the following is most likely to be present in this condition?
    A. Increased very-long-chain fatty acids
    B. A cherry-red spot
    C. Blond hair
    D. Renal tubular acidosis

11. Kernicterus is most likely to cause which of the following?
    A. Dyskinetic cerebral palsy
    B. Spastic diplegia

C. Spastic hemiparesis

D. Spastic quadriparesis

12. **A 3-month-old presents with seizures. The seizures do not respond to phenobarbital, fosphenytoin, or levetiracetam. MRI is normal. Cerebrospinal fluid (CSF) analysis shows 2 white blood cells (WBCs), a normal protein level, and a glucose concentration of 30 mg/dL. The serum glucose level is 90 mg/dL. What is the best treatment?**

A. Lacosamide

B. The ketogenic diet

C. Topiramate

D. Zonisamide

13. **A couple brings a baby they have adopted from Russia to clinic because of poor feeding and excessive sleepiness. He has large fontanelles, a large tongue, a hoarse cry, and a prominent abdomen with an umbilical hernia. Which of the following diagnoses is suspected?**

A. Beckwith-Wiedemann syndrome

B. Congenital hypothyroidism

C. Cornelia de Lange syndrome

D. Cri du chat syndrome

14. **A 4-month-old is referred because of hypotonia and poor feeding. He is alert and smiling but has limited movement. He does not have facial weakness, but he has tongue fasciculations. Deep tendon reflexes are absent. Sensation is intact. What is the most likely cause?**

A. Acid maltase deficiency

B. An imprinting disorder

C. Mutations in the *SMN1* gene

D. Congenital muscular dystrophy

15. **An infant presents with poor feeding and lethargy preceded by constipation. On examination, he has ptosis, his pupils are dilated, and he is weak. The CSF is normal. Which of the following is the best treatment?**

A. Human botulism immune globulin (Baby BIG)

B. Steroids

C. Intravenous immunoglobulin

D. Plasmapheresis

16. **A 9-month-old child presents with rapid eye movements. The family shows a video of him making a nodding motion with his head. On examination, he has nystagmus and a head tilt. Brain MRI is normal. What is the best next step?**

A. Draw blood for measurement of paraneoplastic antibodies.

B. Obtain an MRI of the abdomen.

C. Reassure the family.

D. Arrange for video-EEG monitoring.

17. **A 9-month-old presents with flexor spasms. Hypsarrhythmia is seen on the EEG, and the patient is diagnosed with infantile spasms. Which of the following is a treatable cause of infantile spasms?**

A. Phenylketonuria

B. Maple syrup urine disease

C. Isovaleric acidemia

D. All of the above

18. **A 1-year-old is found to have leukocoria on examination. Which of the following is the most likely diagnosis?**

A. Retinoblastoma

B. Septo-optic-dysplasia

C. Optic glioma

D. Glaucoma

19. **Which of the following statements is *false*?**

A. The most common cause of congenital myasthenic syndromes is defects in the acetylcholine receptor.

B. An incremental response on electromyography (EMG) helps to diagnose congenital myasthenic syndromes.

C. Choline acetyltransferase deficiency can cause sudden apnea triggered by stress.

D. Treatments for some congenital myasthenic syndromes can worsen other types of congenital myasthenic syndromes.

E. Fluoxetine and ephedrine have been used to treat certain congenital myasthenic syndromes.

20. **A 1-year-old boy presents with developmental regression. He is hypotonic and has decreased reflexes on examination. His sister had similar symptoms and progressed to visual impairment and spastic tetraplegia. Her conjunctival, skin, and nerve biopsies showed spheroid bodies. What is the diagnosis?**

A. Infantile neuroaxonal dystrophy

B. Krabbe disease

C. Subacute sclerosing panencephalitis

D. Unverricht-Lundborg disease

21. **An 18-month-old child is brought to the clinic for speech delay. He started babbling at 14 months but does not say any words. He began pointing at objects at 16 months but has not done so in the past few weeks. He has never waved bye-bye. Which of the following steps *would not* be appropriate at this time?**

A. Hearing screen and referral for speech therapy evaluation

B. Lead screening if a history of pica is obtained

C. Lumbar puncture for lactate, amino acids, and neurotransmitters

D. The Checklist for Autism in Toddlers (CHAT) or the Autism Screening Questionnaire

22. **A 4-year-old presents with fever and a 4-minute generalized tonic-clonic seizure. On examination, he has otitis media bilaterally. He has no meningeal signs, and his neurologic examination is normal. Which of the following is recommended?**

A. MRI

B. EEG

C. A comprehensive metabolic profile

D. A lumbar puncture should be considered if the child was pretreated with antibiotics.

23. **A 3-year-old presents with episodes of decreased responsiveness and posturing. They occur most often when the child is sitting in a car seat. During**

an episode, she does not respond the first time her name is called but does respond to touch. The event stops if she is removed from the car seat. The birth history and past medical history are unremarkable. Development is normal. The physical examination is normal. EEG is normal. What is the most likely diagnosis?

A. Childhood absence epilepsy
B. Dystonia
C. Infantile self-gratification syndrome
D. Sandifer syndrome

24. A 4-year-old presents with irritability and difficulty walking about 5 days after spending time in the woods. He develops an ascending paralysis with areflexia. CSF and repetitive nerve stimulation are normal. Which of the following is recommended first?

A. Intravenous immunoglobulin
B. Steroids
C. Plasmapheresis
D. A thorough skin and hair evaluation, especially the scalp

25. A 1-year-old is brought to the clinic because he has episodes of crying to the point of loss of consciousness. The events occur when the patient injures himself. The birth and developmental histories are normal. The physical examination is normal. An electrocardiogram (ECG) is normal. What is the most likely diagnosis?

A. Breath-holding spells
B. Hyperekplexia
C. Periodic paralysis
D. Intermittent explosive disorder

26. A 6-year-old and a 50-year-old are both in the emergency department for stroke. Which of the following statements is *false*?

A. Children with acute stroke usually present with hemiparesis.
B. Most children presenting with acute stroke-like symptoms are found to have a stroke mimic.
C. If a child with stroke presents with a seizure, the stroke is likely to be hemorrhagic.
D. Due to more rapid hepatic clearance, the child is expected to clear tissue plasminogen activator faster than the adult.

27. A child has a left basal ganglia infarction and stenosis at the junction of the distal internal carotid artery, proximal anterior cerebral artery, and proximal middle cerebral artery on the left. Later, repeat imaging indicates that the narrowing is no longer present. The child had a viral illness 3 months before the stroke but otherwise is healthy. Which of the following diagnoses should be suspected?

A. Carotid dissection with emboli
B. Endocarditis with emboli
C. Moyamoya disease
D. Transient cerebral arteriopathy

28. A child presents with fever, confusion, and seizures that are difficult to control. The physical examination is remarkable for cervical lymphadenopathy. CSF, CT, and MRI findings are normal. What is the most likely etiology?

A. *Bartonella henselae*
B. Cytomegalovirus
C. Herpes simplex virus
D. Toxoplasmosis

29. Which of the following diseases is *least* likely to be associated with anterior temporal cysts?

A. Perinatal herpes simplex virus infection
B. Menkes disease
C. Megalencephalic leukodystrophy with subcortical cysts
D. Fabry disease

30. Which of the following diseases is *least* likely to be associated with macrocephaly?

A. Achondroplasia
B. Mowat-Wilson syndrome
C. Neurofibromatosis type 1
D. Sotos syndrome

31. Which of the following diseases is *least* likely to be associated with skeletal abnormalities?

A. Coffin-Lowery syndrome
B. Down syndrome
C. Maple syrup urine disease
D. Rubenstein-Taybi syndrome

32. Which cause of progressive myoclonic epilepsy (PME) results from a dodecamer repeat expansion in the *CSTB* gene?

A. Unverricht-Lundborg disease
B. Lafora body disease
C. Sialidosis type I
D. Infantile neuronal ceroid lipofuscinosis (NCL)

33. A 6-year-old boy presents with repetitive, nonrhythmic shoulder shrugging. He says he usually is not aware of it. He says that he can briefly control it when he realizes it is occurring. His mother states that no one else has noticed the shoulder shrugging and it does not disturb her or the patient. What is the next step?

A. Reassure the mother.
B. Start clonidine.
C. Start risperidone.
D. Start guanfacine.

34. An 8-year-old presents with paroxysmal events. His mother says that the child loses consciousness and then has generalized jerking. These episodes occur when he is exercising or scared. He started having more episodes after being prescribed methylphenidate for attention deficit hyperactivity disorder. His paternal aunt and uncle both had syncope and died suddenly in their twenties. Which of the following is most likely to yield the diagnosis?

A. ECG
B. EEG

C. ECHO

D. Tilt table test

35. An 11-year-old boy presents with recent onset of bilateral leg weakness and urinary incontinence. What is the next diagnostic step?

A. MRI of the spine

B. Electromyography and nerve conduction studies (EMG/NCS)

C. Muscle biopsy

D. Muscular dystrophy genetic panel

36. A 13-year-old girl briefly loses consciousness whenever her blood is drawn. ECG, echocardiogram, and Holter findings are normal. What is the most likely diagnosis?

A. Orthostatic hypotension

B. Psychogenic nonepileptic seizures

C. Postural orthostatic tachycardia syndrome

D. Vasovagal syncope

37. A 15-year-old boy presents with complaints of falls from his skateboard. His examination is unremarkable except for mild ataxia. Imaging demonstrates a cystic mass with an enhancing nodule in the right cerebellar hemisphere. Which of the following is the most likely diagnosis?

A. Ependymoma

B. Medulloblastoma

C. Oligodendroglioma

D. Pilocytic astrocytoma

38. Which of the following is the most common primary cord neoplasm in children?

A. Astrocytoma

B. Ependymoma

C. Hemangioblastoma

D. Ganglioglioma

39. A 15-year-old girl presents with intractable epilepsy. Her seizures started 2 years ago, about 1 month after her father's death. She has generalized shaking for longer than 1 hour. Previous EEGs performed immediately after her seizures have been normal. She has failed treatment with levetiracetam, lamotrigine, topiramate, and lacosamide. She is referred to the epilepsy monitoring unit, where she has an event with asynchronous jerking movements. During the event, her phone rings, and the movements pause briefly and then resume. What is the most likely diagnosis?

A. Frontal lobe epilepsy

B. Juvenile myoclonic epilepsy

C. Temporal lobe epilepsy

D. Psychogenic nonepileptic seizures

40. A 15-year-old patient has been having academic difficulties. His mother says he has not been acting like himself. She has also seen quick jerking movements. EEG shows background slowing and generalized periodic epileptiform discharges occurring every 4 seconds. CSF analysis shows oligoclonal bands. Which of the following is *least* likely to be found in this condition?

A. Cowdry B bodies

B. Demyelination and gliosis

C. Measles antibodies in the CSF

D. Progression to dementia

PEDIATRIC NEUROLOGY

ANSWERS

1. A

There are multiple causes of seizures in the neonate. The most common cause in the first 24 hours of life is hypoxic-ischemic encephalopathy. It is important to exclude sepsis and bacterial meningitis. Intrauterine infection is a less common cause of seizures.

Cytomegalovirus (CMV) is the most common intrauterine viral infection. CMV can cause microcephaly, migration defects, intracerebral calcifications, retinitis, and sensorineural hearing loss. Systemic symptoms of CMV infection include petechiae, an elevated direct hyperbilirubinemia, and hepatosplenomegaly.

The calcifications in patients with CMV infection surround the ventricle. Intracerebral calcifications are also seen in congenital toxoplasmosis, but they tend to be diffuse.

2. A

Erb palsy (upper trunk plexopathy) is the most common brachial plexus injury in the newborn. Large infants with shoulder dystocia are at increased risk. Erb palsy is characterized by a "waiter's tip" posture. C5-, C6-, and sometimes C7-innervated muscles are affected. The child has weakness of the deltoid muscle, affecting abduction; the infraspinatus, affecting external rotation; the biceps and brachioradialis muscles, affecting flexion; and the supinator muscle. Therefore, the arm is adducted and internally rotated, and the elbow is extended and pronated. The biceps reflex is absent.

Klumpke palsy affects muscles innervated by C8 and T1 nerve roots.

A complete brachial plexus palsy may be accompanied by Horner syndrome.

3. A

This patient has Cayler syndrome, which is characterized by hypoplasia of the depressor anguli oris muscle and cardiac defects. An echocardiogram should be performed.

4. C

This patient has classic galactosemia, which is caused by mutations in the *GALT* gene. This gene encodes galactose-1-phosphate uridyltransferase. Classic galactosemia manifests in the newborn period with vomiting, jaundice, lethargy, and a bleeding diathesis after exposure to breast milk or formulas containing lactose. Children with classic galactosemia are prone to *Escherichia coli* sepsis. Cataracts develop. Mental impairment is also a complication of classic galactosemia.

Adrenomyeloneuropathy, arginosuccinase deficiency, and X-linked adrenoleukodystrophy do not usually manifest in the neonatal period.

5. C

This patient has congenital myotonic dystrophy, which is a form of myotonic dystrophy type I. It is usually inherited from the mother. Congenital myotonic dystrophy manifests with hypotonia and weakness at birth. Facial weakness, respiratory insufficiency, poor feeding, clubfoot, and decreased reflexes are also common in neonates with congenital myotonic dystrophy. In this case, the mother's features aid in the diagnosis. Adults with myotonic dystrophy type I tend to have male-pattern baldness, facial weakness, ptosis, and myotonia. The mother's persistent grip is caused by myotonia. Myotonia is not present in newborns. Newborns can be diagnosed with gene testing. Myotonic dystrophy type I is caused by expansion of the CTG repeat in the *DMPK* gene, which is on chromosome 19. Myotonic dystrophy type I is autosomal dominant and demonstrates anticipation.

DNA methylation is one technique used to diagnose Prader-Willi syndrome, which is a cause of neonatal hypotonia. In patients with Prader-Willi syndrome, methylation studies demonstrate the absence of paternally imprinted genes at chromosome 15q11-13.

Neonates born to mothers with myasthenia gravis can have transient neonatal myasthenia gravis due to maternal autoantibodies. These infants have weakness, hypotonia, difficulties with feeding, and respiratory depression.

6. B

This patient has benign sleep myoclonus, which is a normal condition. It is characterized by myoclonic jerks during sleep. If the infant is awakened, they resolve. The EEG is normal in benign sleep myoclonus. Epileptiform activity is seen during myoclonic seizures.

7. A

Most newborns with stroke do *not* have focal deficits at birth. Later in life, the most common presentation for childhood stroke is hemiparesis, but this usually is not seen in the newborn period. Seizures are a common presentation in neonates. Neonatal stroke may also manifest with encephalopathy and/or apnea. Most neonatal strokes involve the left middle cerebral artery (MCA) territory. Although a child who has had a perinatal stroke may not have focal deficits at birth, he or she may later demonstrate early hand preference due to hemiparesis.

In most cases, antithrombotic therapy is not indicated for perinatal stroke. Exceptions include patients with congenital heart disease or an abnormal prothrombotic workup. Abnormal laboratory results should be repeated at least 3 months later and off treatment to determine whether the abnormality is still present.

8. A

This patient has a vein of Galen malformation, which is the most common type of neonatal arteriovenous malformation. Most patients are male. The median prosencephalic vein of Markowski, which normally drains into the vein of Galen, is actually the dilated vein. This vein usually disappears during development but is persistent in patients with a vein of Galen malformation. In the newborn period, vein of Galen malformation typically manifests with congestive heart failure. It can also cause hydrocephalus, ischemia due to a steal phenomenon, or intracranial hemorrhage.

9. B

DiGeorge syndrome is a chromosome 22q11.2 deletion syndrome. Velocardiofacial syndrome and Cayler cardiofacial syndrome are also included in this group of disorders. The 22q11.2 deletion syndrome is usually associated with cardiac and palate abnormalities, developmental delay, and immune dysfunction. The term CATCH-22 has been used for these syndromes; CATCH stands for Cardiac abnormality, Anomalous face, Thymus hypoplasia, Cleft palate, and Hypocalcemia.

DiGeorge syndrome is caused by abnormal development of the third and fourth pharyngeal pouches and the fourth branchial arch. This causes an abnormal thymus and parathyroid glands, resulting in immune dysfunction and hypocalcemia, respectively. DiGeorge syndrome can manifest with tetany or neonatal seizures due to hypocalcemia.

Noonan syndrome is associated with pulmonary valve stenosis.

Turner syndrome can cause coarctation of the aorta or an abnormal aortic valve.

Menkes disease can cause intracranial hemorrhage due to friable blood vessels, but it does not usually cause cardiac disease. Menkes disease can be mistaken for child abuse because of the presence of subdural hygromas and skeletal abnormalities (Wormian bones and spurs at the metaphyses).

10. A

This is Zellweger syndrome, which is a peroxisomal disorder caused by *PEX* mutations. Children with Zellweger syndrome have characteristic facial features, hypotonia, renal cysts, and calcification of the patellae. Zellweger syndrome can cause a number of cortical abnormalities. Increased levels of very-long-chain fatty acids support the diagnosis. Also, phytanic acid, pristanic acid, and pipecolic acid concentrations may be elevated.

11. A

The most common type of cerebral palsy (CP) is spastic CP. Premature infants tend to have spastic diplegia due to periventricular white matter injury. Causes of dyskinetic CP include hypoxic-ischemic injury and kernicterus (bilirubin encephalopathy). Kernicterus is also associated with high-frequency hearing loss and impaired vertical gaze.

American Academy of Neurology (AAN) guidelines regarding assessment of CP recommend neuroimaging if the cause of CP is unknown. Magnetic resonance imaging (MRI) is preferred. If a child has hemiplegic CP due to unexplained infarction, then coagulation studies should be considered. An EEG is not required unless there is concern about seizures. Children with CP should be screened for speech and language disorders, vision and hearing impairments, feeding and swallowing difficulties, and intellectual disability. Metabolic and genetic testing are not required for all children with CP but may be indicated in certain cases. For instance, additional evaluation may be performed in children with CP who have a brain malformation, a family history of neurologic disorders, or clinical worsening.[1]

12. B

This patient has glucose transporter type 1 (Glut-1) deficiency syndrome, also called Glut-1 DS, which results from mutations in the *SLC2A1* gene. *SLC2A1* encodes a glucose transporter in the blood-brain barrier. Glut-1 DS responds to the ketogenic diet.

Mutations in *SLC2A1* cause early-onset absence epilepsy, alternating hemiplegia of childhood, paroxysmal choreoathetosis with episodic ataxia and spasticity (DYT9), and epilepsy with exercise-induced dyskinesia (DYT18).

13. B

This child has congenital hypothyroidism. Congenital hypothyroidism is associated with prolonged physiologic jaundice, poor feeding, increased sleep, constipation, large fontanelles, macroglossia, and an umbilical hernia. Lack of treatment can cause neurologic complications such as intellectual disability.

Down syndrome is also associated with macroglossia and enlarged fontanelles that are slow to close. Hypothyroidism can occur in Down syndrome.

Beckwith-Wiedemann syndrome also causes macroglossia and an umbilical hernia, but it is associated with macrosomia. It is an overgrowth disorder. Growth may be asymmetric, causing hemihyperplasia. Patients with Beckwith-Wiedemann syndrome may be born with an omphalocele. Neonatal hypoglycemia may result from hyperinsulinism. Visceromegaly can occur in this condition. Patients with Beckwith-Wiedemann syndrome are at risk for tumors such as Wilms tumor and hepatoblastoma. Beckwith-Wiedemann syndrome is an imprinting disorder.

Cornelia de Lange syndrome causes intrauterine growth retardation, characteristic facial features, and skeletal abnormalities. Infants have a low-pitched cry similar to a growl.

Cri du chat syndrome is caused by partial deletion of chromosome 5p. It is associated with a high-pitched cry similar to that of a cat, microcephaly, distinctive facial features, and developmental delay.

14. C

This patient has spinal muscular atrophy type 1 (SMA I), which is also known as Werdnig-Hoffman disease. Motor neuron loss occurs in the anterior horn.

SMA is most often caused by mutations in *SMN1* on chromosome 5q. *SMN1* and *SMN2* encode for survival motor neuron protein, but *SMN1* produces more functional protein. *SMN2* is adjacent to *SMN1* and modifies the severity of SMA; more copies of *SMN2* result in less severe disease. SMA is autosomal recessive.

SMA I is the most severe form of SMA. Patients never sit, and they develop aspiration and respiratory insufficiency. Death occurs at about 2 years of age. Patients with SMA II are able to sit but have difficulty walking. Finger tremor may be present. Patients with SMA III (Kugelberg-Welander disease) are able to walk. Onset of symptoms occurs after 1 year of age. SMA IV manifests in adulthood.

Acid maltase deficiency causes Pompe disease, which is glycogen storage disease type 2. Pompe disease causes neonatal hypotonia and weakness. These patients also have macroglossia and congestive heart failure.

Imprinting disorders are responsible for the Prader-Willi, Angelman, Beckwith-Wiedemann, and Russell-Silver syndromes. Prader-Willi syndrome manifests with hypotonia in neonates, but tongue fasciculations do not occur. Newborns with Prader-Willi syndrome tend to be lethargic, not alert.

Congenital muscular dystrophy causes weakness and hypotonia in neonates, but tongue fasciculations are more characteristic of SMA.

15. A

This patient has infantile botulism. Infantile botulism is caused by ingestion of *Clostridium botulinum* spores, which produce toxin in the gastrointestinal tract. Infantile botulism is associated with ingestion of honey, but this is not the only cause. The toxin causes decreased acetylcholine release. Constipation is typically the first symptom. Then a descending weakness occurs. Autonomic dysfunction and respiratory failure can occur. Stool cultures help provide the diagnosis. EMG can also support the diagnosis. Rapid repetitive nerve stimulation can cause an incremental response. Treatment is with human botulism immune globulin (BabyBIG).

In wound botulism, the wound is infected by spores and toxin is produced in the wound.

Foodborne botulism is caused by ingestion of food that contains the botulism toxin, which is produced by the bacteria *C. botulinum*. It is associated with vomiting and diarrhea as well as neurologic symptoms.

Botulism can imitate acute inflammatory demyelinating polyradiculoneuropathy (AIDP), which is the most common type of Guillain-Barré syndrome (GBS). However, in botulism, descending weakness occurs, and the CSF is normal. GBS causes ascending weakness and albuminocytologic dissociation. EMG and nerve conduction studies help to differentiate the conditions.

16. C

This patient most likely has spasmus nutans, which is characterized by nystagmus, head nodding, and a head tilt. Onset is usually during the first year of life. Spasmus nutans self-resolves in a couple of years. An optic nerve glioma, glioma of the chiasm, Leigh disease, Pelizaeus-Merzbacher disease, and vermian hypoplasia are in the differential diagnosis.

17. D

Certain organic acidurias and amino acidopathies can cause infantile spasms (IS). Phenylketonuria, maple syrup urine disease, and isovaleric acidemia can cause IS and are treated with special restricted diets. Patients with infantile spasms due to pyridoxine dependency should be treated with pyridoxine. Likewise, biotinidase deficiency can cause IS and should be treated with biotin. Patients with IS due to glucose transporter type 1 deficiency syndrome benefit from treatment with the ketogenic diet. The developmental delay, epilepsy, neonatal diabetes (DEND) syndrome also causes IS. It results from mutations in a potassium channel gene. These patients benefit from treatment with sulfonylurea. Other metabolic causes of IS are Menkes disease, nonketotic hyperglycinemia (NKH), and, rarely, mitochondrial disease.

18. A

Retinoblastoma is a type of primitive neuroectodermal tumor (PNET) caused by a mutation on chromosome 13. It can manifest with leukocoria or strabismus. Patients with retinoblastoma can also have pineoblastoma or osteosarcoma. Flexner-Wintersteiner rosettes (real rosettes) are seen on histology.

Aniridia can be associated with Wilms tumor. Aniridia and Wilms tumor are seen in the Wilms tumor, aniridia, genitourinary anomalies, and mental retardation (WAGR) syndrome.

19. B

The most common cause of congenital myasthenic syndromes is defects in the acetylcholine receptor, followed by mutations that affect the endplate.

Patients with congenital myasthenic syndromes tend to have fatigable weakness. A decremental response is seen on EMG. Single-fiber EMG may also aid in the diagnosis. Congenital myasthenic syndromes can also manifest with arthrogryposis at birth.

Patients with choline acetyltransferase deficiency, which is one of the presynaptic causes of congenital myasthenic syndrome, can present with apnea after stress. Some patients with choline acetyltransferase deficiency present at birth with hypotonia and apnea.

Pyridostigmine is helpful for some congenital myasthenic syndromes, including choline acetyltransferase deficiency, but it may be harmful for other congenital myasthenic syndromes such as acetylcholinesterase deficiency, slow-channel syndrome, and laminin-β2 deficiency. Some congenital myasthenic syndromes are treated with adrenergic agonists. For instance, laminin-β2 deficiency has been treated with ephedrine. Slow-channel syndrome has been treated with quinine, quinidine, and fluoxetine.[2]

20. A

This patient has infantile neuroaxonal dystrophy, which manifests with developmental delay but then causes regression. It affects the central and peripheral nervous systems. Hypotonia evolves into spasticity, and optic atrophy occurs. Neuropathy may result in limb mutilation. Autonomic dysfunction causes urinary retention and decreased tearing. Hypothalamic dysfunction can result in diabetes insipidus or hypothyroidism. Seizures may occur. MRI shows cerebellar atrophy. Some patients have iron accumulation in the basal ganglia. Spheroid bodies are found on nerve biopsy. Infantile neuroaxonal dystrophy is caused by mutations in the *PLA2G6* gene. This gene encodes A2 phospholipase, which is necessary for metabolizing phospholipids. Mutations in the *PLA2G6* gene also cause neurodegeneration with brain iron accumulation 2B and Parkinson disease 14 (PARK 14).

Krabbe disease, which is also known as globoid cell leukodystrophy, also manifests in infancy and affects the central and peripheral nervous systems. Krabbe disease is a lysosomal storage disease caused by deficiency of galactocerebrosidase (also known as galactosylceramidase or galactosylceramide beta-galactosidase). Krabbe disease usually manifests before 6 months of age with irritability, fever, and sensitivity to external stimuli. It also causes spasticity, optic atrophy, and neuropathy. Nerve conduction velocities are reduced, and nerve biopsy specimens contain deposits of sphingolipids. CSF protein is elevated, and MRI shows increased T2 signal in the white matter.

Subacute sclerosing panencephalitis and Unverricht-Lundborg disease are discussed later.

21. C

This child may have autism. AAN guidelines for screening and diagnosis of autism recommend developmental screening from infancy to school age and when development is a concern. The Denver screens are not believed to be adequate. The AAN guideline recommends the Ages and Stages Questionnaire, the BRIGANCE Screens, the Child Development Inventories, and the Parents' Evaluations of Developmental Status for developmental screening. If a child fails developmental screening, the Checklist for Autism in Toddlers (CHAT) or the Autism Screening Questionnaire should be performed to screen for autism.

If a child does not babble by 12 months, gesture by 12 months, say single words by 16 months, or say spontaneous two-word phrases by 24 months, developmental evaluation is indicated. In addition, loss of language or social skills at any age requires evaluation.

The initial evaluation should include a hearing screen. Lead screening should be performed if there is a history of pica. Lumbar puncture is not part of the initial evaluation.[3]

22. D

This patient most likely had a simple febrile seizure; however, pretreatment with antibiotics can mask the signs of meningitis. Therefore, a lumbar puncture should be considered (see Box 25.1).[4]

Box 25.1 AMERICAN ACADEMY OF PEDIATRICS GUIDELINES REGARDING MANAGEMENT OF A SIMPLE FEBRILE SEIZURE

- The cause of the fever should be investigated. Meningitis should be considered.
- If the child appears ill or the history or physical examination is concerning for meningitis, a lumbar puncture should be performed.
- In a child between 6 and 12 months of age, a lumbar puncture "is an option" if the child could be deficient in immunizations for *Haemophilus influenzae* type b or *Streptococcus pneumoniae*.
- A lumbar puncture "is an option" if the child was pretreated with antibiotics, which can mask signs and symptoms of meningitis.
- Laboratory studies, such as a comprehensive metabolic profile and complete blood count, are not routinely necessary.
- Neuroimaging and electroencephalography are not routinely necessary.

A febrile seizure is a seizure that occurs in a child between 6 and 60 months of age without a central nervous system infection with a temperature of 100.4°F (38°C) or higher by any method. A simple febrile seizure lasts less than 15 minutes, is generalized, and does not recur. A complex febrile seizure is focal, lasts 15 minutes or longer, or recurs within 24 hours.

The consequences of *prolonged* febrile seizures are being investigated. The Consequences of Prolonged Febrile Seizures in Childhood (FEBSTAT) study is a prospective, multicenter study designed to investigate the acute and long-term consequences of febrile status epilepticus, which was defined as a febrile seizure or series of seizures lasting longer than 30 minutes (see Box 25.2).[5,6,7,8,9]

Box 25.2 FINDINGS OF THE CONSEQUENCES OF PROLONGED FEBRILE SEIZURES IN CHILDHOOD (FEBSTAT) STUDY

- Children with febrile status epilepticus (FSE) are at risk for acute hippocampal injury, and a substantial number also have abnormalities in hippocampal development.
- Findings of focal slowing or attenuation are present in EEGs obtained within 72 hours in a substantial proportion of children with FSE and are highly associated with magnetic resonance imaging (MRI) evidence of acute hippocampal injury.
- FSE rarely causes cerebrospinal fluid (CSF) pleocytosis, so CSF pleocytosis should not be attributed to FSE.
- Human herpesvirus type 6 (HHV-6) is a common cause of febrile seizures and can cause FSE. HHV-7 infection is less often associated with FSE. Together, they account for one third of FSE cases.
- Earlier treatment of FSE resulted in shorter seizure duration.

23. C

This patient most likely has infantile self-gratification syndrome, which previously was called infantile masturbation. This is a benign condition.

Sandifer syndrome is posturing caused by gastroesophageal reflux.

Childhood absence epilepsy would manifest with absence seizures in multiple settings, and the EEG would be abnormal.

Improvement with distraction is more characteristic of infantile self-gratification syndrome than of dystonia.

24. D

This patient has tick paralysis. The tick often attaches to the scalp and can be detected by a thorough evaluation. Tick paralysis causes ataxia and an ascending flaccid paralysis. This can progress to cause ptosis, ophthalmoplegia, bulbar paralysis, quadriplegia, and respiratory failure if the tick is not removed. Removal of the tick early in the course results in neurologic improvement within a day or so.

Tick paralysis is in the differential diagnosis for acute inflammatory demyelinating polyradiculoneuropathy (AIDP). AIDP is usually associated with albuminocytologic dissociation (an elevated protein level and normal white blood cells) in the cerebrospinal fluid.

25. A

This patient has breath-holding spells. These occur in infants and improve by school age. The events are typically triggered by fear, pain, or frustration. The child cries and then holds his breath in expiration. He may lose consciousness and become limp. Some children have clonic activity. Patients with breath holding who are iron deficient may respond to iron supplementation. Some children without iron deficiency improve with iron supplementation.

Breath-holding spells have been divided into cyanotic and pallid-type events based on the color of the child during the event. Pallid breath-holding spells may be related to excessive vagal tone.

26. C

Whereas a seizure in an adult suggests there is a higher likelihood that the stroke is hemorrhagic, it is not predictive in the child. Most children with acute stroke present with hemiparesis. However, most children with stroke-like symptoms do not have stroke.

27. D

This child has transient cerebral arteriopathy or focal arteriopathy, which can be seen with varicella-zoster virus and other infectious agents. Varicella tends to affect the M1 segment of the middle cerebral artery.

28. A

This is cat-scratch disease, which is caused by *Bartonella henselae*. Bartonella can cause encephalitis, retinitis, meningitis, transverse myelitis, and a syndrome resembling AIDP. Cervical lymphadenopathy aids in the diagnosis.

29. D

Perinatal herpes simplex virus (HSV) infection, Menkes disease, and megalencephalic leukodystrophy with subcortical cysts all can cause anterior temporal cysts.

30. B

Achondroplasia, neurofibromatosis type 1, and Sotos syndrome cause macrocephaly.

Mowat-Wilson syndrome causes microcephaly. Other features of Mowat-Wilson syndrome are agenesis of the corpus callosum and Hirschsprung disease.

Sotos syndrome causes megalencephaly and gigantism.

Alexander disease, Canavan disease, GM2 gangliosidoses (Tay-Sachs disease and Sandhoff disease), mucopolysaccharidoses, glutaric aciduria type 1, and megalencephalic leukoencephalopathy with subcortical cysts are metabolic causes of megalencephaly.

Linear nevus syndrome and tuberous sclerosis complex can cause hemimegalencephaly. Klippel-Trenaunay syndrome, Proteus syndrome, and hypomelanosis of Ito can cause hemimegalencephaly with somatic hemihypertrophy. Proteus syndrome is caused by a mutation in *PTEN*, which is a tumor suppression gene.

31. C

Maple syrup urine disease is the least likely to be associated with skeletal abnormalities.

Patients with Down syndrome can have atlantoaxial instability.

Rubenstein-Taybi syndrome has also been called broad thumb-hallux syndrome. It is caused by mutations in the gene *CREBBP*, which encodes CREB binding protein. This protein is in the family of chromatin-modifying enzymes and regulates cell growth and division. Rubenstein-Taybi syndrome causes microcephaly, characteristic facial features, micrognathia, a highly arched palate, and broad thumbs and great toes. Some patients have parietal foramina.

Coffin-Lowry syndrome is a cause of X-linked intellectual disability. It results from mutations in the *RSK2* gene, which is in the Ras-MAPK pathway. Patients with Coffin-Lowry syndrome have microcephaly, a thickened calvarium, sensorineural hearing loss, kyphoscoliosis, and beaking of the vertebrae. A pectus deformity may also be present.

32. A

Unverricht-Lundborg disease, Lafora body disease, sialidosis type I, and infantile NCL all cause progressive myoclonic epilepsy.

Unverricht-Lundborg disease (EPM1) typically results from a dodecamer repeat expansion in the *CSTB* gene, which encodes cystatin B. The first symptom in most patients is myoclonic jerks. Generalized tonic-clonic seizures are also a common presentation. The onset is typically between 6 and 15 years. Ataxia occurs later.

33. A

This is a motor tic. Since it is not bothering anyone or causing social problems, no treatment is needed.

34. A

This patient has long QT syndrome, which can be mistaken for epilepsy. Stress and exercise can trigger arrhythmia in these patients, and stimulants should be avoided.

A normal routine ECG does not rule out long QT syndrome.

35. A

Bilateral leg weakness and urinary incontinence suggest a spinal cord lesion, which can be confirmed with MRI.

36. D

This patient has vasovagal syncope, which is characterized by brief loss of consciousness due to a decrease in blood pressure triggered by pain or stress. Accompanying symptoms include dizziness/lightheadedness, nausea, blurred or constricted vision, paleness, and diaphoresis.

37. D

The imaging findings are consistent with pilocytic astrocytoma, which is the most common glioma in children. Most pilocytic astrocytomas occur in the cerebellum, but they can be found in supratentorial sites such as the optic pathway or hypothalamus. Other tumors can also have

the appearance of a cyst with an enhancing mural mass. These include gangliogliomas, pleomorphic xanthoastrocytoma, and hemangioblastomas. If this patient had Von Hippel-Lindau syndrome, his mass would most likely be a hemangioblastoma.

38. A

The most common primary cord neoplasm in children is astrocytoma.

39. D

This patient has psychogenic nonepileptic seizures (PNES). PNES are in the differential for intractable epilepsy. Video-EEG is the gold standard for diagnosis. Often, patients with PNES have suffered significant emotional trauma. Counseling is the treatment.

40. A

This is subacute sclerosing panencephalitis (SSPE), which is a neurodegenerative disease caused by remote measles infection. It manifests with academic deterioration and change in personality. Patients develop seizures and myoclonic jerks. They eventually develop dementia. The EEG shows a characteristic periodic pattern. Elevated anti-measles antibodies (immunoglobulin G) are found in the serum and CSF. Oligoclonal bands can be seen in the CSF. Intranuclear Cowdry A bodies are seen within cells in the brain.

Cowdry B bodies are associated with polio.

REFERENCES

1. Ashwal S, Russman BS, Blasco PA. Practice parameter: Diagnostic assessment of the child with cerebral palsy. *Neurology* 2004;62:851–863.
2. Engel AG, Shen X, Selcen D, Sine SM. Congenital myasthenic syndromes: Pathogenesis, diagnosis, and treatment. *Lancet Neurol* 2015;14:420–434.
3. Filipek PA, Accardo PJ, Ashwal S. Practice parameter: Screening and diagnosis of autism. Report of the Quality Standards Subcommittee of the American Academy of Neurology and the Child Neurology Society. *Neurology* 2000;55:468–479.
4. Subcommittee on Febrile Seizures. Febrile seizures: Guideline for the neurodiagnostic evaluation of the child with a simple febrile seizure. *Pediatrics* 2011;127:389–394.
5. Shinnar S, Bello J, Chan S, et al. MRI abnormalities following febrile status epilepticus in children: The FEBSTAT study. *Neurology* 2012;79:871–877.
6. Nordli DR, Moshe SL, Shinnar S, et al. Acute EEG findings in children with febrile status epilepticus: Results of the FEBSTAT study. *Neurology* 2012;79:2180–2186.
7. Frank LM, Shinnar S, Hesdorffer DC. Cerebrospinal fluid findings in children with fever-associated status epilepticus: Results of the consequences of prolonged febrile seizures (FEBSTAT) study. *J Pediatr* 2012;161:1169–1171.
8. Epstein LG, Shinnar S, Hesdorffer DC, et al. Human herpesvirus 6 and 7 in febrile status epilepticus: The FEBSTAT study. *Epilepsia* 2012;53:1481–1488.
9. Seinfeld S, Shinnar S, Sun S. Emergency management of febrile status epilepticus: Results of the FEBSTAT study. *Epilepsia* 2014;55:388–395.

26.

PSYCHIATRY

Readers are strongly advised to check the American Board of Psychiatry and Neurology (ABPN) website to determine which edition of the *Diagnostic and Statistical Manual of Mental Disorders* (DSM-IV-TR or DSM-5) will be used on their test.

QUESTIONS

1. In the DSM-5, if a physician believes strongly that a patient will meet the full criteria for a diagnosis, the patient can be diagnosed with the condition using which of the following qualifying terms?
   A. Anticipated
   B. Assumed
   C. Predicted
   D. Provisional

2. In the DSM-5, a 7-year-old patient would be diagnosed with which of the following instead of "mental retardation"?
   A. Developmental delay not otherwise specified
   B. Global cognitive impairment
   C. Global developmental delay
   D. Intellectual disability/intellectual developmental disorder

3. In the DSM-5, a patient with impaired social interaction and stereotyped behaviors, who previously would have been diagnosed with Asperger disorder, would be diagnosed with which of the following conditions?
   A. Asperger disorder
   B. Autism spectrum disorder
   C. Pervasive developmental delay not otherwise specified
   D. Pervasive developmental delay spectrum

4. Which of the following statements is *false* regarding the diagnosis of attention deficit hyperactivity disorder (ADHD) in the DSM-5?
   A. Patients with autism spectrum disorder can be diagnosed with ADHD.
   B. Symptoms must begin before the age of 12 years.
   C. Patients ages 17 years and older need to meet more criteria to be diagnosed than younger patients do.
   D. Symptoms need to be present for at least 6 months.

5. A 20-year-old patient believes that his neighbor is a spy. He has been convinced of this for 3 months. Despite this belief, the patient is able to function normally. Apart from avoiding his neighbor, the patient behaves normally. What is the most likely diagnosis?
   A. Brief psychotic disorder
   B. Delusional disorder
   C. Schizophrenia
   D. Schizophreniform disorder

6. Which of the following statements differentiates brief psychotic disorder from schizophreniform disorder and schizophrenia?
   A. Negative symptoms are not part of the criteria for diagnosing brief psychotic disorder.
   B. Hallucinations are not part of the criteria for diagnosing brief psychotic disorder.
   C. Catatonia is an exclusion criterion for brief psychotic disorder.

7. How long must the appropriate symptoms be present to meet criteria for a major depressive episode?
   A. 1 week
   B. 2 weeks
   C. 1 month
   D. 2 months

8. Fill in the blank: In order for an adult to meet criteria for major depressive episode, the patient must have either _____ or _____.
   A. Depressed mood or anhedonia
   B. Depressed mood or thoughts of death
   C. Sleep disturbance or thoughts of death
   D. Decreased energy or depressed mood

9. True or False?
   One major depressive episode is sufficient for the diagnosis of major depressive disorder.

10. Which of the following statements is *false*?
    A. Children tend to have more problems with weight loss when depressed than adults do.
    B. Children with depression may have irritability rather than a depressed mood.
    C. Children withdraw more than adults when depressed.
    D. Children often have somatic complaints when depressed.

11. True or False?
    In the DSM-5, a major depressive episode can be diagnosed in someone who lost a loved one less than 2 months ago.

12. A woman presents with depressed mood for 2 years. She reports poor concentration, difficulty sleeping, and poor energy during most of this time. She denies thoughts of death or feelings of worthlessness or guilt. She has never had symptoms of hypomania or mania. Which of the following diagnoses is most likely?
    A. Persistent depressive disorder (formerly dysthymia)
    B. Cyclothymic disorder
    C. Bipolar II disorder
    D. Restricted affectivity

13. **True or False?**
    In certain circumstances, one may be diagnosed with a manic episode even if it appears to have been triggered by medication, such as starting an antidepressant.

14. **True or False?**
    Psychosis is an exclusion criterion for hypomania.

15. **True or False?**
    To be diagnosed with bipolar I disorder, one must have had a major depressive episode.

16. **True or False?**
    Mania is an exclusion criterion for bipolar II disorder.

17. **Which of the following statements is *false*?**
    A. Risk factors for panic attacks include a tendency to experience negative emotions and smoking.
    B. The tendency to consider anxiety symptoms harmful is a risk factor for panic attacks.
    C. Cannabis can trigger a panic attack.
    D. Repeated panic attacks are sufficient to meet criteria for panic disorder.

18. **A 10-year-old boy is brought to the clinic for rages and aggression at school and at home. These outbursts have been occurring multiple times per week for the past 2 years with minor provocation. He is chronically irritable. What is the most likely diagnosis?**
    A. Disruptive mood dysregulation disorder
    B. Conduct disorder
    C. Oppositional defiant disorder
    D. Bipolar II disorder
    E. Intermittent explosive disorder

19. **Which of the following statements is *false*?**
    A. Mood dysregulation is more severe in conduct disorder than in oppositional defiant disorder.
    B. Aggression toward animals is characteristic of conduct disorder but not of oppositional defiant disorder.
    C. Theft is characteristic of conduct disorder but not of oppositional defiant disorder.
    D. Destruction with the intent of to intimidate, or to acquire power or money, is characteristic of conduct disorder but not of oppositional defiant disorder.

20. **A 29-year-old woman has seen six gastroenterologists in the past 7 months for severe abdominal pain and nausea. She cannot sleep because she is concerned about the pain. She spends hours on the Internet researching this condition. She has undergone has an extensive workup, and no abnormalities were found. Which of the following diagnoses is most likely?**
    A. Conversion disorder
    B. Illness anxiety disorder
    C. Body dysmorphic disorder
    D. Factitious disorder
    E. Somatic symptom disorder

21. **True or False?**
    In the DSM-5, amenorrhea is required for the diagnosis of anorexia nervosa.

22. **True or False?**
    Flashbacks are required for the diagnosis of PTSD.

23. **What is the term for the inability to remember information about one's life, especially traumatic events?**
    A. Depersonalization
    B. Derealization
    C. Dissociative identity disorder
    D. Dissociative amnesia

24. **Fill in the blank: A child must be at least _____ years old to be diagnosed with enuresis.**
    A. 3 years old
    B. 5 years old
    C. 8 years old
    D. 10 years old

25. **True or False?**
    Paraphilia is a mental disorder.

26. **Which of the following disorders is *least* likely to be treated with ECT?**
    A. Catatonia
    B. Depression
    C. Post-traumatic stress disorder (PTSD)
    D. Psychosis

27. **A 30-year-old woman reports that she is having difficulty completing tasks at work despite long hours and dedication to the organization. Her coworkers offer to assist, but she does not trust them to do the work as it should be done. She says she is very detail oriented and believes strongly in obeying rules. What is her diagnosis?**
    A. Obsessive-compulsive disorder
    B. Obsessive-compulsive personality disorder
    C. Histrionic personality disorder
    D. Narcissistic personality disorder

28. **True or False?**
    It is possible to have both obsessive-compulsive disorder and obsessive-compulsive personality disorder.

29. **Fill in the blank: Patients with avoidant, dependent, or obsessive-compulsive personality disorders tend to be _____.**
    A. Dramatic
    B. Eccentric
    C. Anxious
    D. Suspicious
    E. Impulsive

30. **Patients with which of the following personality disorders do not desire relationships, prefer solitude, and appear detached?**
    A. Avoidant
    B. Narcissistic
    C. Schizoid
    D. Schizotypal

31. **Which of the following is most characteristic of borderline personality disorder?**
    A. Deceitfulness
    B. Lack of remorse

C. Mood instability
D. Arrogance

32. A patient is diagnosed with an inoperable brain tumor. Instead of grieving, he researches investigational treatments. Which psychological defense is this?
   A. Denial
   B. Intellectualization
   C. Rationalization
   D. Undoing

33. True or False?
   There are situations in which patient confidentiality should be breached.

34. A patient with Parkinson disease is diagnosed with depression. A serotonergic medication should *not* be prescribed if the patient is taking which of the following medications?
   A. Pramipexole
   B. Ropinirole
   C. Selegiline

35. Which selective serotonin reuptake inhibitor (SSRI) has a short half-life, increasing the risk for a withdrawal syndrome?
   A. Citalopram
   B. Fluoxetine
   C. Paroxetine
   D. Sertraline

36. What is the mechanism of action of bupropion?
   A. It is a opamine reuptake inhibitor.
   B. It is a norepinephrine reuptake inhibitor.
   C. It is a serotonin reuptake inhibitor.
   D. A and B
   E. B and C

37. A 20-year-old woman with bulimia is diagnosed with depression. Which of the following antidepressants should be avoided?
   A. Fluoxetine
   B. Sertraline
   C. Bupropion
   D. Escitalopram

38. Which of the following is a serotonin antagonist and reuptake inhibitor (SARI)?
   A. Duloxetine
   B. Mirtazapine
   C. Phenelzine
   D. Trazodone

39. Which of the following is *not* usually a side effect of tricyclic antidepressants (TCAs)?
   A. Dry mouth and urinary retention
   B. Orthostatic hypotension
   C. Memory impairment and delirium
   D. QT-interval prolongation on the ECG
   E. Insomnia

40. A 26-year-old man presents with priapism. He says that his psychiatrist warned him that this could occur when he prescribed the medication. Which medication is most likely responsible?
   A. Venlafaxine
   B. Bupropion
   C. Nefazodone
   D. Trazodone

41. Neuroleptics/conventional antipsychotics treat psychosis by blocking which receptor in the mesolimbic pathway?
   A. D1
   B. D2
   C. D3
   D. D4
   E. D5

42. Which of the following medications is a partial agonist at the D2 and 5-HT$_{1A}$ receptors?
   A. Aripiprazole
   B. Olanzapine
   C. Quetiapine
   D. Ziprasidone

43. Which antipsychotic demonstrates potent α_1-antagonism and causes dose-dependent lengthening of the QT interval?
   A. Iloperidone
   B. Lurasidone
   C. Paliperidone

44. Which of the following statements about clozapine is *false*?
   A. Clozapine can be used to treat psychosis in patients with Parkinson disease.
   B. Clozapine is associated with a risk for agranulocytosis.
   C. Clozapine has a high risk of tardive dyskinesia.
   D. Clozapine lowers the seizure threshold.

45. Which of the following is preferred for short-term treatment of tardive dyskinesia symptoms?
   A. Botulinum toxin
   B. Bromocriptine
   C. Clonazepam
   D. Galantamine

46. Which of the following is *not* usually a side effect of lithium?
   A. Hypokalemia
   B. Polyuria
   C. Hypothyroidism
   D. Weight loss

47. An 18-year-old patient presents with altered mental status, mydriasis, tachycardia, dry mucous membranes, and decreased bowel sounds. Which of the following medications is most likely responsible?
   A. Amitriptyline
   B. Cocaine
   C. Fentanyl
   D. Meperidine

PSYCHIATRY

ANSWERS

1. D

In the DSM-5, the patient can be given a provisional diagnosis if a physician believes strongly that the patient will ultimately meet full criteria for the diagnosis but not enough information is available to make a firm diagnosis.

2. D

The terms *intellectual disability* and *intellectual developmental disorder* have replaced the term mental retardation. To be diagnosed with this condition, the onset must be in the developmental period, and the patient must have intellectual and adaptive functioning deficits. Severity is determined by performance in conceptual, social, and practical domains.

The term global developmental delay is used for individuals younger than 5 years of age when severity cannot be determined. If a child older than 5 years cannot be accurately assessed, the term unspecified intellectual disability (intellectual developmental disorder) can be used.

3. B

Autism spectrum disorder is characterized by deficits in social communication and interaction and limited, repetitive interests and behaviors. Symptoms start early in development and cause difficulties in functioning. The severity of autism spectrum disorder is classified by the level of support needed, which is determined by the individual's social communication level and behaviors. Language delay is *not* required for the diagnosis of autism spectrum disorder in the DSM-5.

Children diagnosed with autistic disorder, Asperger disorder, or pervasive developmental delay not otherwise specified based on DSM-IV criteria will most likely be diagnosed with autism spectrum disorder under the DSM-5 criteria.

If a patient has impaired social communication but does not meet the full criteria for autism spectrum disorder, the diagnosis of social (pragmatic) communication disorder should be considered. These patients have difficulty with verbal and nonverbal social communication but do not have restricted interests and behaviors.

Children with impaired speech production or comprehension, such as decreased vocabulary or difficulty forming sentences, beginning in early development are diagnosed with language disorder.

Autism spectrum disorder can be diagnosed in a patient with intellectual disability if the child's social communication is less developed than would be expected for his or her level of intellectual functioning.

4. C

Patients age 17 years and older need to meet fewer criteria to be diagnosed than younger patients do.

For children younger than 17 years of age, at least six symptoms of either inattention or hyperactivity and impulsivity, lasting at least 6 months, are still needed for the diagnosis. For patients 17 years and older, only five symptoms are needed in the DSM-5. In the DSM-5, ADHD symptoms need to start before age 12 years (instead of age 7 years in the DSM-IV). Patients with autism spectrum disorder can be diagnosed with ADHD.

5. B

This patient has delusional disorder, which is characterized by the presence of a delusion for at least 1 month with normal functioning and behavior (except in relation to the delusion). In DSM-IV, delusional disorder was diagnosed if a patient had a nonbizarre delusion for 1 month (and did not meet the criteria for schizophrenia). In the DSM-5, one can be diagnosed with delusional disorder even if the delusion is bizarre.

6. A

To be diagnosed with brief psychotic disorder, one must have at least one of the following: delusions, hallucinations, and disorganized speech. One may also have disorganized or catatonic behavior. Symptoms are present for longer than 1 day but less than 1 month and then resolve. Negative symptoms are not one of the criteria. Negative symptoms are included in the diagnostic criteria for schizophrenia and schizophreniform disorder.

Duration of symptoms is the main difference between schizophrenia and schizophreniform disorder. In schizophrenia, symptoms have been present for at least 6 months. In schizophreniform disorder, symptoms have been present for at least 1 month but less than 6 months.

Criterion A for diagnosis of schizophrenia or schizophreniform disorder is the presence of at least two of the following for most of 1 month: delusions, hallucinations, disorganized speech, grossly disorganized behavior or catatonia, and negative symptoms. In DSM-IV, only one of these features was required if the delusions were bizarre or the patient experienced hallucinations in which a voice gave running commentary on the patient or two or more voices spoke to each other. In DSM-5, this caveat was removed. A new requirement in DSM-5 is that at least one of the two symptoms required for a diagnosis of schizophrenia must be delusions, hallucinations, or disorganized speech. Also in DSM-5, the subtypes of schizophrenia (e.g. paranoid, disorganized, catatonic) were removed.

Schizoaffective disorder is diagnosed if there is a major mood disturbance concurrent with Criterion A for schizophrenia and if delusions or hallucinations occur for at least 2 weeks independently of mood disturbance. Symptoms that meet the criteria for a major mood episode are present for the majority of the illness.

7. B

Appropriate symptoms must be present for 2 weeks to meet criteria for a major depressive episode.

8. A

Five of the appropriate symptoms are required for an adult to meet criteria for a major depressive episode, but one of those symptoms must be depressed mood or anhedonia. Children and adolescents may have an irritable mood instead of a depressed mood. Other symptoms include weight or appetite changes, sleep disturbance, psychomotor agitation or retardation, decreased energy, guilt or feelings of worthlessness, difficulties with attention or decision making, and thoughts of death. Individuals are considered to have a higher risk for suicide during the 2 years after a suicide attempt.

9. True

One major depressive episode is sufficient for the diagnosis of major depressive disorder, but an episode of hypomania or mania excludes this diagnosis.

10. A

Children tend to have fewer problems with weight loss when depressed than adults do. In children, consider failure to make expected weight gains.

11. True

In the DSM-5, a major depressive episode can be diagnosed in someone who lost a loved one less than 2 months ago (see Table 26.1).

Table 26.1 COMPARISON OF BEREAVEMENT AND MAJOR DEPRESSIVE EPISODE

GRIEF/BEREAVEMENT	MAJOR DEPRESSIVE EPISODE
Feelings of emptiness/loss	Depressed mood, anhedonia
Decreases with time, "pangs of grief" (waves of feelings when thinking of the deceased)	More persistent depressed mood
May have some positive emotions, humor	Self-critical ruminations
Self-esteem preserved	Feelings of worthlessness, self-loathing
Thoughts of death revolve around joining the deceased	Thoughts of death due to worthlessness, thoughts that death will end one's suffering

12. A

This patient most likely has persistent depressive disorder. This term replaces the terms dysthymia and chronic major depressive disorder in the DSM-5. To make the diagnosis, mood must have been depressed most of the time for 2 years in adults. In children, the duration is 1 year, and the mood may be irritable rather than depressed (see Boxes 26.1 and 26.2).

Box 26.1 FEATURES COMMON TO PERSISTENT DEPRESSIVE DISORDER AND MAJOR DEPRESSIVE DISORDER

- Depressed mood
- Change in appetite
- Change in sleep
- Decreased energy
- Poor self-esteem
- Decreased concentration
- Feelings of hopelessness

Box 26.2 CRITERIA FOR MAJOR DEPRESSIVE EPISODE BUT NOT PERSISTENT DEPRESSIVE DISORDER

- Anhedonia
- Psychomotor agitation or retardation
- Feelings of worthlessness or guilt
- Recurrent thoughts of death, suicidal ideation, or suicide attempt or plan

In cyclothymic disorder, the patient has a history of symptoms of hypomania and symptoms of depression lasting for at least 2 years in an adult (or 1 year in a child or adolescent) but has never met criteria for a major depressive, manic, or hypomanic episode.

This patient does not meet criteria for bipolar II disorder because she has never had an episode of hypomania.

Restricted affectivity refers to a decreased emotional response.

13. True

If the patient's symptoms meet the criteria for mania after the physiologic effect of the medication has worn off, then mania can be diagnosed even if it began with starting an antidepressant.

14. True

If a patient is psychotic, he or she has mania, not hypomania (see Box 26.3).

Both mania and hypomania are characterized by mood change and change in energy/activity. Also, both diagnoses require four of the other symptoms if the mood is irritable, or three if it is not.

For a diagnosis of hypomania, the symptoms must have been present for at least 4 days, and the patient must not have marked impairment in functioning or require hospitalization.

For a diagnosis of mania, the symptoms must have been present for 1 week or the patient must have been hospitalized for any duration. Also, the symptoms must cause marked impairment in functioning or require hospitalization. Psychosis also fulfills this requirement.

15. False

One does not have to have had a major depressive episode to be diagnosed with bipolar I disorder, only a manic episode.

16. True

To be diagnosed with bipolar II disorder, the patient must have had a hypomanic episode and a major depressive episode. A manic episode indicates that the patient has bipolar I disorder, not bipolar II disorder.

17. D

To meet criteria for panic disorder, a patient must have, in addition to recurrent, unexpected panic attacks, fear of an attack or the consequences of an attack, or a maladaptive change in behavior to avoid an attack, for at least 1 month.

18. A

This patient has disruptive mood dysregulation disorder, which is a new diagnosis in the DSM-5. The core feature of this diagnosis is chronic and severe irritability. It is characterized by persistent, recurrent temper outbursts that are grossly out of proportion to the situation. The temper outbursts must occur an average of three times a week over the course of a year in at least two settings. The age at onset is less than 10 years, but the diagnosis should not be made in children younger than 6 years of age. Also, the diagnosis of disruptive mood dysregulation disorder should not be made initially after age 18 years. A patient with disruptive mood dysregulation disorder may also be diagnosed with anxiety, depression, or ADHD if they meet criteria. This diagnosis cannot coexist with that of oppositional defiant disorder (ODD), bipolar disorder, or

intermittent explosive disorder. Children with disruptive mood dysregulation disorder are at risk for depression and anxiety, and the diagnosis is listed among the depressive disorders in DSM-5.

ODD is characterized by irritability, defiant behavior, or vindictiveness. Like patients with disruptive mood dysregulation disorder, patients with ODD have irritability and outbursts; however, in patients with ODD, these outbursts are less frequent and less severe.

The absence of hypomania in disruptive mood dysregulation disorder aids in its differentiation from bipolar II disorder. It is hoped that the ability to diagnose disruptive mood dysregulation disorder will prevent overdiagnosis of bipolar disorder.

A patient with intermittent explosive disorder is unable to control outbursts or aggressive behaviors triggered by a minimal stimulus. Patients with intermittent explosive disorder lack the enduring negative mood symptoms found in patients with disruptive mood dysregulation disorder.

Conduct disorder is characterized by premeditated aggression and destruction. Destruction in disruptive mood dysregulation disorder and in intermittent explosive disorder is not premeditated or goal oriented.

19. A

Aggression toward animals or individuals, theft, destruction of property, and deceitfulness help to differentiate conduct disorder from oppositional defiant disorder (ODD). Also, mood dysregulation is characteristic of ODD, not conduct disorder. The absence of mood symptoms in conduct disorder also helps to differentiate it from disruptive mood dysregulation disorder.

20. E

This patient has somatic symptom disorder, which is characterized by excessive concern about somatic symptoms lasting at least 6 months.

The DSM-5 refers to somatoform disorders as somatic symptom and related disorders. The number of disorders has decreased compared with DSM-IV. Hypochondriasis, pain disorder, somatization disorder, and undifferentiated somatoform disorder are not included in DSM-5. Factitious disorder and conversion disorder are included.

In DSM-5, the focus of these disorders is the distress or impairment caused by somatic symptoms. Less emphasis is placed on the lack of medical explanation for the symptoms.

Most of the patients who previously were diagnosed with hypochondriasis will now meet criteria for somatic symptom disorder. Some of the patients who would have been diagnosed with hypochondriasis will now be diagnosed with illness anxiety disorder. These patients have excessive anxiety about their health but do not have somatic symptoms or have only mild symptoms. Patients with more severe somatic symptoms are diagnosed with somatic symptom disorder.

Conversion disorder is also known as functional neurologic symptom disorder. The patient has neurologic symptoms that cannot be explained.

Patients with body dysmorphic disorder are focused on a perceived defect in their appearance.

Factitious disorder is diagnosed when symptoms are consciously feigned, even if there is no obvious reward.

21. False

The criteria for anorexia are restricted intake to the point that the patient has a significantly low weight, fear of gaining weight or behavior that interferes with weight gain, and disturbance in body image. In the DSM-5, amenorrhea is not required for the diagnosis.

There was also a change in the criteria for bulimia nervosa. The minimum frequency of binge-eating and compensatory behavior was reduced from twice weekly to once weekly for 3 months.

22. False

The presence of recurring, distressing dreams or memories can be used to meet criteria for intrusion symptoms, which occur in posttraumatic stress disorder (PTSD). Alternatively, physiologic reactions or psychological distress on exposure to reminders of the trauma can be used to meet criteria for intrusion symptoms. Flashbacks, which are a type of dissociative reaction, are *not* required to meet criteria for PTSD.

23. D

This is dissociative amnesia, which is characterized by inability to recall information about one's life, particularly an event that was stressful. Dissociative amnesia can be a stand-alone diagnosis, or it can be present as a part of other disorders, for example in dissociative identity disorder, which is defined as the presence of at least two personality states.

Depersonalization is the feeling of being detached from one's self, such as feeling as if one is observing one's self from outside one's body.

Derealization is characterized by feeling detached from one's environment or feeling that one's surroundings are distorted or dream-like.

Depersonalization and derealization can occur in depersonalization/derealization disorder, or they can occur in acute stress disorder or PTSD (but are not necessary for diagnosis of those disorders). Acute stress disorder is similar to PTSD, but the duration of the symptoms is 3 days to 1 month. To meet criteria for PTSD, symptoms must last for at least 1 month.

24. B

A child must be at least 5 years old (chronologically or developmentally) to be diagnosed with enuresis. Encopresis can be diagnosed at age 4 years.

25. False

A paraphilia, in itself, is not a mental disorder according to the DSM-5. If it causes distress or impairment, then it is a mental disorder.

26. C

The major use of electroconvulsive therapy (ECT) is for depression. A generalized seizure is needed for ECT to have antidepressive effect. Other uses are for mania, psychosis, and catatonia.

Lithium increases the risk for delirium after the procedure and the risk for prolonged seizure activity. Bupropion and clozapine also lower the seizure threshold. Benzodiazepines increase the seizure threshold.

Headache and muscle soreness are the most common side effects of ECT. Postictal confusion is a concern. Older age, cognitive deficits, and neurologic disease are risk factors for postictal confusion, as are increased ECT intensity, bilateral treatment, greater number of treatments, and more frequent treatments. The impact of ECT on memory is also a concern.

27. B

This patient has obsessive-compulsive personality disorder, which is characterized by inflexibility and perfectionism at the expense of productivity.

Obsessive-compulsive disorder (OCD) is characterized by obsessions and/or compulsions, which do not occur in obsessive-compulsive personality disorder.

Histrionic personality disorder is characterized by increased emotionality and the desire for attention.

28. True

OCD is characterized by obsessions and/or compulsions that consume time and cause distress. Obsessions are recurrent, distressing, intrusive thoughts. The patient may try to negate them by performing repetitive behaviors (compulsions) with rigid requirements.

Obsessions and compulsions are not required for the diagnosis of obsessive-compulsive personality disorder. The essential feature of obsessive-compulsive personality disorder is a preoccupation with orderliness and control at the expense of flexibility and efficiency. Some characteristics of this disorder are preoccupation with rules and schedules, perfectionism that interferes with task completion, extreme devotion to work, inflexibility regarding morals or values, inability to discard useless items, reluctance to delegate tasks, aversion to spending money, and rigidity or stubbornness.

In the DSM-5, obsessive-compulsive personality disorder is not included in the chapter about OCD and related disorders but in the chapter about personality disorders. The chapter about OCD and related disorders includes the diagnoses of OCD, body dysmorphic disorder, and some new diagnoses such as hoarding disorder and excoriation (skin-picking) disorder. Trichotillomania was moved from the chapter on impulse-control disorder in DSM-IV to the chapter on OCD and related disorders in DSM-5.

29. C

Patients with cluster C personality disorders (avoidant, dependent, and obsessive-compulsive personality disorders) tend to be anxious.

Patients with cluster A personality disorders (paranoid, schizoid, and schizotypal personality disorders) tend to be eccentric.

Patients with cluster B personality disorders (antisocial, borderline, histrionic, and narcissistic personality disorders) tend to be dramatic and emotional.

30. C

Patients with schizoid personality disorder do not care about forming relationships, choose to be alone, and seem emotionally cold.

Patients with avoidant personality disorder feel inferior and avoid new relationships and situations because of fear of rejection.

Patients with narcissistic personality disorder have an exaggerated sense of worth, need admiration, and lack empathy.

Patients with schizotypal personality disorder have unusual beliefs and behaviors and do not have close friends.

31. C

Patients with borderline personality disorder have mood instability, a fear of abandonment, and unstable relationships. They are impulsive and may demonstrate suicidal behaviors or self-mutilate. They have disturbance of identity, chronic feelings of emptiness, trouble with anger, and transient stress-related paranoia or dissociative symptoms.

Deceitfulness and lack of remorse are features of antisocial personality disorder.

Arrogance is a feature of narcissistic personality disorder.

32. B

This is intellectualization. Rather than addressing his grief, he is distancing himself from the problem through his research.

Denial is a primitive defense mechanism. If he were using denial as a psychological defense, he would not be able to accept or believe that he had a brain tumor.

Rationalization is an unconscious defense mechanism in which the individual attempts to provide a logical justification for an unacceptable behavior or feeling. The result is giving a false, more acceptable reason for one's behavior.

Undoing is a primitive defense mechanism in which an action is performed to counteract a prior behavior for which one feels guilty.

33. True

The Tarasoff rule indicates that there is a duty to protect a person from injury if a psychiatric patient has indicated that he or she plans to harm the person. In such a case, confidentiality may be breached.

34. C

Selegiline is a monoamine oxidase B (MAO-B) inhibitor. However, at higher doses, it can also inhibit monoamine oxidase A (MAO-A). The combination of an MAO-A inhibitor and a serotonergic medication can result in serotonin syndrome.

35. C

Paroxetine has a short half-life, which results in an increased risk for withdrawal symptoms. Abrupt discontinuation of an SSRI can cause discontinuation syndrome, which is characterized by dizziness, anxiety, nausea, headache, and irritability. Its withdrawal effects may also be related to the fact that it inhibits its own metabolism. When the drug is withdrawn, its rate of decline in the body can become faster because this self-inhibition ends.

Fluoxetine has a long half-life, as does its major metabolite. Therefore, there is a low risk for discontinuation syndrome. However, one must wait a long time (at least 5 weeks) between discontinuing fluoxetine and starting a monoamine oxidase inhibitor.

36. D

Bupropion (Wellbutrin) is a norepinephrine-dopamine reuptake inhibitor (NDRI). It does not have serotonergic activity. Its structure is similar to that of a stimulant. As a result, a patient taking bupropion who undergoes urine drug screening can test positive for amphetamines, depending on the screen used.

37. C

Bupropion lowers the seizure threshold and should not be used in patients with bulimia. It is much less likely than SSRIs to have sexual side effects. It has been used to treat ADHD and for smoking cessation.

38. D

Trazodone is a serotonin antagonist and reuptake inhibitor (SARI). It is an antagonist to the serotonin 5-HT$_2$ receptor.

Duloxetine, venlafaxine, and desvenlafaxine are serotonin-norepinephrine reuptake inhibitors (SNRIs). In addition to treating anxiety and depression, duloxetine has been used to treat diabetic peripheral neuropathy. It can cause nausea. SNRIs and tricyclic antidepressants, such as imipramine, bind the serotonin transporter (SERT) and the norepinephrine transporter (NET).

Mirtazapine (Remeron) is a noradrenergic and specific serotonergic antidepressant (NaSSA). It increases release of serotonin and norepinephrine It does not inhibit serotonin reuptake. Mirtazapine causes sedation, so it is used to treat patients with concomitant insomnia. It also causes weight gain.

Phenelzine, tranylcypromine, and selegiline are monoamine oxidase inhibitors.

39. E

TCAs tend to cause sedation and weight gain because of their antihistamine (anti-H1) effect. TCAs include amitriptyline, nortriptyline, imipramine, desipramine, clomipramine, amoxapine, and doxepin. TCAs have anticholinergic side effects, such as dry mouth and urinary retention. TCAs can cause cardiac arrhythmias and can be lethal in overdose (see Box 26.4).

Box 26.4 MECHANISMS OF ACTION OF TRICYCLIC ANTIDEPRESSANTS

- Serotonin reuptake inhibition
- Norepinephrine reuptake inhibition
- Anticholinergic effects (central and peripheral)
- Antihistamine effects (central and peripheral)
- Peripheral α_1-antagonism
- Fast sodium channel blockade

---

40. D

Trazodone rarely can cause priapism. It is indicated for major depression and is used for insomnia because it is sedating.

Trazodone can cause a false-positive test for amphetamines on urine drug screening.

41. B

Neuroleptics treat psychosis by blocking D2 receptors in the mesolimbic pathway.

Blockage of D2 receptors in the tuberoinfundibular pathway can cause hyperprolactinemia, and blockage of D2 receptors in the nigrostriatal pathway can cause extrapyramidal symptoms. Atypical antipsychotics (with the exception of risperidone) tend to have less risk for extrapyramidal side effects and hyperprolactinemia than conventional antipsychotics.

Most atypical antipsychotics (also referred to as second-generation antipsychotics) are serotonin-dopamine antagonists; they antagonize the 5-HT$_{2A}$ receptor as well as the D2 receptor. The atypical antipsychotics also act more specifically on the mesolimbic rather than striatal pathways. An antipsychotic that is a partial agonist at the 5-HT$_{1A}$ receptor or at the D2 receptor is also called atypical.

Antipsychotics also act at multiple other receptors. Some have anticholinergic side effects such as dry mouth, urinary retention, constipation, and blurred vision. The neuroleptics with potent anticholinergic effects tend to have less extrapyramidal symptoms.

Alpha-adrenergic blockade can cause orthostatic hypotension and drowsiness. Blockage of histamine H1 receptors causes sedation.

Low-potency neuroleptics tend to have more anticholinergic, antihistaminic, and α_1-antagonist properties than high-potency neuroleptics; therefore, they tend to be more sedating and to cause more weight gain. They also cause orthostatic hypotension more frequently. Chlorpromazine (Thorazine) and thioridazine (Mellaril) are low-potency antipsychotics. Haloperidol and pimozide (Orap) are high-potency neuroleptics.

42. A

As discussed earlier, atypical antipsychotics may be antagonists at the 5-HT$_{2A}$ receptor, partial agonists at the D2 receptor, or partial agonists at the 5-HT$_{1A}$ receptor. Most are antagonists at the 5-HT$_{2A}$ receptor. Aripiprazole (Abilify) is a partial agonist at the D2 and 5-HT$_{1A}$ receptors, as well as an antagonist of the 5-HT$_{2A}$ receptor. It has a relatively lower risk for extrapyramidal symptoms than most antipsychotics. Antagonism of the 5-HT$_{2A}$ receptor may improve negative symptoms of schizophrenia. Aripiprazole does not have significant anticholinergic activity but does have antihistaminergic and antiadrenergic activity. There is a relatively low risk of dyslipidemia.

In addition to antagonizing multiple receptors, including the D2 and 5HT$_{2A}$ receptors, Ziprasidone (Geodon) also inhibits norepinephrine and serotonin reuptake. There is a lower risk compared with other antipsychotics for weight gain, insulin resistance, and dyslipidemia.

43. A

Iloperidone, lurasidone, and paliperidone are all atypical antipsychotics; they are antagonists at the D2 and 5-HT$_{2A}$ receptors.

Iloperidone (Fanapt) demonstrates potent α_1-antagonism. It has a low metabolic risk and a low risk for extrapyramidal symptoms, but it does cause dose-dependent lengthening of the QT interval. It is metabolized by CYP2D6 and CYP3A4.

Lurasidone (Latuda) is a strong antagonist of the 5-HT$_7$ receptor. It does not significantly increase glucose or lipids and does not affect the QT interval as much as many other antipsychotics do.

Paliperidone (Invega) is an active metabolite of risperidone; however, it is not metabolized in the liver.

44. C

Clozapine, which is a weak D2 antagonist and a strong 5-HT$_{2A}$ antagonist, can be used for psychotic patients who are at increased risk of extrapyramidal side effects (EPS), including patients with Parkinson disease who develop psychosis. It has a lower risk for EPS and tardive dyskinesia than most antipsychotics. It is one of the most effective treatments for psychosis in patients for whom other antipsychotic medications have failed. However, it lowers the seizure threshold and can cause agranulocytosis. It does not increase prolactin. Relative to other atypical antipsychotics, it has more anticholinergic side effects and tends to cause more weight gain.

Olanzapine (Zyprexa) is structurally similar to clozapine; however, it has less risk for agranulocytosis and seizures. Similar to clozapine, olanzapine has less risk for EPS than most antipsychotics. Both clozapine and olanzapine carry a very high risk for weight gain.

Quetiapine (Seroquel), which has structural similarities to olanzapine and clozapine, also has a low risk for EPS. Quetiapine's receptor binding properties depend on the dose. The immediate-release formulation blocks H1 receptors quickly, causing sedation. In order to bind D2 receptors for a full day without high dosing, twice-daily doses of the immediate formulation of quetiapine or once-daily doses of the extended-release formulation may be needed. Quetiapine is unlikely to increase prolactin levels.

CYP1A2, which metabolizes olanzapine and clozapine, is induced by smoking. Therefore, smokers may need higher doses of these medications. Fluvoxamine inhibits CYP1A2 and can raise the level of clozapine, which can increase the risk for seizures.

45. C

Of the options listed, clonazepam is preferred for short-term treatment of tardive dyskinesia symptoms. Evidence does not support the use of diltiazem, eicosapentaenoic acid, or galantamine for this purpose, and there is insufficient evidence to support the use of botulinum toxin, bromocriptine, vitamin E, vitamin B6, α-methyldopa, or reserpine.

There is some evidence that ginkgo biloba is useful in the treatment of tardive syndromes in inpatients with schizophrenia. There is weak evidence that amantadine decreases tardive syndromes when given with neuroleptics in the short term. Tetrabenazine may possibly decrease tardive symptoms. Clozapine has been effective in decreasing severe tardive dyskinesia, but symptoms often recur if it is discontinued.[1]

46. D

Lithium can cause weight gain. It can also cause diarrhea, tremor, edema, acne, and nephrogenic diabetes insipidus. Lithium toxicity can result in seizures and arrhythmias.

The cardiac effects of lithium resemble those of hypokalemia on the ECG (i.e., T-wave flattening or inversion). Lithium can be teratogenic.

Most diuretics and angiotensin-conversion enzyme (ACE) inhibitors increase the risk of lithium toxicity. An encephalopathic syndrome has been reported in patients who received the combination of lithium and haloperidol. Dehydration can also lead to increased levels of lithium, which can result in toxicity.

47. A

Cocaine, amphetamines, anticholinergics, antihistamines, sympathomimetics, thyroid hormone, and theophylline can produce tachycardia. Decreased bowel sounds are characteristic of anticholinergic medications. This patient most likely ingested amitriptyline, which is a tricyclic antidepressant (TCA). TCAs produce anticholinergic side effects, such as mydriasis and dry mucous membranes, in addition to tachycardia and absent bowel sounds. Sodium bicarbonate is sometimes used in treatment of TCA poisoning.

Fentanyl and meperidine are opioids. Opiate toxicity causes somnolence, pupillary miosis, respiratory depression, and decreased bowel sounds. Opiates can also cause flash pulmonary edema. Meperidine also can cause seizures.

SUPPLEMENTARY INFORMATION

Table 26.2 CHARACTERISTIC FEATURES OF SELECTIVE SEROTONIN REUPTAKE INHIBITORS (SSRIS)

SSRI	CHARACTERISTIC FEATURES
Citalopram	Risk for QTc prolongation at higher doses, mild antihistaminergic activity
Escitalopram	Low risk of CYP-mediated drug interactions, no antihistaminergic activity
Fluoxetine	Long half-life, $5\text{-}HT_{2C}$ antagonist, tends to be activating
Fluvoxamine	Sigma-1 receptor binding
Paroxetine	Short half-life, high risk for withdrawal reaction, muscarinic anticholinergic activity and norepinephrine transporter inhibition
Sertraline	Dopamine transporter inhibition and sigma-1 receptor binding can be activating

Table 26.3   CHARACTERISTIC FEATURES OF ANTIPSYCHOTICS

ANTIPSYCHOTIC	CHARACTERISTIC FEATURES
Aripiprazole (Abilify)	Partial agonist at the D2 and 5-HT$_{1A}$ receptors
Clozapine (Clozaril)	Agranulocytosis, seizure risk, weight gain, anticholinergic side effects
Iloperidone (Fanapt)	Dose related QT prolongation, potent α_1-antagonism
Lurasidone (Latuda)	Antagonist at 5-HT$_7$ receptor, low risk of weight gain, low risk of QT prolongation
Olanzapine (Zyprexa)	Strong potency at H1 and 5-HT$_{2A}$ receptors, weight gain
Quetiapine (Seroquel)	Binding properties depend on the dose
Paliperidone (Invega)	Active metabolite of risperidone, not hepatically metabolized
Risperidone (Risperdal)	At higher doses can cause extrapyramidal symptoms, similar to conventional antipsychotics.
Ziprasidone (Geodon)	Inhibits norepinephrine and serotonin reuptake; weight gain and dyslipidemia are not commonly an issue

REFERENCE

1. Bhidayasiri R, Fahn S, Weiner WJ, et al. Evidence-based guideline: Treatment of tardive syndromes. Report of the Guideline Development Subcommittee of the American Academy of Neurology. *Neurology* 2013;81:463–469.

27.

SLEEP DISORDERS

QUESTIONS

1. Which of the following statements is *false*?
   A. Infants spend a greater amount of time asleep than adults do, and they spend a greater portion of the time in REM sleep.
   B. Sleep efficiency decreases with age.
   C. The elderly spend more time in stage N3 sleep than younger adults do.
   D. Neonates enter sleep through the REM stage.

2. Which of the following statements is *false*?
   A. Excessive daytime sleepiness is noted when a person sleeps in an atypical setting or falls asleep unintentionally.
   B. Alcohol and sleep deprivation increase snoring.
   C. The STOP-BANG questions are a method of screening for obstructive sleep apnea.
   D. Portable polysomnogram monitoring should be considered for all patients who are being evaluated for classic polysomnograms.

3. Which of the following symptoms is *least* suggestive of obstructive sleep apnea (OSA)?
   A. Arousals due to choking
   B. Awakening diaphoretic
   C. Morning headaches
   D. Morning vomiting

4. Which of the following statements is *false*?
   A. A sleep study should be done for OSA only if the patient's teacher or parent reports that the patient appears sleepy.
   B. Children with OSA are more likely to have partial obstruction than complete obstruction.
   C. Adenotonsillar enlargement frequently is found in children with OSA.
   D. Pediatric criteria for OSA require fewer respiratory disturbances per hour than the adult criteria do.

5. Which of the following statements is *false*?
   A. Paradoxical insomnia occurs when patients have slept but think they have been awake.
   B. In order to diagnose insomnia, there should be an impact on daytime activities.
   C. Circadian rhythm disorders may be mistaken for insomnia or excessive sleepiness.
   D. With chronic sleep deprivation, one's perception of sleepiness is impaired.
   E. A polysomnogram should not be ordered for OSA unless there is at least mild snoring.

6. A 20-year-old patient presents with sleepiness. He is afraid he's going to lose his job because he falls asleep at work. When he awakens in the morning, he feels refreshed but for a brief period feels as if he can't move. Also, he's been falling when he laughs. Which abnormality of the cerebrospinal fluid (CSF) is most closely associated with this condition?
   A. Increased protein
   B. Decreased glucose
   C. Decreased orexin
   D. Increased hypocretin
   E. Decreased serotonin

7. True or False?
   Patients with narcolepsy are instructed to avoid naps in the daytime to improve sleep quality at night.

8. A 60-year-old man is brought to the office by his wife. The wife reports that her husband has been awakening from sleep and tackling her and the furniture. Afterward, he tells her he's been dreaming of football. What is the most likely diagnosis?
   A. Confusional arousals
   B. REM sleep behavior disorder
   C. Sleepwalking
   D. Sleep terrors

9. A 30-year-old patient presents with difficulty sleeping due to an uncomfortable feeling in her legs. The feeling makes her want to move her legs and is worse in the evening. Which of the following laboratory tests should be performed?
   A. Vitamin B12 level
   B. Ferritin level
   C. Folate level
   D. Hemoglobin electrophoresis

10. Which of the following medications is used *least often* to treat restless leg syndrome?
    A. Benzodiazepines
    B. Calcium channel alpha-2-delta ligands
    C. Dopaminergic agents
    D. Opioids
    E. Selective serotonin reuptake inhibitors (SSRIs)

11. A mother brings her 6-year-old son to the clinic because of events that happen at night. The patient wakes up about 2 hours after going to sleep and screams. He appears scared. He is tachycardic and diaphoretic. His mother cannot console him. In the morning, he

has no memory of the event. What is the most likely diagnosis?

A. Sleep terror disorder
B. Nightmares
C. REM sleep behavior disorder
D. Restless leg syndrome

12. Which of the following is *not* a risk factor for somnambulism (sleep walking)?

A. Sleep deprivation
B. Zolpidem
C. Stress
D. Genetic susceptibility
E. Clonazepam

13. A 16-year-old boy is brought to clinic because of sleepiness during the day. He says he does not become sleepy until 2 A.M. School starts at 7:30 A.M. He has been chastised for falling asleep in school. On weekends, he sleeps until 4 P.M. He says he sleeps well once he falls asleep. He denies caffeine intake in the afternoon. Which of the following diagnoses should be considered?

A. Advanced sleep phase disorder
B. Delayed sleep phase disorder
C. Irregular sleep-wake rhythm disorder

14. What is the mechanism of action of ramelteon?

A. Benzodiazepine receptor agonist
B. Selective histamine H1 receptor antagonist
C. Selective melatonin receptor agonist
D. Glutamate agonist

15. Which of the following medications does *not* increase slow-wave sleep?

A. Zolpidem
B. Gabapentin
C. Mirtazapine
D. Pregabalin
E. Trazodone

16. Which of the following medications is most helpful in treating sleep maintenance insomnia?

A. Doxepin
B. Ramelteon
C. Zaleplon
D. Zolpidem oral spray

17. Which of the following is the best description of hypersomnia in an adult?

A. Sleeping more than 10 hours per night
B. Sleeping more than 12 hours per night
C. Excessive daytime sleepiness and difficulty maintaining alertness when awake
D. Feeling fatigued

18. Which of the following is *not* characteristic of REM sleep?

A. Low muscle tone on submental EMG
B. Sawtooth waves
C. Low-amplitude, mixed-frequency EEG

D. Increase in epileptiform activity
E. Irregular breathing

19. Which of the following is *least* likely to cause sleep-onset REM?

A. Circadian rhythm disorder
B. Deprivation of REM sleep
C. Withdrawal of medications that suppress REM
D. Fluoxetine

20. Which of the following statements is *false*?

A. Central apnea is the absence of effort to breathe.
B. In exploding head syndrome, one hears an explosion sound as one falls asleep.
C. Sleep drunkenness is unsteadiness caused by severe sleep deprivation.
D. Hypnic headaches occur outside of REM sleep.

21. Which of the following statements is *false*?

A. Tricyclic antidepressants (TCAs), monoamine oxidase inhibitors (MAOIs), and SSRIs can cause behavior similar to that seen with REM sleep behavior disorder.
B. Cognitive behavioral therapy is not helpful in treating insomnia.
C. Melatonin at night and bright light in the morning can be used to treat circadian rhythm disturbances.
D. Treatment of restless leg syndrome with dopamine agonists can result in worsening of symptoms earlier in the day or symptoms in the morning.

22. Which of the following statements is *false*?

A. Sleep-disordered breathing is a risk factor for stroke.
B. The majority of patients with resistant hypertension have OSA.
C. Sleep disturbance occurs in the majority of patients with Huntington disease.
D. Patients with cluster headache do not have an increased risk of OSA.

23. To be diagnosed with enuresis, a child should be at least _____ years old.

A. Three
B. Five
C. Seven
D. Eight

24. Which of the following statements regarding the comparison of nocturnal frontal lobe seizures and non-REM parasomnias is *false*?

A. Seizures are more stereotyped.
B. Seizures may occur many times in the night.
C. Seizures tend to be shorter.
D. Non-REM parasomnias usually occur during the few hours before the patient awakens.

25. Which of the following is *not* a non-REM sleep disorder?

A. Confusional arousals
B. Sleepwalking
C. Sleep terrors
D. Recurrent isolated sleep paralysis

26. **Which of the following symptoms is most helpful in differentiating sleep terrors from other parasomnias?**
    A. Sympathetic activation
    B. Confusion after the event
    C. Duration

27. **Where are circadian rhythms generated?**
    A. Pulvinar nucleus of the thalamus
    B. Anterior nucleus of the thalamus
    C. Suprachiasmatic nucleus of the hypothalamus
    D. Arcuate nucleus of the hypothalamus

28. **Why do patients with Alzheimer disease have sleep-wake disturbances?**
    A. There is damage to cholinergic neurons in the suprachiasmatic nucleus and the ventrolateral preoptic nucleus.
    B. There is damage to the ventral arcuate nucleus and the pre-Bötzinger complex of the medulla.
    C. There is damage to the sublaterodorsal tegmental nucleus.

29. **During sleep, neurons in the arousal system are inhibited by which neurotransmitter?**
    A. Dopamine
    B. GABA
    C. Glycine
    D. Histamine
    E. Serotonin

30. **Which of the following inhibit the arousal system during sleep?**
    A. Parabrachial nucleus
    B. Ventral periaqueductal gray matter
    C. Ventrolateral preoptic nuclei and median preoptic nuclei (VLPO and MNPO)

31. **Where are the neurons that generate REM sleep?**
    A. Dorsal raphe
    B. Locus coeruleus
    C. Subcoeruleus area/sublaterodorsal nucleus and precoeruleus region of the pons
    D. Tuberomammillary nucleus

32. **Which areas of the brain are responsible for stopping REM, acting as the REM-off center?**
    A. Ventrolateral periaqueductal gray matter and lateral pontine tegmentum (vlPAG/LPT)
    B. Ventrolateral preoptic nuclei (VLPO)
    C. Laterodorsal tegmental nuclei (LDT)
    D. Pedunculopontine tegmental nuclei (PPT)

33. **Sleep diaries are most helpful for diagnosing which of the following conditions?**
    A. Circadian rhythm disorders
    B. Obstructive sleep apnea
    C. Restless leg syndrome
    D. REM sleep behavior disorder

34. **Actigraphy is most helpful for diagnosing which of the following conditions?**
    A. Circadian rhythm disorders
    B. Obstructive sleep apnea
    C. REM sleep behavior disorder
    D. Restless leg syndrome

35. **Which of the following statements is *false*?**
    A. The Multiple Sleep Latency Test (MSLT) is helpful in any age group.
    B. A mean sleep latency of less than 8 minutes plus at least two sleep-onset REM events is consistent with the diagnosis of narcolepsy.
    C. A polysomnogram is done the night before an MSLT; however, a polysomnogram is not required the night before a maintenance of wakefulness test.

36. **The parents of a 15-year-old boy report that for the past week he has awakened only to eat, and during that time he eats an extremely large amount. On further questioning, they state that this behavior has occurred on two other occasions in the past year. During the episodes, he is confused and apathetic. What is his diagnosis?**
    A. Narcolepsy
    B. Kleine-Levin syndrome
    C. Ondine's curse
    D. Advanced sleep phase syndrome

SLEEP DISORDERS

ANSWERS

1. C

Newborns sleep for approximately 16 to 20 hours per day. They spend about 50% of the time asleep in rapid-eye-movement (REM) sleep, and they enter sleep through REM. Adults usually enter sleep through stage N1, and REM does not occur until approximately 60 to 90 minutes after sleep onset.

Sleep efficiency decreases with age. There is an increase in the number of awakenings as one becomes older.

The elderly spend more time in stage N2 sleep than younger adults do. They spend little time in stage N3.

2. D

Patients with excessive daytime sleepiness may fall asleep in an atypical setting or fall asleep unintentionally. There are a multitude of etiologies, such as medical (including psychiatric) disorders, disorders related to medications or other substances, and sleep-related disorders. The cause may be too little sleep, poor-quality sleep, or a primary hypersomnia.

Obstructive sleep apnea (OSA) is a common cause of excessive daytime sleepiness. The STOP-BANG questionnaire screens for OSA. Snoring is just one criterion (see Box 27.1).[1] In addition to anatomic features, a number of other factors can contribute to snoring, including sleep deprivation and alcohol use. Polysomnography is used to diagnose OSA. Some patients are eligible for portable polysomnography. However, patients with certain pulmonary, cardiac, and neuromuscular diseases are not eligible.

Box 27.1 THE STOP-BANG QUESTIONNAIRE (SCREEN FOR OBSTRUCTIVE SLEEP APNEA) CRITERIA

- **S**noring loudly
- **T**iredness during the day
- **O**bserved apnea
- **P**ressure (blood) is elevated.
- **B**ody mass index (BMI) >35
- **A**ge >50 years
- **N**eck circumference >40 cm
- **G**ender is male.

3. D

Morning vomiting is concerning for increased intracranial pressure.

Symptoms of OSA include diaphoresis, a dry mouth on awakening, morning headaches, and arousals due to choking.

OSA is associated with cognitive impairment; cardiovascular, cerebrovascular, and endocrine diseases; pulmonary hypertension; and increased mortality.

4. A

Children with OSA may not appear sleepy. They may be hyperactive.

Adenotonsillar enlargement is common in children with OSA. Often, children continue to have some degree of OSA after tonsillectomy and adenoidectomy.

Allergies are a more common cause of OSA in children than in adults. Craniofacial abnormalities and decreased upper airway tone also contribute to OSA in children. For instance, patients with Pierre Robin syndrome, which causes micrognathia, are at increased risk. Patients with Down syndrome have a number of anatomic abnormalities that contribute to OSA, such as macroglossia, upper airway hypotonia, and micrognathia. Patients with cleft palate, choanal atresia, achondroplasia, Prader-Willi syndrome, mucopolysaccharidoses, Apert syndrome, Crouzon syndrome, hypothyroidism, or Chiari malformations are also at increased risk for OSA.

In children with OSA, intermittent or prolonged partial obstruction is more common than the recurrent obstruction seen in adults. The diagnosis of adult OSA requires an apnea-hypopnea index (AHI) of at least 5 events per hour, but for children the diagnosis requires an AHI greater than 1.

5. E

Some patients cannot snore. For instance, some patients with neuromuscular conditions are unable to produce enough force to cause snoring. Therefore, lack of snoring does not rule out OSA.

Insomnia is difficulty falling asleep or staying asleep to the point that there is daytime impairment. Multiple factors contribute to insomnia.

Paradoxical insomnia occurs when patients believe they have been awake but actually have been sleeping. Actigraphy and polysomnography can aid in this diagnosis.

6. C

This patient most likely has narcolepsy, which is associated with low levels of hypocretin/orexin in the CSF.

Narcolepsy is accompanied by the following symptoms: excessive daytime sleepiness, cataplexy, hypnagogic or hypnopompic hallucinations, and sleep paralysis. Patients do not have to have all of the symptoms. To meet criteria, the duration of excessive daytime sleepiness should be at least 3 months.

Patients with narcolepsy can have disrupted sleep at night, including difficulty going to sleep. Most patients who have narcolepsy with cataplexy, now called narcolepsy type 1, are positive for the HLA-DQB1*0602 genotype. Narcolepsy is diagnosed with a sleep study that includes a Multiple Sleep Latency Test (MSLT), looking for mean sleep latency of 8 minutes or less and two or more sleep-onset REM episodes during naps. A decreased CSF hypocretin level can verify the diagnosis of narcolepsy type 1.

7. False

Treatment for narcolepsy includes trying to improve sleep at night and, if possible, taking short naps in the afternoon.

Stimulants have been used to promote wakefulness in patients with narcolepsy, but modafinil and armodafinil have fewer cardiac side effects. Sodium oxybate (β-hydroxybutyrate, or GHB), selective serotonin reuptake inhibitors (SSRIs), serotonin-norepinephrine reuptake inhibitors (SNRIs), and tricyclic antidepressants (TCAs) are helpful for cataplexy.

8. B

This patient has REM sleep behavior disorder (RBD), which is characterized by recurrent episodes of dream-enactment. In contrast to sleep walking, the eyes are usually closed with RBD. Since the events occur during REM sleep, they are more common in the second half of the night, when REM sleep is more prominent (unless the patient also has narcolepsy). The normal atonia characteristic of REM sleep is not present in patients with RBD.

RBD is much more prominent in men than in women. It tends to occur in patients older than 55 years of age. Patients with synucleinopathies (e.g., Parkinson disease) are at risk for RBD. Likewise, patients with RBD are at risk for synucleinopathies.

Patients with RBD should be prevented from hurting themselves or their bed partners. Melatonin and clonazepam are useful in treating RBD. Pramipexole has also been used.

Medications can also trigger RBD. These include serotonin-norepinephrine reuptake inhibitors (SNRIs) such as venlafaxine, tricyclic antidepressants (TCAs), selective serotonin reuptake inhibitors (SSRIs), and monoamine oxidase inhibitors (MAOIs). Withdrawal of REM-suppressing medications can also produce RBD. Alcohol, drugs, and caffeine can contribute to RBD.

9. B

This patient most likely has restless leg syndrome (RLS), which may be caused by iron deficiency. The patient's ferritin level should be checked. If it is low, an iron supplement should be prescribed.

RLS is characterized by a need to move the legs, especially in the evening. The patient may have an uncomfortable sensation in the legs. Symptoms are worse when the patient is at rest and improve with activity.

RLS is more common in women than in men. Multiple genes have been linked to RLS, most commonly *BTBD9* on chromosome 6. Conditions associated with RLS include pregnancy, peripheral neuropathy, and end-stage renal disease. Caffeine, nicotine, and alcohol worsen RLS. Also, dopamine antagonists, opioid withdrawal, and benzodiazepine withdrawal can worsen it.

RLS is frequently associated with increased periodic limb movements in sleep, but polysomnography is not required to diagnose RLS.

10. E

Benzodiazepines, calcium channel alpha-2-delta ligands, dopaminergic agents, and opioids are used to treat restless leg syndrome (RLS). SSRIs can worsen RLS. Bupropion does not.

Calcium channel alpha-2-delta ligands include gabapentin and pregabalin. They can cause sleepiness and weight gain.

Dopaminergic agents such as pramipexole and ropinirole can cause nausea, sudden sleepiness, postural hypotension, leg edema, and impulse-control disorders such as compulsive gambling or shopping. Augmentation can also occur with dopaminergic agents. For instance, symptoms may begin earlier in the evening, involve additional areas of the body, or worsen.

11. A

This patient has sleep terrors disorder, which occurs most frequently between 4 and 12 years of age and usually resolves during adolescence. It can occur in adulthood, most often between 20 and 30 years of age. Sleep terrors occur out of slow-wave sleep and are more common during the first half of the night. Patients with sleep terrors appear terrified; demonstrate autonomic activation such as tachycardia, tachypnea, or diaphoresis; and cannot be consoled. If they are awakened, they are confused. They do not have memory of the event.

12. E

Clonazepam is a treatment for severe cases of somnambulism.

Somnambulism usually begins during the first decade of life, but it can begin in adulthood. It typically occurs out of slow-wave sleep; therefore, it is more prominent in the first third of the night. Patients appear confused when getting out of bed and are confused if awakened. Their eyes are open during the event.

Genetics may contribute. If one or both parents have a history of somnambulism, the child is at increased risk. Sleep deprivation is one of the most common risk factors for somnambulism. Alcohol and stress also increase one's risk. Medications that can precipitate somnambulism include hypnotics, antihistamines, anticholinergics, sodium oxybate, stimulants, and lithium. Zolpidem can cause amnesia, sleep walking, sleep driving, and sleep eating.

Sleep hygiene and stress management are used to treat sleep walking. For severe cases, benzodiazepines may be used.

13. B

Circadian rhythm sleep disorders are characterized by chronic difficulty being awake or asleep at appropriate times. Examples include advanced sleep phase disorder, delayed sleep phase disorder, jet lag disorder, non-24-hour sleep-wake disorder, irregular sleep-wake rhythm disorder, and shift work disorder. Patients with advanced sleep phase disorder fall asleep early in the evening and wake up early in the morning. Patients with delayed sleep phase disorder cannot fall asleep until late at night and then sleep late. Patients with irregular sleep-wake rhythm disorder have disorganized sleep. They have multiple sleep and wake periods within 24 hours.

Treatments for circadian rhythm sleep disorder include chronotherapy, in which the time at which one goes to sleep is gradually changed; carefully timed phototherapy; and melatonin. In addition, night shift workers should nap before their shift and may benefit from stimulants such as caffeine or modafinil during their shift.

14. C

Ramelteon is a treatment for sleep-onset insomnia. It is a selective melatonin receptor agonist. Melatonin receptors are prevalent in the suprachiasmatic nucleus. Ramelteon should not be prescribed to patients who are taking fluvoxamine.

15. A

Zolpidem (Ambien) does not increase slow-wave sleep. Gabapentin, mirtazapine, pregabalin, and trazodone do increase slow-wave sleep.

16. A

Doxepin is a selective histamine H1 receptor antagonist. It is used for sleep maintenance. It should be avoided in patients who are taking monoamine oxidase inhibitors (MAOIs).

Ramelteon is a selective melatonin receptor agonist. It is used for sleep-onset insomnia. Zaleplon and zolpidem are benzodiazepine receptor agonists that are not themselves benzodiazepines. They are also useful for sleep initiation. There is an extended-release formulation of zolpidem that is more helpful for sleep maintenance than the oral spray formulation.

Diphenhydramine is in many over-the-counter sleep aids. It is an antihistamine and has anticholinergic side effects.

17. C

The number of required hours of sleep varies from person to person. Therefore, the definition of hypersomnia is not based on the duration of time asleep. Hypersomnia refers to the inability to maintain alertness during waking hours.

Fatigue is not synonymous with sleepiness. It more indicative of lack of energy.

18. D

Usually there is less epileptiform activity during REM sleep than during other stages of sleep (see Box 27.2).

Box 27.2 FEATURES OF REM SLEEP

- Low or absent muscle tone on submental electromyography (EMG)
- Rapid eye movements
- Sawtooth waves (sharply-contoured waves over the central leads in the theta frequency range)
- Low voltage, mixed frequency electroencephalography (EEG)
- Irregular breathing
- Decrease in epileptiform activity
- Somatic muscle atonia

---

19. D

There are a number of conditions or situations in which a patient without narcolepsy can have sleep-onset REM. Examples include sleep deprivation or deprivation of REM sleep, circadian rhythm disorder, and withdrawal of medications that suppress REM.

SSRIs such as fluoxetine; TCAs such as protriptyline and imipramine; and the SNRI venlafaxine suppress REM. They have been used in the treatment of cataplexy.

20. C

Sleep drunkenness is difficulty being alert after a long period of sleep.

Hypnic headache is a primary headache disorder that occurs in older adults. Patients describe a throbbing headache, which may be unilateral or bilateral. Hypnic headaches begin during REM sleep.

21. B

Cognitive-behavioral therapy is helpful in treating insomnia. There are a number of different types of behavioral therapy, such as sleep restriction therapy, relaxation therapy, and stimulus control therapy. During sleep restriction therapy, the patient limits the amount of time spent in bed in order to reduce the time to sleep onset. During stimulus control therapy, the bed is used almost exclusively for sleep, and the patient lies down on it only when sleepy.

22. D

Patients with cluster headache do have an increased risk of OSA. The risk is even greater if the patient is overweight. Treatment of OSA in these patients may result in improvement in their cluster headaches.

Patients who have had a transient ischemic attack (TIA) or stroke should be assessed for sleep-disordered breathing, which is a risk factor for stroke.

23. B

To be diagnosed with enuresis, the child should be at least 5 years of age.

There is a link between OSA and enuresis. Enuresis may have a genetic component.

24. D

Non-REM parasomnias usually occur in the first half of the night, when non-REM sleep predominates.

Most nocturnal frontal lobe seizures occur outside of non-REM sleep, usually in stage N2, but they can occur at any time of the night. They are brief, are stereotyped, may occur multiple times per night, and are not typically associated with postevent confusion. These features aid in distinguishing them from non-REM parasomnias. Sometimes no EEG correlate is seen with nocturnal frontal lobe seizures, so EEG does not always differentiate the entities.

25. D

Recurrent isolated sleep paralysis is a REM sleep disorder (see Boxes 27.3 and 27.4).

Box 27.3 NON-REM SLEEP DISORDERS

- Confusional arousals
- Sleep terrors
- Sleepwalking

Box 27.4 REM SLEEP DISORDERS

- REM sleep behavior disorder
- Recurrent isolated sleep paralysis
- Nightmare disorder

---

26. A

Sympathetic activation is helpful in differentiating sleep terrors from other parasomnias.

27. C

The suprachiasmatic nucleus of the hypothalamus, which is in the ventral-anterior region of the hypothalamus, controls circadian rhythms. Lesions here cause abnormal sleep-wake, eating, and temperature rhythms.

28. A

Patients with Alzheimer's disease may have sleep-wake disturbances due to damage to cholinergic neurons in the suprachiasmatic nucleus and ventrolateral preoptic nucleus.

Damage to the sublaterodorsal tegmental nucleus is associated with REM sleep behavior disorder (RBD).[2]

29. B

During sleep, neurons in the arousal system are inhibited by GABA and galanin.

There are two branches of the ascending arousal system. Both start in the upper pons and activate the cerebral cortex. There are monoaminergic and cholinergic neurons in the ascending arousal system.

The dorsal pathway is from the pons to the thalamus. Specifically, cholinergic neurons in the pedunculopontine tegmental nucleus (PPT) and the laterodorsal tegmental nucleus (LDT) innervate the thalamus, including the reticular nucleus. The final result is thalamocortical transmission and cortical activation.

The ventral pathway is from the pons through the hypothalamus to the basal forebrain and cortex. It consists primarily of monoaminergic neurons—neurons in the locus coeruleus (norepinephrine), dorsal and median raphe nuclei (serotonin), parabrachial nucleus and precoeruleus area (glutamate), periaqueductal gray matter (dopamine), and tuberomammillary nucleus (histamine).

Neurons in the lateral hypothalamus that produce orexin/hypocretin are also involved in wakefulness. They innervate the components of the ascending arousal system and the cerebral cortex. Loss of orexin neurons causes narcolepsy (Box 27.5 and Table 27.1).[2]

Box 27.5 NEUROTRANSMITTERS AND NEUROPEPTIDES INVOLVED IN WAKEFULNESS

- Acetylcholine
- Dopamine
- Glutamate
- Histamine
- Hypocretin/orexin
- Norepinephrine
- Serotonin

Table 27.1 LOCATION OF SPECIFIC NEUROTRANSMITTERS/NEUROPEPTIDES

NEUROTRANSMITTER/ NEUROPEPTIDE	LOCATION OF NEURONS
Acetylcholine	Pedunculopontine tegmental nucleus (PPT) and laterodorsal tegmental nucleus (LDT)
Dopamine	Substantia nigra
Glutamate	Parabrachial nucleus and precoeruleus area
Histamine	Tuberomammillary nucleus
Hypocretin/orexin	Lateral hypothalamus
Norepinephrine	Locus coeruleus
Serotonin	Dorsal and median raphe

30. C

The ventrolateral preoptic nuclei (VLPO) and median preoptic nuclei (MNPO) inhibit the arousal system during sleep. Neurons of the VLPO release galanin and GABA; those of the MNPO release GABA (see Box 27.6).

Caffeine promotes wakefulness by blocking the adenosine receptor.[2]

Box 27.6 NEUROTRANSMITTERS INVOLVED IN SLEEP

- Acetylcholine (REM sleep)
- Adenosine
- GABA
- Galanin

---

31. C

Neurons in the pons cause REM sleep. They are inhibited by neurons in the lower midbrain, which act as REM-off neurons. Specifically, neurons in the subcoeruleus area/sublaterodorsal nucleus and precoeruleus region of the pons generate REM sleep. These neurons are glutamatergic. Neurons in this region promote atonia, rapid eye movements, and EEG desynchronization during REM sleep. For instance, atonia is caused by descending projections from this region to medullary and spinal interneurons that hyperpolarize alpha motor neurons. Neurons in the laterodorsal tegmental nuclei (LDT) and the pedunculopontine tegmental nuclei (PPT), which are cholinergic, are also thought to promote REM.

The dorsal raphe, locus coeruleus, and tuberomammillary nucleus are involved in the arousal system, which is inhibited during sleep.[2]

32. A

The vlPAG/LPT areas stop REM. They inhibit the sublateraldorsal nucleus (SLD)/precoeruleus (PC) neurons and are inhibited by them.

The VLPO, LDT, and PPT promote REM.[2]

33. A

Sleep diaries are a means of documenting sleep and wake times. They are helpful in the diagnosis of circadian rhythm disorders.

34. A

An actigraph measures movement and acts an indirect measure of alertness. Actigraphy is helpful in diagnosis of circadian rhythm disorder; insomnia, including paradoxical insomnia; and periodic limb movements. It also is useful in assessing the effectiveness of treatment of these conditions.

35. A

The MSLT and the maintenance of wakefulness test (MWT) are not validated in young children.

MSLT is helpful in the assessment of daytime sleepiness and in the diagnosis of narcolepsy. A polysomnogram is performed the night before an MSLT. The patient is instructed to try to fall asleep during five naps at 2-hour intervals. A mean sleep latency of less than 8 minutes is indicative of excessive daytime sleepiness. This finding plus two sleep-onset REM periods can be used to diagnose narcolepsy in the appropriate clinical setting.

An MWT is an objective, structured test that is used to determine whether a patient can remain awake. The patient tries to stay awake during four 40-minute trials. A mean sleep latency of less than 8 minutes suggests excessive daytime sleepiness. A polysomnogram is not required the night before an MWT.

36. B

This patient has Kleine-Levin syndrome, which is characterized by episodes of hypersomnia lasting for 2 days to 4 weeks that recur at least once per year. Patients may sleep for 15 to 21 hours per day. They are normal between episodes. During the episodes, patients are confused and have unusual behavior. Apathy is common. Hyperphagia, hypersexuality, hallucinations, or derealization may occur. The first episode may be triggered by an infection. EEG typically shows background slowing. Single-photon emission computed tomography (SPECT) shows dysfunction of the frontal and temporal lobes, thalamus, and hypothalamus during the episodes.[3]

REFERENCES

1. Chung F, Yegneswaran B, Liao P, et al. STOP questionnaire: A tool to screen patients for obstructive sleep apnea. *Anesthesiology* 2008;108:812–821.
2. Saper CB. The neurobiology of sleep. *Continuum (Minneap Minn)* 2013;19(1 Sleep Disorders):19–31.
3. Arnulf I, Rico TJ, Mignot E. Diagnosis, disease course, and management of patients with Klein-Levin syndrome. *Lancet Neurol* 2012;11:918–928.

28.

SUBSTANCE-RELATED DISORDERS

QUESTIONS

1. For which of the following substances does the *Diagnostic and Statistical Manual of Mental Disorders* (DSM-5) *not* include a substance use diagnosis?
   A. Alcohol
   B. Caffeine
   C. Cannabis
   D. Tobacco

2. True or False?
   According to the DSM-5, a patient who experiences tolerance and withdrawal to a substance is addicted to that substance.

3. Which of the following medications inhibits aldehyde dehydrogenase and has been used to treat alcohol dependence but requires abstention from alcohol in medicines and desserts in order to avoid unpleasant symptoms?
   A. Naloxone
   B. Naltrexone
   C. Flumazenil
   D. Methadone
   E. Disulfiram

4. A 56-year-old woman presents with confusion, wide-based gait, and dysconjugate gaze. She smells of alcohol. What is the best treatment?
   A. Ativan
   B. Valium
   C. Thiamine
   D. Disulfiram

5. A 40-year-old man presents to the emergency department with confusion. His family reports recent problems with diarrhea and a history of alcoholism. On examination, he is thin and appears to have a sunburn on his face, chest, and hands, but the family denies significant sun exposure. Which of the following diagnoses should be considered?
   A. Beriberi
   B. Lupus
   C. Pellagra
   D. Dermatomyositis

6. A 50-year-old man is admitted for confusion. The family reports a long history of alcoholism. Every day he re-introduces himself. When asked the date, he says, "Time flies doesn't it?" He seems to invent answers to

questions. Which of the following diagnoses is most likely?
   A. Early-onset Alzheimer disease
   B. Korsakoff syndrome
   C. Wet beriberi
   D. Alcohol-induced fugue state

7. As a result of decreasing ethanol levels, patients can have which of the following signs of withdrawal even while still intoxicated?
   A. Autonomic hyperactivity
   B. Seizure
   C. Tremor

8. Which of the following can occur with chronic alcohol use?
   A. Demyelination of the corpus callosum
   B. Myopathy
   C. Neuropathy
   D. All of the above

9. Which of the following features is characteristic of fetal alcohol syndrome?
   A. Short palpebral fissures, thin upper lip, and smooth philtrum
   B. Growth deficiency
   C. Hyperactivity, inattention, and cognitive impairment
   D. All of the above

10. Which of the following medications is most dangerous to use in a patient with acute cocaine intoxication?
    A. Benzodiazepines
    B. Beta-blockers
    C. Calcium channel blockers
    D. Diuretics

11. Which of the following statements correctly describes a difference between 3,4-methylenedioxymethamphetamine (MDMA) and cocaine?
    A. MDMA does not cause hallucinations.
    B. MDMA has more dopaminergic activity than cocaine.
    C. MDMA has more serotonergic activity than cocaine.
    D. MDMA does not have long-term side effects.

12. At which receptor does lysergic acid diethylamide (LSD) primarily act?
    A. Norepinephrine
    B. Epinephrine
    C. Dopamine
    D. Serotonin
    E. Glutamate

13. **Which of the following is *least* likely to cause stroke?**
    A. γ-Hydroxybutyrate (GHB)
    B. Heroin
    C. Lysergic acid diethylamide (LSD)
    D. Phencyclidine (PCP)
    E. Marijuana

14. **Which inhalant is most likely to cause myeloneuropathy?**
    A. Gasoline
    B. Hexane
    C. Nitrous oxide
    D. Toluene
    E. Trichloroethylene

15. **A 20-year-old postoperative patient is difficult to arouse. On examination, his pupils are pinpoint and he has slowed respirations. Which of the following medications is most likely to be diagnostic and therapeutic?**
    A. Diphenhydramine
    B. Dopamine
    C. Epinephrine
    D. Naloxone

16. **Which of the following is *least* likely to occur during opioid intoxication?**
    A. Hypersexuality
    B. Hypothermia
    C. Postural hypotension
    D. Vomiting

17. **Which of the following statements about heroin use is true?**
    A. Heroin is metabolized to morphine.
    B. Heroin can cause a myelopathy resembling anterior spinal artery syndrome.
    C. Heroin can be associated with vertebral osteomyelitis.
    D. Heating heroin and inhaling the vapor can cause spongiform encephalopathy.
    E. All of the above.

18. **Which of the following is *least* likely to cause agitated delirium in adults?**
    A. Anticholinergic medications
    B. Opioid withdrawal
    C. Nicotine
    D. Phencyclidine (PCP)

19. **Which of the following medications is most useful in blocking the side effects of opioid withdrawal?**
    A. Clonidine
    B. Diphenhydramine
    C. Propranolol
    D. Verapamil

20. **Which of the following is most likely to cause seizures, delirium, myoclonus, and tremor?**
    A. Fentanyl
    B. Meperidine
    C. Morphine
    D. Oxycodone

21. **What is the mechanism of action for phencyclidine (PCP)?**
    A. It is an α-amino-3-hydroxyl-5-methyl-4-isoxazole-propionate (AMPA) agonist.
    B. It is an *N*-methyl-D-aspartate (NMDA) antagonist.
    C. It is a serotonin receptor agonist.
    D. It is a dopamine receptor agonist.

22. **Which of the following statements is *false*?**
    A. PCP can cause a schizophrenia-like syndrome.
    B. PCP intoxication can cause rhabdomyolysis.
    C. PCP intoxication can cause severe agitation.
    D. PCP raises the seizure threshold.

23. **A child presents with altered mental status, diaphoresis, salivation, vomiting, and diarrhea. Which of the following is the most likely cause?**
    A. Belladonna
    B. *Datura stramonium*
    C. Nitrous oxide
    D. Tobacco

SUBSTANCE-RELATED DISORDERS

1. B

In the DSM-5, substance abuse and substance dependence are not differentiated. The DSM-5 uses the term *substance use disorder*. Gambling disorder is also included among the substance-related and addictive disorders.

For diagnosis of a substance use disorder, there must be evidence of pathologic behaviors regarding the substance, such as impaired control, effects on relationships or obligations, or continued use despite risk. Tolerance and withdrawal are also among the criteria, but they are not required for the diagnosis.

Caffeine intoxication and caffeine withdrawal are diagnoses in DSM-5, but there is no caffeine use disorder diagnosis.

In addition to substance use disorders, the DSM-5 lists substance-induced disorders such as intoxication, withdrawal, sexual dysfunction, mood disorders (psychotic, bipolar, depressive, obsessive-compulsive), sleep disorders, delirium, and neurocognitive disorders.

2. False

The term "addiction" is not used in the DSM-5. The need for increasing doses to achieve the same effect indicates tolerance. Most substances have a typical withdrawal syndrome.

3. E

Ethanol is metabolized by alcohol dehydrogenase to acetaldehyde, which is metabolized by aldehyde dehydrogenase to acetic acid.

Disulfiram (Antabuse) inhibits aldehyde dehydrogenase, resulting in the accumulation of acetaldehyde if alcohol is ingested. This causes flushing, nausea, and vomiting.

4. C

This patient has symptoms concerning for Wernicke encephalopathy (cognitive changes, ataxia, disturbances in extraocular movements), which occurs in patients with thiamine deficiency. Patients who abuse alcohol are at risk for thiamine deficiency. To avoid Wernicke encephalopathy in patients who might be at risk for the condition, thiamine should be administered before intravenous fluids with glucose.

Wernicke encephalopathy causes magnetic resonance imaging (MRI) changes such as fluid-attenuated inversion recovery (FLAIR) abnormalities in the thalamus, mammillary bodies, periaqueductal gray region, and tectum.

5. C

Patients who abuse alcohol are at risk for niacin deficiency, which manifests as pellagra. Patients with pellagra have characteristic skin findings, dementia, and diarrhea.

6. B

Korsakoff syndrome is an amnestic syndrome that is caused by thiamine deficiency and characterized by both retrograde and anterograde amnesia. Confabulation is characteristic.

7. B

Seizures and tremor are typically the earliest signs of alcohol withdrawal. Patients can have a seizure due to decreasing ethanol levels while still intoxicated.

Patients can develop delirium tremens without having earlier signs of withdrawal. Delirium tremens is characterized by agitation, altered mental status, hallucinations, and autonomic hyperactivity. Benzodiazepines are the treatment of choice.

8. D

Chronic alcohol use can cause multiple neurologic problems. It can cause dementia characterized by global impairment. Alcohol can cause both an acute and a chronic myopathy. It can cause neuropathy directly or as a result of nutritional deficiencies. Alcohol intoxication is a risk factor for compressive neuropathies. In addition, chronic alcohol use causes cerebellar degeneration; typically the superior vermis is most affected. Less commonly, chronic alcohol use can cause Marchiafava-Bignami disease, which is characterized by corpus callosum demyelination. Liver damage due to chronic alcohol use also has neurologic complications.

In addition to affecting the cardiovascular and gastrointestinal systems, alcohol suppresses the immune system. Alcohol is a risk factor for infection with *Streptococcus pneumoniae*, which can cause endocarditis, pneumonia, and meningitis. Alcohol is also a risk factor for *Listeria monocytogenes* meningitis.

9. D

Fetal alcohol syndrome causes craniofacial abnormalities, growth deficiency, and cognitive impairment. Children with fetal alcohol syndrome often have microcephaly as well as short palpebral fissures, a smooth philtrum, and a thin upper lip. They have impaired growth and developmental delay. They often demonstrate hyperactivity, inattention, impaired executive function, and intellectual disability.

10. B

Beta-blockers should be avoided in patients with acute cocaine intoxication because they can cause paradoxical hypertension due to unopposed alpha stimulation.

11. C

MDMA, also known as Ecstasy, has properties similar to those of an amphetamine and a hallucinogen. Compared with cocaine or methamphetamine, MDMA has more serotonergic activity. Cocaine and methamphetamine have more dopaminergic activity than MDMA. Cognitive impairment occurs with long-term use of either cocaine or MDMA.

12. D

LSD acts at the serotonin receptor.

13. A

Of the substances listed, GHB is least likely to cause stroke.

Cocaine can cause hypertension; hemorrhagic, ischemic, or cardioembolic stroke; and vasculitis.

LSD is an ergot and can cause vasoconstriction and ischemic stroke. PCP also causes vasoconstriction. Heroin and marijuana can also cause stroke.

14. C

Nitrous oxide causes myeloneuropathy. It causes a clinical picture similar to that of vitamin B12 deficiency, possibly because it interferes with methionine synthetase (see Table 28.1).

Table 28.1 NEUROLOGIC COMPLICATIONS OF COMMON INHALANTS

INHALANT	NEUROLOGIC COMPLICATION
Gasoline	Lead encephalopathy
Hexane	Peripheral neuropathy
Nitrite	Methemoglobinemia
Nitrous oxide	Myeloneuropathy
Toluene	Dementia, leukoencephalopathy, ataxia
Trichloroethylene	Trigeminal neuropathy

15. D

Opioid overdose produces coma with miosis and respiratory depression. Flash pulmonary edema may occur.

Opioid intoxication is treated with naloxone. Naloxone can precipitate opioid withdrawal in patients who are dependent on opioids.

16. A

Opioid intoxication tends to cause decreased libido, not hypersexuality. It also is accompanied by euphoria, hypothermia, vomiting, constipation, and postural hypotension. Pruritus may occur as a result of histamine release.

17. E

Heroin, which is metabolized to morphine, is immunosuppressive. Injection of heroin increases the patient's risk for a number of infections such as abscess, endocarditis, joint infections, and osteomyelitis in addition to parenterally acquired infections. Heroin can also cause a myelopathy that resembles anterior spinal artery syndrome.

Heating heroin and inhaling the vapor, which has been referred to as "chasing the dragon," can cause spongiform encephalopathy.

18. B

Opioid withdrawal causes yawning, rhinorrhea, tearing, and diaphoresis followed by abdominal cramping, vomiting, diarrhea, piloerection, and mydriasis. Seizures and delirium are atypical in opioid withdrawal in adults and should raise suspicion that another substance was ingested.

19. A

Methadone helps prevent opioid withdrawal symptoms. Clonidine treats the autonomic symptoms.

20. B

Normeperidine, which is the metabolite of meperidine, can cause altered mental status, seizures, myoclonus, and tremor. High doses of other opioids can also cause myoclonus.

21. B

PCP is an NMDA antagonist.

Ketamine and dextromethorphan are also NMDA receptor antagonists. Ketamine has similar but milder effects than PCP and has been used for anesthesia in veterinary practices. The combination of dextromethorphan and quinidine has been used to treat pseudobulbar palsy. Dextromethorphan can cause a urine drug screen to be falsely positive for PCP.

22. D

PCP lowers the seizure threshold; it can cause seizures. In addition, it can cause myoclonus, hypertensive encephalopathy, and ischemic and hemorrhagic stroke.

PCP was originally used as a dissociative anesthetic; however, it was discontinued as an anesthetic because it produced symptoms of psychosis. PCP can cause symptoms of schizophrenia, both positive and negative. It can cause paranoia, hallucinations, flat affect, and catatonic posturing. PCP can cause nystagmus, hyperthermia, tachycardia, hypertension, and respiratory depression at higher doses.

Benzodiazepines are used for sedation in patients who have taken PCP. Before using an antipsychotic agent, it should be remembered that neuroleptics can lower the seizure threshold, can worsen myoglobinuria, and can have anticholinergic side effects such as tachycardia.

23. D

Tobacco ingestion can cause cholinergic symptoms such as altered mental status, salivation, vomiting, and diarrhea. Atropine can treat the parasympathetic symptoms.

Belladonna and *D. stramonium* (Jimson weed) can cause symptoms of anticholinergic poisoning. Anticholinergic poisoning may be treated with physostigmine. Neuroleptics have anticholinergic properties and should be avoided in anticholinergic poisoning.

Nitrous oxide is a dissociative anesthetic.

29.

VITAMIN DEFICIENCY AND EXCESS

QUESTIONS

1. A homeless man is brought to the emergency department by the police. They say that he is confused and unsteady. On examination, you notice nystagmus and lateral rectus weakness. Which of the following vitamins is deficient in this condition?
   A. Folate
   B. Pyridoxine
   C. Thiamine
   D. Vitamin B12

2. The combination of dementia with diarrhea and a scaly rash is concerning for deficiency of which vitamin?
   A. Niacin
   B. Thiamine
   C. Vitamin B12
   D. Vitamin E

3. A 23-year-old woman presents with falls when walking in the dark. She also reports a tingling sensation from her neck down her back with neck flexion. On examination, she has decreased reflexes and decreased sensation to all modalities in the upper and lower extremities. She denies medications except for a vitamin "to give her energy and help her lose weight." Which of the following best explains her symptoms?
   A. Pyridoxine toxicity
   B. Hypervitaminosis A
   C. Hypervitaminosis D
   D. Hypervitaminosis E

4. Fill in the blank: Isoniazid (INH) causes _____ _____deficiency.
   A. Vitamin B12
   B. Pyridoxine (vitamin B6)

   C. Riboflavin
   D. Thiamine

5. Night blindness may occur with which of the following?
   A. Hypervitaminosis A
   B. Pantothenic acid deficiency
   C. Riboflavin deficiency
   D. Vitamin A deficiency

6. A patient with inflammatory bowel disease presents with leg paresthesias and falls. On examination, the patient has impaired vibration and position sense, a positive Babinski sign bilaterally, ankle areflexia, and a positive Romberg sign. Which of the following is the most likely cause?
   A. Selenium deficiency
   B. Vitamin B12 deficiency
   C. Vitamin E deficiency
   D. Vitamin K deficiency

7. Fill in the blank: Excess intake of _____ causes myeloneuropathy due to copper deficiency.
   A. Cadmium
   B. Cobalt
   C. Lead
   D. Zinc

8. After undergoing bariatric surgery, a 40-year-old woman develops myelopathy. You suspect a vitamin deficiency. Which of the following vitamins is *least* likely to be the culprit?
   A. Copper
   B. Vitamin A
   C. Vitamin B12
   D. Vitamin E

VITAMIN DEFICIENCY AND EXCESS

ANSWERS

1. C

Wernicke encephalopathy is associated with a triad of ophthalmoparesis (with nystagmus), ataxia, and confusion. It is caused by thiamine (vitamin B1) deficiency and is classically seen in alcoholics. Thiamine is given in the emergency department to prevent Wernicke disease. It also can occur in other patients with malnutrition, such as patients with acquired immune deficiency syndrome (AIDS), cancer, or hyperemesis gravidarum; patients on long-term parenteral nutrition; and patients who have undergone bariatric surgery.

Pathologic findings in Wernicke encephalopathy are symmetric lesions of the mammillary bodies, periventricular regions of the thalamus and hypothalamus, periaqueductal gray, and superior cerebellar vermis.

If a patient with Wernicke disease is not responding to thiamine, consider hypomagnesemia.

If there is a chronic problem with memory, the patient has Wernicke-Korsakoff syndrome. Classically, Korsakoff psychosis has been associated with confabulation.

2. A

Niacin deficiency causes pellagra, which is characterized by dementia, diarrhea, and a characteristic rash (dermatitis).

3. A

Pyridoxine causes an axonal sensory neuropathy and Lhermitte's phenomenon in high doses.

Hypervitaminosis A can cause pseudotumor cerebri/intracranial hypertension. The structure of isotretinoin (Accutane) resembles that of vitamin A, so it can cause similar symptoms. Isotretinoin is also a teratogen.

Hypervitaminosis D causes hypercalcemia.

Hypervitaminosis E can cause increased bleeding (because of its effect on vitamin K).

4. B

INH increases pyridoxine excretion and can cause pyridoxine deficiency, which is associated with a sensory polyneuropathy (see Box 29.1). Severe pyridoxine deficiency can cause seizures. There is a neonatal form of pyridoxine deficiency characterized by refractory seizures.

5. D

Vitamin A deficiency can result in night blindness.

Vitamin E deficiency can cause retinitis pigmentosa, which manifests with night blindness. Other neurologic causes of retinitis pigmentosa include Refsum disease, abetalipoproteinemia, and mitochondrial diseases such as Kearns-Sayre syndrome and NARP syndrome (neuropathy, ataxia, and retinitis pigmentosa).

6. B

This patient has vitamin B12 deficiency, which predominantly affects the posterior columns and corticospinal tract in the spinal cord. The regions of the spinal cord that are first affected are the posterior columns of the cervical and thoracic segments (see Boxes 29.2 and 29.3).

In addition, vitamin B12 deficiency causes megaloblastic anemia; autonomic dysfunction (postural hypotension, infertility, incontinence); and glossitis.

Nitrous oxide toxicity causes symptoms similar to those of vitamin B12 deficiency. Nitrous oxide interferes with methionine synthetase, a vitamin B12-dependent enzyme that converts homocysteine to methionine. Vitamin B12 is also a cofactor for methylmalonyl–coenzyme A mutase. Therefore, vitamin B12 deficiency is associated with elevated levels of homocysteine and methylmalonic acid. If vitamin B12 deficiency is suspected but the B12 level is normal, determination of the

---

Box 29.1 B VITAMINS THAT CAUSE POLYNEUROPATHY

- Thiamine (deficiency)
- Pyridoxine (deficiency *and* toxicity)
- Pantothenic acid (deficiency)
- Vitamin B12 (deficiency)

Box 29.2 CAUSES OF VITAMIN B12 DEFICIENCY

- Poor nutrition (e.g. vegan diet)
- Impaired absorption: autoimmune atrophic gastritis/pernicious anemia (due to lack of intrinsic factor), gastrectomy, gastric bypass, inflammatory bowel disease, ileal resection, blind loop syndrome
- Increased metabolism (neoplasm, thyrotoxicosis)

Box 29.3 NEUROLOGIC COMPLICATIONS OF B12 DEFICIENCY

- Dementia
- Myelopathy
- Optic neuropathy

homocysteine and methylmalonic acid levels may aid in the diagnosis.

Selenium deficiency can cause myopathy.

Vitamin E deficiency causes peripheral neuropathy and a spinocerebellar syndrome.

7. D

Zinc excess causes myeloneuropathy due to copper deficiency. Copper deficiency resembles vitamin B12 deficiency. It causes paresthesias, loss of vibration and position sense, a sensory ataxia, hyperreflexia, extensor plantar responses, and a spastic gait.

8. B

Deficiency of copper, vitamin B12, or vitamin E can cause myelopathy.

Deficiency of copper or vitamin B12 can occur after gastric bypass surgery. In addition, vitamin D, calcium, folate, iron, thiamine, and zinc deficiencies may be present. Loss of fat-soluble vitamins (e.g., vitamin E), may also follow gastric bypass; this is less of an issue with gastric banding.

Table 29.1 COMPARISON OF VITAMIN B12 DEFICIENCY, VITAMIN E DEFICIENCY, AND FRIEDREICH ATAXIA

REGION AFFECTED	VITAMIN B12 DEFICIENCY	VITAMIN E DEFICIENCY	FRIEDREICH ATAXIA
Corticospinal tract	Yes	No	Yes
Posterior columns	Yes	Yes	Yes
Spinocerebellar tracts	No	Yes	Yes
Dorsal root ganglia	No	Yes	Yes

Vitamin E deficiency can occur with fat malabsorption. It is also associated with ataxia with vitamin E deficiency, homozygous hypobetalipoproteinemia, and abetalipoproteinemia (Bassen-Kornzweig disease). The symptoms of vitamin E deficiency resemble those of Friedreich ataxia. Patients with vitamin E deficiency have decreased reflexes, a sensory ataxia, and loss of joint and position sense (see Table 29.1).

INDEX

Page numbers followed by *f* indicate a figure; page numbers followed by *t* indicate a table

CPSIA information can be obtained
at www.ICGtesting.com
Printed in the USA
BVHW011548250322
632225BV00004B/15